T0263436

Rhinoplasty: Current Concepts

Guest Editors

RONALD P. GRUBER, MD
DAVID STEPNICK, MD, FACS

CLINICS IN PLASTIC SURGERY

www.plasticsurgery.theclinics.com

April 2010 • Volume 37 • Number 2

SAUNDERS an imprint of ELSEVIER, Inc.

W.B. SAUNDERS COMPANY
A Division of Elsevier Inc.

1600 John F. Kennedy Boulevard • Suite 1800 • Philadelphia, Pennsylvania 19103-2899

http://www.theclinics.com

CLINICS IN PLASTIC SURGERY Volume 37, Number 2
April 2010 ISSN 0094-1298, ISBN-13: 978-1-4377-1862-1

Editor: Barbara Cohen-Kligerman

Clinics in Plastic Surgery (ISSN 0094-1298) is published quarterly by Elsevier Inc., 360 Park Avenue South, New York, NY 10010-1710. Months of issue are January, April, July, and October. Business and Editorial Offices: 1600 John F. Kennedy Blvd., Suite 1800, Philadelphia, PA 19103-2899. Periodicals postage paid at New York, NY and additional mailing offices. Subscription prices are $384.00 per year for US individuals, $551.00 per year for US institutions, $193.00 per year for US students and residents, $436.00 per year for Canadian individuals, $644.00 per year for Canadian institutions, $495.00 per year for international individuals, $644.00 per year for international institutions, and $244.00 per year for Canadian and foreign students/residents. To receive student/resident rate, orders must be accompanied by name of affiliated institution, date of term, and the *signature* of program/residency coordinator on institution letterhead. Orders will be billed at individual rate until proof of status is received. Foreign air speed delivery is included in all *Clinics* subscription prices. All prices are subject to change without notice. **POSTMASTER:** Send address changes to *Clinics in Plastic Surgery*, Elsevier Health Sciences Division, Subscription Customer Service, 3251 Riverport Lane, Maryland Heights, MO 63043. **Customer Service: 1-800-654-2452 (US and Canada). From outside of the United States and Canada, call 314-447-8871. Fax: 314-447-8029. E-mail: JournalsCustomerService-usa@elsevier.com (for print support); JournalsOnlineSupport-usa@elsevier.com (for online support).**

Reprints. For copies of 100 or more of articles in this publication, please contact the Commercial Reprints Department, Elsevier Inc., 360 Park Avenue South, New York, New York 10010-1710. Tel.: (+1) 212-633-3812; Fax: (+1) 212-462-1935; E-mail: reprints@elsevier.com.

Clinics in Plastic Surgery is covered in *Current Contents, EMBASE/Excerpta Medica, Science Citation Index, MEDLINE/ PubMed (Index Medicus), ASCA, and ISI/BIOMED.*

Contributors

GUEST EDITORS

RONALD P. GRUBER, MD
Adjunct Clinical Assistant Professor, Division of Plastic & Reconstructive Surgery, Stanford University, Stanford; Clinical Assistant Professor, Division of Plastic & Reconstructive Surgery, University of California, San Francisco, Oakland, California

DAVID STEPNICK, MD, FACS
Associate Professor of Otolaryngology-Head and Neck Surgery, Case Western Reserve University; Center for Aesthetic Facial Surgery, Department of Plastic and Reconstructive Surgery, University Hospitals, Cleveland, Ohio

AUTHORS

WILLIAM P. ADAMS, MD
Associate Clinical Professor of Plastic Surgery, Department of Plastic Surgery, University of Texas Southwestern Medical Center, Dallas, Texas

SHAN R. BAKER, MD
Professor, Division of Facial Plastic and Reconstructive Surgery, Department of Otolaryngology-Head and Neck Surgery, University of Michigan Medical Center, Ann Arbor, Michigan

RICHARD J. BEIL, MD
Adjunct Clinical Instructor, Department of Surgery, University of Michigan; Center for Plastic and Reconstructive Surgery, St. Joseph Mercy Hospital, Ann Arbor, Michigan

KELLY BOLDEN, MD
Resident, Department of Plastic Surgery, University of Texas Southwestern Medical Center, Dallas, Texas

EDWARD BUCHANAN, MD
Division of Plastic & Reconstructive Surgery, University of California, San Francisco, Oakland, California

JAMAL M. BULLOCKS, MD
Assistant Professor, Division of Plastic Surgery, Department of Surgery, Baylor College of Medicine, Houston, Texas

EDWARD CHANG, MD
Division of Plastic & Reconstructive Surgery, University of California, San Francisco, Oakland, California

C. SPENCER COCHRAN, MD
Clinical Assistant Professor, Department of Otolaryngology-Head and Neck Surgery, University of Texas Southwestern Medical Center at Dallas; Gunter Center for Aesthetics and Cosmetic Surgery, Dallas, Texas

ROLLIN K. DANIEL, MD
Clinical Professor, Aesthetic and Plastic Surgery Institute, University of California, Irvine, Irvine, California

ERIC J. DOBRATZ, MD
Assistant Professor, Department of Otolaryngology-Head and Neck Surgery; Director, Division of Facial Plastic and Reconstructive Surgery, Eastern Virginia Medical School, Norfolk, Virginia

RYAN M. GREENE, MD, PhD
Advanced Facial Plastic Surgery & Laser Center, Fort Lauderdale, Florida

RONALD P. GRUBER, MD
Adjunct Clinical Assistant Professor, Division of Plastic & Reconstructive Surgery, Stanford University, Stanford; Clinical Assistant Professor, Division of Plastic & Reconstructive Surgery, University of California, San Francisco, Oakland, California

JOSEPH M. GRYSKIEWICZ, MD
Clinical Professor, Cleft Palate and Craniofacial Clinics, University of Minnesota, Academic Health Center School of Dentistry, Minneapolis, Minnesota

JACK P. GUNTER, MD
Clinical Professor, Departments of Plastic Surgery and Otolaryngology-Head and Neck Surgery, University of Texas Southwestern Medical Center at Dallas, Dallas, Texas

BAHMAN GUYURON, MD, FACS
The Kiehn-DesPrez Professor and Chair, Case Western Reserve University; Center for Aesthetic Facial Surgery, Department of Plastic and Reconstructive Surgery, University Hospitals, Cleveland, Ohio

FRED L. HACKNEY, MD, DDS
Dallas, Texas

DANIEL A. HATEF, MD
Resident, Division of Plastic Surgery, Department of Surgery, Baylor College of Medicine, Houston, Texas

PETER A. HILGER, MD
Professor, Department of Otolaryngology-Head and Neck Surgery; Director, Division of Facial Plastic Surgery, University of Minnesota, Minneapolis, Minnesota

P. CRAIG HOBAR, MD, FRCS
Associate Clinical Professor of Plastic Surgery, Department of Plastic Surgery, University of Texas Southwestern Medical Center, Dallas, Texas

C. ALEJANDRA MITCHELL, MD
Clinical Plastic Surgeon and Director of International Surgical Development, LEAP Foundation, Clinical Faculty, Department of Plastic Surgery, University of Texas Southwestern Medical Center, Dallas, Texas

SAM P. MOST, MD
Division of Facial Plastic and Reconstructive Surgery, Stanford University School of Medicine, Stanford, California

ROBERT M. ONEAL, MD
Adjunct Clinical Professor, Department of Surgery, University of Michigan; Center for Plastic and Reconstructive Surgery, St. Joseph Mercy Hospital, Ann Arbor, Michigan

STEPHEN S. PARK, MD
Professor, Vice Chairman, and Director, Division of Facial Plastic & Reconstructive Surgery, Department of Otolaryngology-Head & Neck Surgery, University of Virginia Health Systems, Charlottesville, Virginia

STEPHEN W. PERKINS, MD, FACS
President, Meridian Plastic Surgeons; President, Meridian Plastic Surgery Center; Clinical Associate Professor, Department of Otolaryngology-Head and Neck Surgery, Indiana University School of Medicine, Indianapolis, Indiana

COLIN D. PERO, MD
Clinical Assistant Professor, Division of Facial Plastic and Reconstructive Surgery, Department of Otolaryngology-Head and Neck Surgery, University of Texas-Southwestern Medical School, Dallas, Texas; Private Practice, Plano, Texas

DIANA PONSKY, MD
Assistant Professor, Department of Otolaryngology and Plastic Surgery, University Hospitals-Case Medical Center, Cleveland, Ohio

ROD J. ROHRICH, MD, FACS
Professor and Chairman, Department of Plastic Surgery, University of Texas Southwestern Medical Center, Dallas, Texas

ROBERT L. SIMONS, MD, FACS
Clinical Professor Voluntary, Division of Facial Plastic and Reconstructive Surgery, Department of Otolaryngology-Head and Neck Surgery, University of Miami School of Medicine; Medical Board Chairman, The Miami Institute for Age Management and Intervention, Miami, Florida

SAMUEL STAL, MD
Professor and Chairman, Division of Plastic Surgery, Department of Plastic Surgery, Baylor College of Medicine, Houston, Texas

DAVID STEPNICK, MD, FACS
Associate Professor of Otolaryngology-Head and Neck Surgery, Case Western Reserve University; Center for Aesthetic Facial Surgery, Department of Plastic and Reconstructive Surgery, University Hospitals, Cleveland, Ohio

RAVI S. SWAMY, MD, MPH
Division of Facial Plastic and Reconstructive Surgery, Stanford University School of Medicine, Stanford, California

JONATHAN M. SYKES, MD
Professor and Director of Facial Plastic and Reconstructive Surgery, University of California, Davis Medical Center, Sacramento, California

DEAN M. TORIUMI, MD
Professor, Division of Facial Plastic and Reconstructive Surgery, Department of Otolaryngology-Head and Neck Surgery, University of Illinois at Chicago Medical School, Chicago, Illinois

TOM D. WANG, MD, FACS
Professor, Division of Facial Plastic and Reconstructive Surgery, Department of Otolaryngology-Head and Neck Surgery, Oregon Health & Science University, Portland, Oregon

STEPHEN M. WEBER, MD, PhD
Assistant Professor, Division of Facial Plastic and Reconstructive Surgery, Department of Otolaryngology-Head & Neck Surgery, Oregon Health & Science University, Portland, Oregon

CHARLES R. WOODARD, MD
Resident, Department of Otolaryngology-Head & Neck Surgery, University of Virginia Health Systems, Charlottesville, Virginia

Contents

Erratum xi

Preface xiii

Ronald P. Gruber and David Stepnick

Nasal and Facial Analysis 181

Charles R. Woodard and Stephen S. Park

Rhinoplasty remains one of the most challenging aesthetic procedures to master. Astute surgeons must consider a continually evolving societal perception of beauty with their own sense of aesthetic proportion when planning surgical intervention. Optimal results are achieved when the outcome is anticipated and satisfying to patient and surgeon. This requires a careful, thoughtful, systematic approach to preoperative analysis. Patients should leave with a clear understanding of the surgeon's perspective of their nose, aesthetically and anatomically. Understanding the interplay of surface deformities and their underlying anatomic counterpart is critical, involving a systematic analysis to create a surgical plan that avoids landmines leading to a suboptimal result.

Surgical Anatomy of the Nose 191

Robert M. Oneal and Richard J. Beil

A detailed understanding of nasal anatomy is essential when undertaking rhinoplasty surgery. This article describes the nasal anatomy, careful study of which makes for a more confident, prepared practitioner.

Principles of Photography in Rhinoplasty for the Digital Photographer 213

Ravi S. Swamy, Jonathan M. Sykes, and Sam P. Most

The art and technology of photography can be overwhelming to the facial plastic surgeon. Photographic documentation of patients undergoing rhinoplasty is essential for patient consultation, perioperative planning, and postsurgical evaluation. Possession of a basic understanding of photographic principles, technique, equipment, as well as consideration regarding consistency of patient positioning is essential for producing the best photographic results. This article reviews the basic principles of photography and discusses their application to facial plastic surgery practice, and rhinoplasty in particular.

Diagnosis and Correction of Alar Rim Deformities in Rhinoplasty 223

Fred L. Hackney

Recognition of alar rim deformities is an important component of the preoperative analysis of the nose. Correction of these deformities improves the esthetic balance of the nose and has an added benefit of improving the function of the external nasal valve. Classification systems have been proposed to enable surgeons to more accurately diagnose alar deformities. These classification systems help guide surgeons as to the appropriate surgical procedure to correct a problem. The purpose of this article is to review the proposed classification systems for alar rim deformities and review the specific surgical techniques that have been proposed for each of the deformities.

Suture Techniques in Rhinoplasty 231

Ronald P. Gruber, Edward Chang, and Edward Buchanan

Suture techniques are an indispensable means to biologically sculpt the cartilage of the nose. Here the authors review their use in tip-plasty and present a 4-suture algorithm that allows for simple, complete control in sculpting the shape of all nasal tips in primary rhinoplasty. After a standard cephalic trim of the lateral crus leaving it 6 mm wide, one or more of the four suture techniques are applied. One of the newest techniques that has yielded excellent results is the hemi-transdomal suture, a variation of the conventional transdomal suture. This technique narrows the dome but also everts the lateral crus slightly to avoid concavities of the nostril rim. The 4-suture algorithm is useful in both the open and closed approaches. A more general use of sutures is described and referred to as the "universal horizontal mattress suture," which can be applied to remove all unwanted convexities or concavities and can be used not only to straighten the cartilage but also strengthen it. This suture has applications for the crooked septum, the collapsed lateral crus (external valve), and the collapsed internal valve, as well as for converting ear cartilage grafts into straighter, stronger grafts than previously thought possible.

Alar Base Disharmonies 245

Diana Ponsky and Bahman Guyuron

The nasal base is often overlooked during the initial planning of rhinoplasty. Poor surgical planning or improper correction of alar base disharmonies can be irreversible and can have significant functional consequences. This article simplifies the recognition of common alar base disharmonies. The classification system is intended to facilitate choosing the best surgical technique to correct the alar base flaws.

Alar Cartilage Grafts 253

Stephen M. Weber and Shan R. Baker

The alar cartilages provide the contour and structural support of the nasal tip. Current rhinoplasty concepts support preservation of alar structure with suture techniques or judicious cephalic trim indicated for tip deformities. In many primary cases and some revisions, adequate alar structure exists to achieve the desired aesthetic and functional results with conservative surgical methods. In some primary and most revision cases, however, the existing tip structure is inadequate to create a structurally sound and aesthetically pleasing nasal tip without adding structure. In these cases, alar cartilage grafting techniques are indicated to recapitulate nasal tip contour and structure.

Rhinoplasty[5] Pearls: Value of the Endonasal Approach and Vertical Dome Division 265

Robert L. Simons and Ryan M. Greene

Successful outcomes in rhinoplasty depend more on diagnosis than on approach or technique. When the needs of each patient are assessed on multiple occasions, operative performance improves and revision rates decline. The evolutionary track from an endonasal and excisional operation to the more commonly preferred external and restructuring technique is outlined in this article. The senior author's rationale and preference for the endonasal approach and the repositioning of cartilage in the tip using vertical dome division techniques is emphasized.

Humpectomy and Spreader Flaps **285**

Ronald P. Gruber and Stephen W. Perkins

In a primary rhinoplasty that requires a humpectomy, the dorsal aspect of the upper lateral cartilages is commonly discarded. Many of these patients need spreader grafts to reconstruct the middle third of the nose. However, it is possible to reconstruct the upper lateral cartilages into "spreader flaps" that act much like spreader grafts. In the process of making spreader flaps, an incremental humpectomy is performed on the dorsal septum and bony hump. This humpectomy procedure is more accurate than the conventional humpectomy that involves resection of the bone, and septum as a single unit. The open and closed approaches of this technique are discussed in this article.

Rhinoplasty: Dorsal Grafts and the Designer Dorsum **293**

Rollin K. Daniel

Over the last 2 decades, many of the difficulties in shaping primary tips and rebuilding destroyed secondary tips have been solved through the use of tip sutures and grafts. Dorsal grafts, which are a highly visible determinant of the nasal profile and contour, have become the greatest challenge in rhinoplasty surgery. This article reviews the author's different approaches to dorsal grafts using fascia and diced cartilage, either separately or in combination.

Osteotomies **301**

Eric J. Dobratz and Peter A. Hilger

The most challenging and instrumental step in achieving harmonious form and function during rhinoplasty is the successful completion of osteotomies. Osteotomies are performed to correct deformities of the bony nasal vault. Successful treatment of deformity of the bony vault is achieved through organized thinking, comprehensive knowledge of nasal anatomy, and thorough preoperative and intraoperative planning. In this review the authors discuss the pertinent anatomy, technical considerations, and complications that rhinoplasty surgeons should be aware of to optimize the correction of deformities of the nasal bony vault.

Surgical Treatment of the Crooked Nose **313**

David Stepnick and Bahman Guyuron

One-stage septorhinoplasty has become a surgical standard of care because many surgeons in the mid-twentieth century recognized that septal surgery played an essential role in the management of the crooked nose and therefore combined septoplasty and rhinoplasty into a single operation. Definitive predictable correction of the crooked nose is one of the most exigent aspects of this operation. The surgeon should methodically analyze the anatomy and aesthetics of a patient's nose, as a unique structure and as part of the overall face, and must have an understanding of the interrelationships of the structural components of the nose and of the dynamics of change that result from altering these various structures. This article discusses the general principles and the surgical details of septorhinoplasty.

Lengthening the Short Nose 327

P. Craig Hobar, William P. Adams, and C. Alejandra Mitchell

Lengthening the short nose is a challenging area of rhinoplasty. The short nose can be a naturally occurring aesthetic disproportion, or the result of a congenital abnormality or traumatic deformity. The surgical approach depends mostly on the quality of the lining, skeleton, overlying skin, and the amount of correction desired.

Asian Rhinoplasty 335

Dean M. Toriumi and Colin D. Pero

Asian rhinoplasty differs from traditional rhinoplasty approaches in preoperative analysis, patient expectations, nasal anatomy, and surgical techniques used. Platyrrhine nasal characteristics are common, with low dorsum, weak lower lateral cartilages, columellar retraction, and thick sebaceous skin often noted. Typically, patients seek augmentation of these existing structures rather than reductive procedures. Autologous cartilage, in particular use of costal cartilage, has been shown to be a reliable technique, which, when executed properly, produces excellent long-term results. An understanding of cultural perspectives, knowledge of the nasal anatomy unique to Asian patients, and proficiency with augmentation techniques are prerequisites in attaining the desired results for patient and surgeon.

Ethnic Rhinoplasty 353

Rod J. Rohrich and Kelly Bolden

As the United States becomes more racially and ethnically diverse, the number of non-Caucasian patients seeking rhinoplasty is increasing. The non-Caucasian, or ethnic, rhinoplasty patient can be a surgical challenge due to the significant anatomic variability from the standard European nose as well as variability within each ethnicity. Becoming familiar with the common anatomic differences as well as the aesthetic goals in the ethnic rhinoplasty patient will assist the surgeon in attaining consistent, ethnically congruent, and aesthetically pleasing results.

Secondary Rhinoplasty and the Use of Autogenous Rib Cartilage Grafts 371

C. Spencer Cochran and Jack P. Gunter

Postoperative rhinoplasty deformities—such as displacement or distortion of anatomic structures, inadequate surgery resulting in under-resection of the nasal framework, or over-resection caused by overzealous surgery—require a secondary rhinoplasty. Success in secondary rhinoplasty, therefore, relies on an accurate clinical diagnosis and analysis of the nasal deformities, a thorough operative plan to address each abnormality, and a meticulous surgical technique. Septal cartilage is the grafting material of choice for rhinoplasty; however, auricular cartilage and rib cartilage are used in secondary rhinoplasty. This article discusses the steps involved in the external approach to secondary rhinoplasty.

Secondary Rhinoplasty in Unilateral Cleft Nasal Deformity 383

Tom D. Wang

The cleft-lip nasal deformity presents a formidable challenge in rhinoplasty surgery. A wide variety of techniques have been proposed for the correction of this problem, which is proof of the difficulty of this reconstructive problem. The approach outlined in this article amalgamates many cleft-lip rhinoplasty concepts into a single unified technique. This technique is designed to address the deficiencies present on the cleft side of the nose.

Problems in Rhinoplasty **389**

Joseph M. Gryskiewicz, Daniel A. Hatef, Jamal M. Bullocks, and Samuel Stal

In this review, the complications of rhinoplasty are examined in terms of their timing of presentation. An algorithmic approach to postoperative problems is discussed. Complications can frequently be avoided by meticulous technique, recognition of pitfalls, and early attention to perioperative morbidity. Reoperative rates can be minimized with good patient education and proper command of the postoperative situation, so that unnecessary procedures are not undertaken.

Index **401**

Erratum

In the October 2009 issue of *Clinics in Plastic Surgery*, Volume 36, Number 4, in the article by Drs Basil A. Pruitt Jr and Steven E. Wolf titled "An Historical Perspective on Advances in Burn Care Over the Past 100 Years," an error was made in the formula for calculating insensible water loss, which appeared on page 530, in the last paragraph in the right-hand column. The sentence with the correct formula should read as follows: "This loss of water can be estimated as: total insensible water loss (mL/h) = (25+% total body surface area burned) $\times$ m^2, where m^2 is total body surface area in square meters.[28]"

Clinics in Plastic Surgery

FORTHCOMING ISSUES

July 2010

Abdominoplasty
Al Aly, MD, FACS, *Guest Editor*

October 2010

Perforator Flaps
Peter C. Neligan, MB, FRCS(I), FRCSC, FACS, *Guest Editor*

January 2010

Vascular Malformations
Chad Perlyn, MD, PhD, and Arin K. Greene, MD, MMSc, *Guest Editors*

RECENT ISSUES

January 2010

Cutaneous Melanoma
William Dzwierzynski, MD, FACS, *Guest Editor*

October 2009

Burns
Robert Cartotto, MD, FACS, *Guest Editor*

July 2009

Aesthetic Facial Reconstruction
Stefan O.P. Hofer, MD, PhD, FRCS(C) *Guest Editor*

ISSUES OF RELATED INTEREST

Dermatologic Clinics October 2009 (Vol. 27, No. 4)
Cosmetic Dermatology
Vic A. Narurkar, MD, FAAD, *Guest Editor*
Available at: http://www.derm.theclinics.com

Facial Plastic Surgery Clinics of North America November 2009 (Vol. 17, No. 4)
Facelift: Current Approaches
Stephen Prendiville, MD, *Guest Editor*
Available at: http://www.facialplastic.theclinics.com

Preface

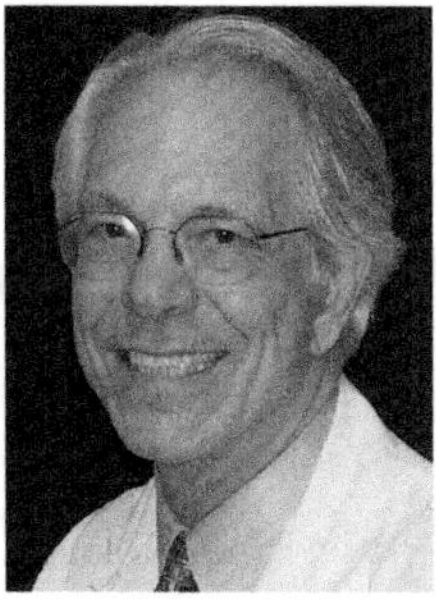

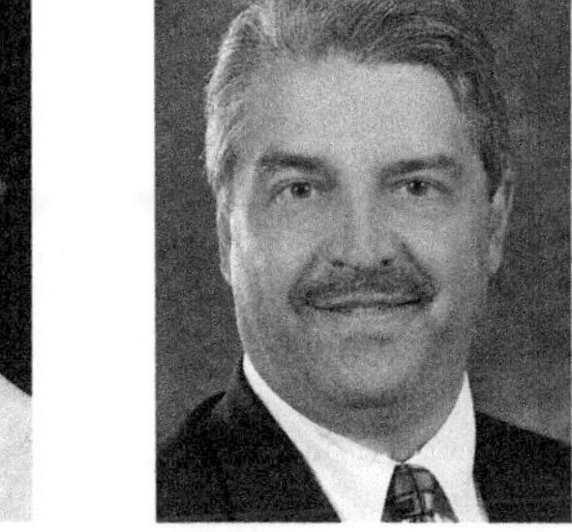

Ronald P. Gruber, MD David Stepnick, MD, FACS
Guest Editors

For a number of reasons, rhinoplasty is arguably the most intricate and challenging operation in all of aesthetic plastic surgery. Because the nose is a relatively small structure, a millimeter change makes a discernible difference in its aesthetics. It is located in the middle of the face, constantly available for inspection by the patient and others. The magnitude of the effects of the healing process often equals and occasionally exceeds the magnitude of the changes that the surgeon is seeking to make. Indeed, the healing process can completely distort the sculptured result the surgeon has achieved. Furthermore, almost every surgeon knows what an aesthetically pleasing nose looks like when he or she sees it. However, not every surgeon intuitively understands what components of the nose are responsible for the unaesthetic appearance and knows what components should be altered to achieve an aesthetic nose.

This issue of *Clinics in Plastic Surgery*, therefore, is devoted to providing surgeons with a better appreciation of the solutions to these problems. Some of the very best rhinoplasty surgeons from a plastic surgery or facial plastic surgery background were asked to share their experience on topics with which they have special expertise. As a result, this issue of *Clinics* is what we believe to be a state-of-the-art compendium of modern rhinoplasty.

The issue begins with a discussion of facial analysis and imaging. The statement that analysis is responsible for 50% of the final result is a cliché for good reason. Not knowing precisely what aspects of the nasal form will benefit from surgical modification is a recipe for a very unsatisfactory result. The use of imaging facilitates that analysis and that point is strongly emphasized here. Anatomy is vital to the decision-making process because the nasal framework is a complicated structure that does not relate directly to its outside appearance. Consequently, it is the focus of discussion as well.

We then provide individual articles that deal with the actual surgical techniques for specific surgical problems. One often-debated topic is the approach for accomplishing the rhinoplasty: endonasal versus external. One article is devoted entirely to one of the most important means of controlling nasal shape: cartilage grafts. A discussion of the various grafts, such as ear, rib, septum, and diced cartilage, is provided. Suture techniques to sculpture the cartilaginous framework are also presented because they are equally important in controlling nasal shape.

Specific parts of the nose demand special variations in the operative procedure. Therefore, an article has been devoted to the dorsum and its augmentation. Yet another has been dedicated to the alar rim and the special challenges it presents. Osteotomies have been a challenge, as evidenced by complaints from too many surgeons about the difficulty of achieving precise control of the nasal bones. Consequently, a section is devoted to this topic. Even a seemingly mundane issue, such as "humpectomy," has received its own special coverage because it has become apparent in recent years that an aesthetic dorsum with a proper functioning internal valve is just as important to a successful rhinoplasty result as a high quality "tip-plasty."

As rhinoplasty is the most difficult aesthetic operation, lengthening the short nose is possibly the most difficult aspect of a rhinoplasty. Consequently one article is devoted to techniques for lengthening a nose that is too short. The same

Clin Plastic Surg 37 (2010) xiii–xiv
doi:10.1016/j.cps.2009.12.012

may be said for straightening the crooked nose; it has had a notoriously high recurrence over the decades. Consequently, this is the topic of an article. As any surgeon knows, having to reoperate on a patient poses a unique set of problems. The tissues of such a nose are simply not as compliant, and the procedure is prone to even more scar tissue deposition than occurred with the first operation: an article specifically addresses this subject.

Special problems require individual discussion. These challenges include Asian and other ethic noses with their complicated problems related, in part, to thick skin. Patients with cleft lip nasal deformities require even greater care in that anatomical distortions beyond the nose affect the nose itself and need to be addressed. The final article provides an overview of the complications seen following rhinoplasty.

We feel that this issue of the *Clinics* has covered virtually every aspect of rhinoplasty, so that today's surgeon will have a completely up-to-date accounting of all the thought processes, caveats, modalities, techniques, and prognostications for providing patients with the best possible outcome.

Ronald P. Gruber, MD
3318 Elm Street
Oakland, CA 94609, USA

Divisions of Plastic & Reconstructive Surgery
Stanford University
University of California, San Francisco

David Stepnick, MD, FACS
Case Western Reserve University
Brainard Medical Building
29001 Cedar Road, Suite 203
Lyndhurst, OH 44124, USA

E-mail addresses:
rgrubermd@hotmail.com (R.P. Gruber)
David.Stepnick@UHhospitals.org (D. Stepnick)

Nasal and Facial Analysis

Charles R. Woodard, MD[a], Stephen S. Park, MD[b,*]

KEYWORDS

- Rhinoplasty • Preoperative analysis • Nasal deformity
- Aesthetics

Rhinoplasty remains one of the most challenging aesthetic procedures to master. Astute surgeons must consider a continually evolving societal perception of beauty with their own sense of aesthetic proportion when planning surgical intervention. An optimal result is achieved when the outcome is anticipated and satisfying to the patient and surgeon. This requires a careful, thoughtful, systematic approach to preoperative analysis.

HISTORY

A focused history and physical examination is required to design a mutually agreeable operative plan. Information regarding past medical history, past surgical history (especially previous nasal surgery), medications (including herbals), allergies, social habits, and a personal or family history of coagulopathy is important. During the preoperative rhinoplasty history, it is essential to determine the patient's motivation for surgery, expectations, and psychosocial stability.

Patients seeking rhinoplasty are motivated by several different factors. It is the surgeon's responsibility to decide whether or not the factors have a positive or negative impact on a patient's decision-making process. Those who desire surgery secondary to external pressures (ie, want to please others, are in a time of crisis, to salvage a relationship) are poor operative candidates.[1] Patients who are self-motivated to change a nasal deformity are more likely to have a satisfactory outcome.

Expectations must be realistic. This involves clear communication between surgeon and patient, often in front of a mirror. Goals between surgeon and patient must be congruent.

Establishing a patient's baseline psychological status may uncover red flags in surgical intervention. Personality disorders affect up to 10% to 15% of the United States adult population.[2] Knowledge of these disorders assists with the psychological work-up (**Table 1**). Obvious psychopathology necessitates a psychiatric evaluation.

Special consideration is given to the pediatric and elderly population. In general, rhinoplasty is delayed until after pubertal growth, age 15 in girls and age 17 in boys.[3] This is not a steadfast rule and many exceptions exist, particularly when the nose is clearly the adult size. Most warnings against early intervention are anecdotal. Minor functional changes may be appropriate at a younger age on a case-by-case basis. Teenagers are particularly susceptible to external pressures. Therefore, an in-depth discussion of their motivation is essential. Interviewing a patient without parental presence may be necessary to gather this information. Older patients, alternatively, have lived with a nasal deformity for a longer period of time, and it has become ingrained as part of their identity. Dramatic changes to their nose may have an untoward psychological impact. From an anatomic standpoint, their skin is thinner, nasal bones are fragile, and tip-supporting mechanisms are weaker.[3] Conservative surgery is a rule for middle-aged patients.

[a] Department of Otolaryngology - Head & Neck Surgery, University of Virginia Health Systems, 1 Hospital Drive, 2nd Floor OMS, Charlottesville, VA 22908, USA

[b] Division of Facial Plastic & Reconstructive Surgery, Department of Otolaryngology - Head & Neck Surgery, University of Virginia Health Systems, 1 Hospital Drive, 2nd Floor OMS, Room 2747, Charlottesville, VA 22908, USA

* Corresponding author.

E-mail address: SSP8A@hscmail.mcc.virginia.edu (S.S. Park).

Clin Plastic Surg 37 (2010) 181–189
doi:10.1016/j.cps.2009.12.006

plasticsurgery.theclinics.com

Table 1
Personality disorders

Disorder	Description
Dependent personality	Overly compliant, physician seen as a parental figure
Passive-aggressive	Willful incompetence, seeks to prove the physician wrong
Obsessive-compulsive	Rigid and precise, excessive attention to details
Histrionic	Seductive and narcissistic, overreaction to disappointment
Paranoid	Distrustful, expectation of disappointment
Schizoid	Distant and aloof, actions are socially inappropriate
Cyclothymic	Mood swings between mania and depression

Adapted from Correa AJ, Sykes JM, Ries WR. Considerations before rhinoplasty. Otolaryngol Clin North Am 1999;32(1):7–14.

Preoperative photoimaging assists with an accurate facial analysis. Pictures taken in the frontal, right and left lateral, right and left oblique, and basal views are useful in surgical planning. Standardizing these views allows for accurate comparison of the preoperative deformity and postoperative correction. They are another means of effective communication and preoperative counseling. The advent of computerized imaging has added yet another tool to the armamentarium of the rhinoplasty surgeon. The specifics of photographic and computerized imaging are discussed elsewhere.[4,5]

Once an adequate history is obtained, an analysis is performed for the purpose of identifying the underlying anatomic abnormalities that result in the observed cutaneous deformities. Function must be considered when determining the desired aesthetic outcome.

ANATOMY

The quality of the skin-soft tissue envelope varies among individuals and within the same individual. Thin skin leaves little room for error as even the most minor irregularities become visible. Conversely, very thick skin can hinder all attempts to refine the nasal tip and make a narrow and elegant contour nearly impossible. Skin is thinnest over the rhinion and thick over the lower third and nasion where a variable amount of fibroadipose tissue is found.

The underlying superficial musculoaponeurotic system is continuous with the mimetic nasal muscles and a critical surgical landmark. The avascular plane deep to this layer is the correct plane for dissection during any degloving of the nose.

The upper third of the nose consists of paired nasal bones that attach laterally to the ascending process of the maxilla, superiorly to the frontal bone, and posteriorly to the perpendicular plate of the ethmoid bone. They are thinnest along their caudal aspect, at the junction with the upper lateral cartilages (ULC). The periosteum insinuates into the internasal suture line, requiring sharp dissection to tease the tissue out during elevation.

The lower two-thirds of the nose are comprised of cartilaginous structures that include the ULC, lower lateral cartilages (LLC), sesamoid cartilage, and quadrilateral septal cartilage. Cephalically, the paired ULCs attach to the caudal aspect of the nasal bones. Medially, they attach to the septum and are free floating laterally. The paired LLCs may be divided into the medial, intermediate, and lateral crura. Medial crura form the pods, contributing anteriorly to the shape of the infratip lobule. Intermediate crura form the dome, within which are the tip-defining points. Lateral crura are responsible for the overall width of the tip and help form the supra-alar creases. The paired sesamoid cartilages are lateral to the ULCs, providing support to the fibromuscular tissue between the ULCs and pyriform aperture. The quadrilateral septal cartilage attaches to the vomer posteriorly and nasal spine inferiorly. An important landmark is the anterior septal angle, identified in the supratip as the edge of the dorsal septal cartilage. The posterior septal angle is located at the attachment of the septum to the nasal spine. The internal nasal valve represents the space between the caudal end of the ULC and the dorsal septum. The external nasal valve is defined as the area within the nasal vestibule, under the alar lobule. It is lined with vibrissae and is bordered by the alar lobule, anterior nasal spine, membranous septum, and caudal septum. The intervalve area is under the nasal sidewall corresponding to the lateral aspect of the lateral crus and the lateral fibroareolar tissue extending to the bony pyriform aperture. It is here that a majority of functional problems arise.

The skin and soft tissue of the nose are supplied by the dorsal nasal, lateral nasal, angular, and columellar arteries. The septum and nasal mucosa are supplied by branches of the external (sphenopalatine, greater palatine, and superior labial) and internal (anterior and posterior ethmoidal) carotid arteries.

Tip support mechanisms delineate important anatomic relationships that provide structure to the tip. They are divided into major and minor mechanisms.[6]

ANALYSIS

Although this issue of *Clinics in Plastic Surgery* is dedicated to rhinoplasty, it is essential that surgeons analyze the entire face. Analysis should be based on accepted cultural standards; different aesthetic facial proportions exist in patients of different ethnic descent. The goals of analysis, alternatively, remain the same: define external deformities, predict the underlying anatomic variations, and determine the appropriate surgical intervention.[6] Preoperative evaluation includes observation, inspection, and certainly palpation, in a systematic fashion. Completing this comprehensive assessment prior to surgical planning helps avoid pitfalls and assists in identifying common nasal deformities that require surgical intervention (**Table 2**).

General

Determine patient age, height, and weight, as these variables effect overall proportion. Patients who are planning significant weight loss should have their surgery delayed. Assess the skin quality (ie, solar lentigo) and thickness. Recall, that thin skin provides less camouflage for grafts, whereas thick skin obscures subtle refinement. Identify acquired deformities from trauma or prior surgery and congenital malformations.

Table 2
Nasal deformities by view

View	Deformity
Frontal	Inverted V Twisted dorsum Bifid tip Pinched tip Parenthetic tip
Lateral	Low or high radix Inadequately positioned nasion Dorsal hump Saddle nose Pollybeak Under- or overprojection Alar notching Ptotic tip Tension nose
Base	Boxy tip Bulbous tip Bifid tip Amorphous tip Caudal septal deviation

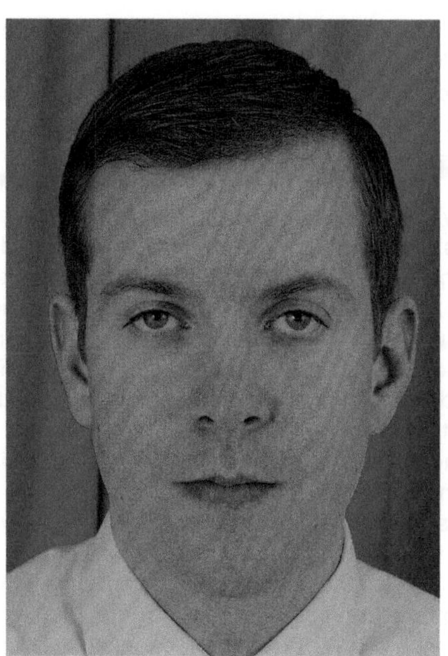

Fig. 1. Frontal view. Key points to identify are listed in **Box 1**.

Frontal View

Information gathered in the frontal view should include assessment of symmetry, balance, shape, and tip coutour (**Fig. 1**) (**Box 1**).

Box 1
Frontal view: key points to identify

Vertical fifth

Horizontal third

Upper third

- Width
- Symmetry
- Midline deviations/distortions

Middle third

- Width
- ULC symmetry
- Septal deviation

Lower third

- Width
- LLC symmetry
- Anterior septal angle position
- Shape and definition

Brow-tip aesthetic line

Tip/lobule

- Bulbosity
- Tip-defining points
- Alar shape
- Nostril size and shape

Imagine a vertical line in the midsagittal plane. Evaluating the facial halves may uncover slight facial asymmetry, which may effect the perception of a straight dorsum. Creating a perfectly straight nose on an asymmetric face appears unnatural. The assistance of a straight object in the midline may help to identify the direction of the deviation. This aids in identification of even subtle dorsal irregularities. Divide the nose into horizontal thirds and inspect each third independently. Deviation of the upper third indicates malposition of the nasal bones. A C-shaped deformity occurs if the middle third is deviated and indicates a problem with the septum or ULCs. Tip deviation in the lower third is the result of asymmetry of the LLCs or deviation at the anterior septal angle.

Assessment of balance is achieved by dividing the face into horizontal thirds and vertical fifths (**Fig. 2**). The nose should represent one-third the length of the face and one-fifth the width. In the absence of any other imperfection, an unbalanced nose remains aesthetically unpleasing.

The ideal shape of the nose is dictated by the brow-tip aesthetic line (**Fig. 3**). It is a gently sweeping line from the medial brow, along the lateral nasal wall, to the tip-defining points. Although it may seem arbitrary, the purpose of the brow-tip aesthetic line is to call attention to any contour irregularities that may stand out. The female nose should assume an unbroken hourglass shape; the aesthetic shape is narrow at the middle third and slightly wider at the radix and tip. Alar base width should lie just inside vertical lines extending from the medial canthi, representing the intercanthal distance.[7] An ill-defined brow-tip aesthetic line may result from a decrease in shadowing across the dorsum from an underprojected nose. Collapse of the middle vault leads to a pinched appearance in the middle third. Its anatomic etiologies include collapse of the ULCs from the dorsal septum, incomplete infracture of nasal bones, or cephalic orientation of ULCs.

The anterior view is used for assessing tip shape. The tip-defining points represent the anterior most projection of the intermediate crura and should have balance with respect to the entire nose. Reflections of light at the apex of the tip lobule often help identify them.[8] The medial and

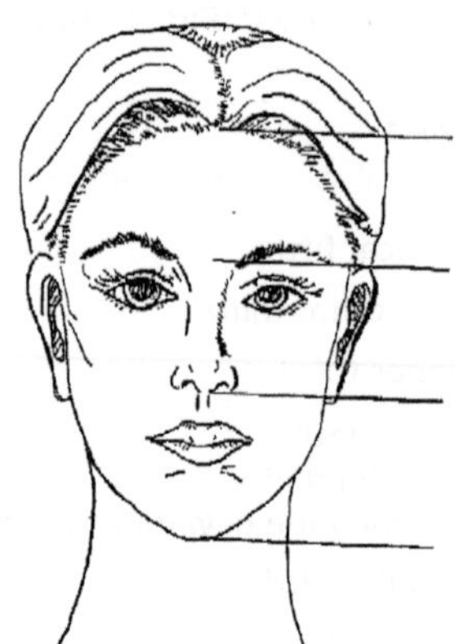

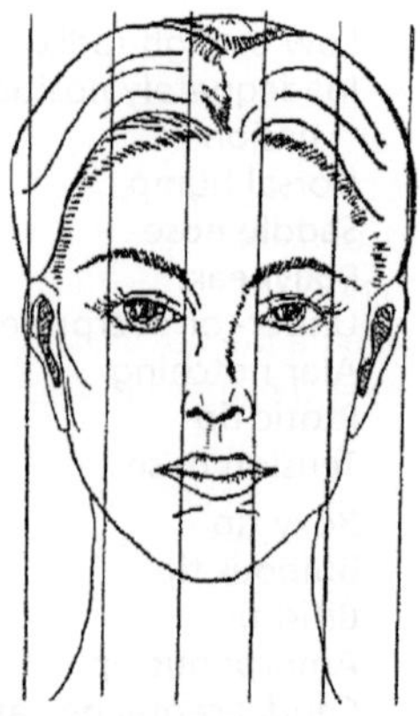

Fig. 2. Horizontal thirds and vertical fifths.

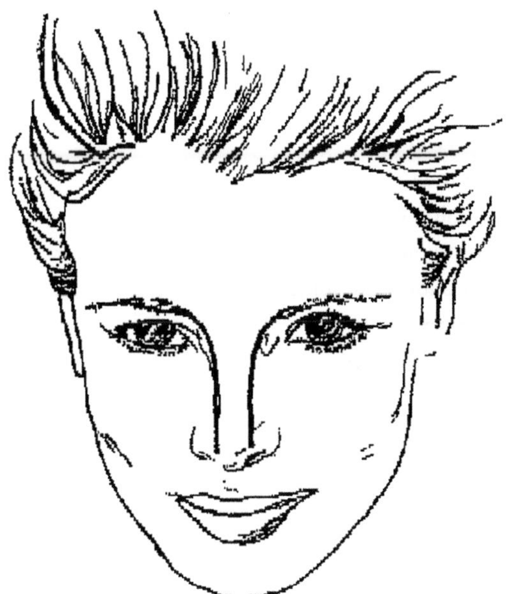

Fig. 3. Brow-tip aesthetic line.

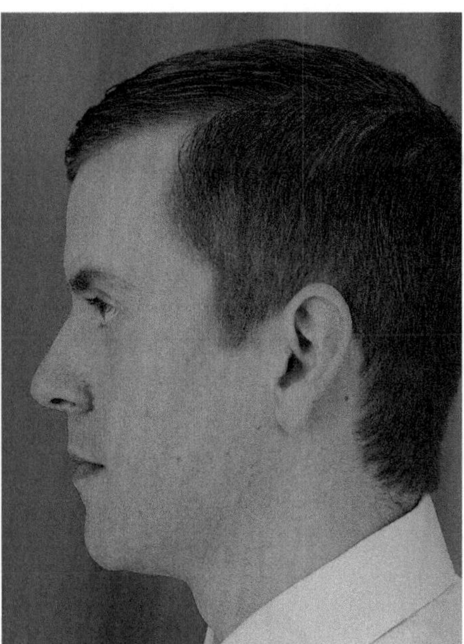

Fig. 4. Lateral view. Key points to identify are listed in Box 2.

lateral crura usually meet at roughly 30° and the tip can appear unnaturally sharp and narrow with increased acuity of the angle.[9] A bulbous, amorphous tip may result from sebaceous skin, wide lateral crura, dome divergence, or increased interdomal distance.[10] Irregular tip morphology is often the result of atypical convexity.[11] A boxy tip results from wide lateral crura that blunt the appearance of the domes. The columella hangs below the alar rims, giving shape to the infratip lobule.

Lateral View

On lateral view, with the head position in the Frankfort horizontal plane, it is possible to assess nasal length, projection, and rotation **(Fig. 4)** (**Box 2**). Attention to the alar-columellar relationship is also important. In addition, a comprehensive evaluation includes analysis of the radix and chin position. Standard anthropomorphic landmarks are vital to accurate analysis in profile (**Fig. 5**) (**Box 3**).

To maintain harmony between the horizontal thirds, it is critical to assess the relationship of the nose to the remainder of the face in profile. The forehead shape affects the nasal appearance. A sloping forehead from the hairline anteriorly to the brow gives the illusion of an over-projected nose, whereas a flat or protruding forehead may appear to shorten or deproject the nose.[12] Likewise, an underprojected chin may lead to the perception of an overprojected nose and vice versa. Several methods have been described to determine the ideal chin position. A simple technique was proposed by Goode, where an imaginary line is drawn perpendicular to the Frankfort horizontal plane at the alar-facial groove (**Fig. 6**).[12] The pogonion should approximate or lie just posterior to this line.

Determination of nasal length requires identification of the starting point or root of the nose (ie, the nasion). Most rhinoplasty surgeons portend this to be at the supratarsal crease. This point represents the deepest portion of the nasofrontal angle, which is approximately 120° between the

Box 2
Lateral view: key points to identify

Chin projection

Radix height

Nasion position

Nasal length

Nasofrontal angle

Nasolabial angle

Dorsum

- Hump or pseudohump
- Supratip break
- Projection

Tip

- Projection
- Rotation
- Double break
- Columellar show/hooding

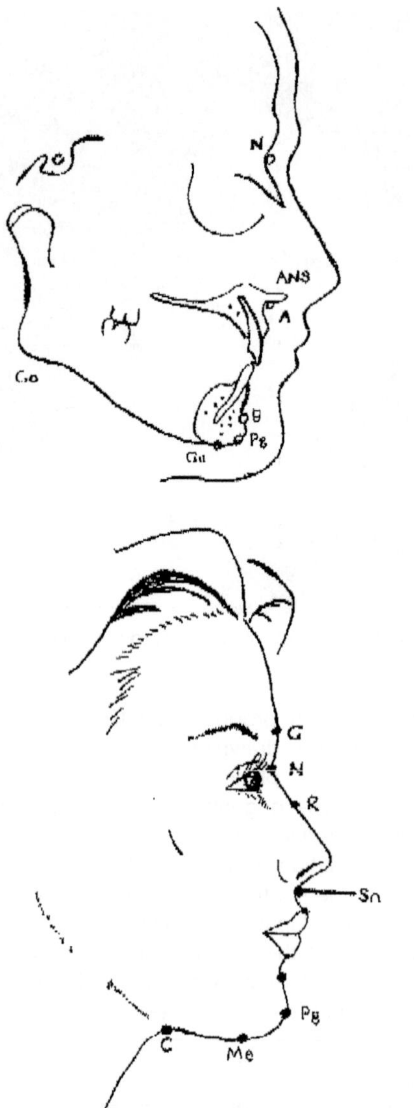

Fig. 5. Facial landmarks. Definitions are listed in **Box 3**.

Box 3
Facial landmarks with definitions

Landmark	*Definition*
Glabella (G)	Most prominent point of forehead in midsaggital plane
Nasion (N)	Deepest point of frontonasal angle
Rhinion (R)	Midline point of junction of nasal bones and ULCs
Subspinale (A)	Deepest point on premaxilla
Anterior nasal spine (ANS)	Tip of most prominent point of superior premaxilla
Supramentale (B)	Deepest point on outer cortex of mandible
Pogonion (Pg)	Most anterior point of chin
Gnathion (Gn)	Most inferior point of chin
Gonion (Go)	Most inferior/posterior point of mandible
Menton (Me)	Lowest point of mandibular symphysis
Cervical point (C)	Innermost point between submental area and neck
Subnasale (Sn)	Junction of columella and upper lip in midsaggital plane

glabella and nasal tip. The radix, centered over the nasion extending inferiorly to a horizontal plane at the level of the lateral canthus, should be evaluated independent of and prior to dorsal assessment. Its position is measured as the vertical distance between the corneal plane and radix plane. The corneal plane is a line tangent to the corneal surface, and the radix plane is a line tangent to the deepest point of the radix. The aesthetic range of radix position should fall between 9 and 14 mm.[13] A low radix creates the perception of decreased nasal length and a dorsal pseudohump. Ideal nasal length is two-thirds of the midfacial height, where midfacial height is measured from the most prominent point of the glabella to the alar base.[13]

Several methods are described for determining nasal projection. Crumley and Lanser describe a 3:4:5 right angle triangle, where the hypotenuse is represented by a line from the nasion to the tip.[14] Ideal projection is 60% of nasal length measured from the alar crease to the tip in a line parallel to the Frankfort horizontal plane. Goode defines ideal nasal projection as 0.55 to 0.6 of the distance from the nasion to the tip-defining points.[12] An underprojected tip generates the illusion of a dorsal pseudo-hump in the supratip region, also known as a pollybeak. Etiologies of overprojection include tension from the anterior septal angle, large anterior nasal spine, or

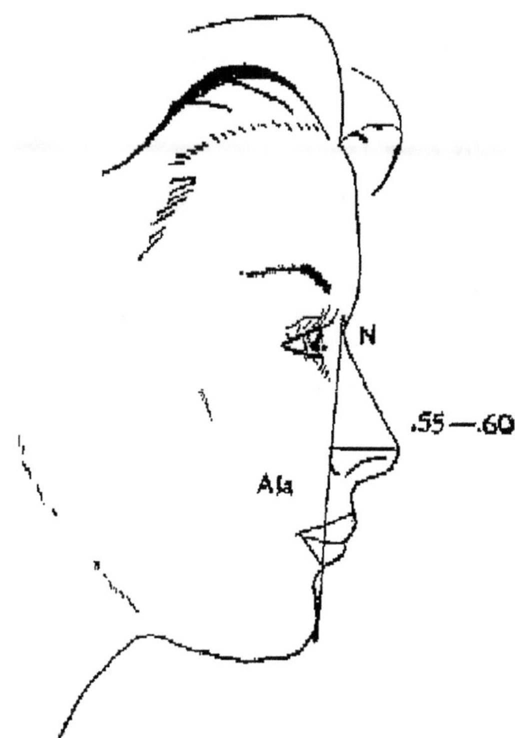

Fig. 6. Goode method of ideal chin projection.

overdevelopment of the LLCs.[3] Adequate projection confers a refined appearance on frontal view.

After determining aesthetic length, projection, and radix position, the dorsum is evaluated. It should lie at or slightly posterior to a line from the nasion to the tip at ideal nasal projection. Reduction is indicated anterior to the line in the absence of a pseudohump. The female dorsum in not perfectly straight, where a slight supratip break is desirable to distinguish the tip from the dorsum. Inadequate support of the dorsum leads to collapse of the middle third (saddle nose deformity) and nasal obstruction. This condition is seen most often after trauma, accidental or iatrogenic.

Nasal tip rotation is defined as movement about an arc with its radius centered at the nasolabial angle extending to the tip. The nasolabial angle is formed by the junction of the columella and subnasale. In women, the aesthetic angle is 90° to 100°, whereas a more acute angle of approximately 90° is sought after in men. The patient's height must be considered, as it is inversely proportional to the desired rotation. In shorter individuals cephalic rotation with an obtuse angle is more acceptable than their taller counterparts, regardless of gender.

Cephalic or caudal repositioning of the tip leads to a corresponding change in nasal length and columellar inclination. This concept is best illustrated by the tripod theory originally described by Anderson.[15] The paired LLCs are compared to a tripod, where the conjoined medial crura represent one leg and the lateral crura correspond to the remaining two legs. Loss of integrity of one limb changes the position of the tripod, affecting rotation and projection. For example, shortening of the medial crura derotates and deprojects the tip, giving the tip a ptotic appearance.

The relationship of the ala and columella is assessed on profile. Acceptable columellar show is between 2 and 4 mm. If greater than 4 mm, a distinction must be made between alar retraction and a hanging columella. A hanging columella may result from a prominent nasal spine, overdevelopment of the caudal septum, or enlarged medial crura. Alar retraction, or notching, is typically the result of an unfavorable outcome from prior rhinoplasty. It may also be present, however, as a normal variant in patients with cephalically positioned lateral crura and certain tension noses. If columellar show is less than 2 mm, the surgeon should suspect a retracted columella or dependent alar lobule. A double break of the columella is desirable, with the first break at the point where the tip begins its descent along the infratip lobule and the second break at the meeting of the medial and intermediate crura.

Base View

The base view allows for a thorough examination of nostril shape/size, columellar width, alar base width, length of medial crura, recurvature of lateral crura, and alar lobule thickness (**Fig. 7**) (**Box 4**). The nose should appear as an isosceles triangle with the upper third representing the tip lobule and the lower two-thirds corresponding to the columella (**Fig. 8**).[16]

It is critical to determine whether or not recurvature of the lateral crura is present (**Fig. 9**). If noted, the surgeon must recognize the risk of iatrogenic nasal obstruction if tip narrowing is performed.

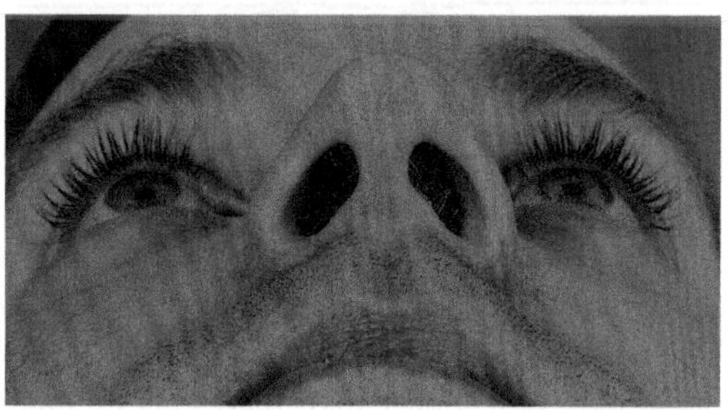

Fig. 7. Base view. Key points to identify are listed in **Box 4**.

Box 4
Base view: key points to identify

Shape of LLC (recurvature?)
Length of medial crura and position of pods
Tip lobule/shape
Nostril shape and position
Septal position
Base width

The length and symmetry of the medial crura contribute to the position of the tip-defining points and projection and rotation, based on the aforementioned tripod theory. The shape of the lateral crura contributes to overall tip appearance and if abnormal, may lead to a bulbous, boxy, or parenthetic tip as previously described. The nostrils are pear shaped and should be symmetric and widest at the nasal sill. The columella is narrowest at its midpoint, corresponding to the inferior break point on lateral view. It flares anterior and posterior to this point. The ideal alar base width is just inside vertical lines from the medial canthi.

Palpation

Determine skin elasticity and texture through palpation. It is essential to identify the intrinsic strength of the lower third of the nose, as weak LLCs may require a different surgical approach. This is accomplished through the tip recoil test, where the tip is depressed toward the upper lip and released.[17] Bimanual palpation of the LLCs provides important information on the size, strength, and shape of the cartilages. The nasal bones should be palpated to determine size, position, and presence of bony step-offs.

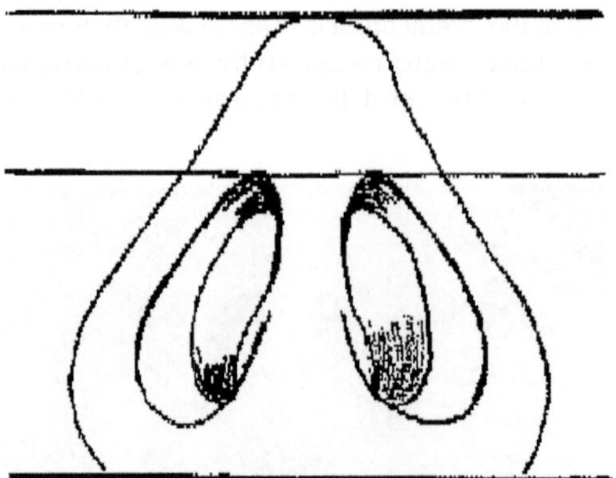

Fig. 8. Base view. Upper third represents tip lobule and lower two-thirds demonstrate columella and nostrils.

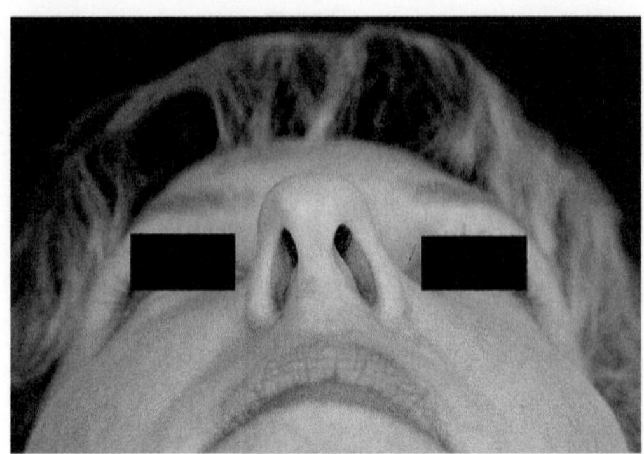

Fig. 9. Recurvature of the lower lateral crura.

Intranasal Inspection

Analysis is incomplete without intranasal inspection to identify possible areas that would predispose a patient to nasal obstruction. The external and internal components of the nasal valve and the intervalve area, which corresponds to the lateral margin of the lateral crus, all should be examined independently. The cartilaginous and bony portions of the septum are examined for any deviation, perforation, or deformity. Determination of the amount of septal cartilage present is critical as it is an important source of autologous material for reconstruction. The size and position of the turbinates is noteworthy. If lateral wall collapse is suspected, a Cottle maneuver may identify the precise area of involvement.

SUMMARY

Preoperative analysis lays the foundation for a successful surgical outcome. On completion of analysis, patients should leave with a clear understanding of the surgeon's perspective of their nose, aesthetically and anatomically. Understanding the interplay of surface deformities and their underlying anatomic counterpart is critical. This involves a systematic analysis to create a surgical plan that avoids landmines leading to a suboptimal result.

REFERENCES

1. Correa AJ, Sykes JM, Ries WR. Considerations before rhinoplasty. Otolaryngol Clin North Am 1999;32(1):7–14.
2. Widiger TA, Sanderson CJ. Personality disorders. In: Tasman A, Kay J, Lieberman JA, editors. Psychiatry. New York: Harcourt Brace & Co; 1997. p. 1291–317.
3. Bradley DT, Park SS. Preoperative analysis and diagnosis for rhinoplasty. Facial Plast Surg Clin North Am 2003;11(3):377–90.

4. Tardy ME, Brown M. Principles of photography in facial plastic surgery. New York: Thieme; 1992.
5. Mühlbauer W, Holm C. Computer imaging and surgical reality in aesthetic rhinoplasty. Plast Reconstr Surg 2005;115(7):2098–104.
6. Toriumi DM. Rhinoplasty. In: Park SS, editor. Facial plastic surgery: the essential guide. New York: Thieme Medical Publishers; 2005. p. 223–53.
7. Larrabee WF. Facial analysis for rhinoplasty. Otolaryngol Clin North Am 1987;20(4):653–74.
8. Burres S. Tip points: defining the tip. Aesthetic Plast Surg 1999;23(2):113–8.
9. Sheen JH, Sheen JP. Aesthetic rhinoplasty. 2nd edition. St Louis (MO): Mosby; 1987.
10. Ellis DA, McDonald DA. Narrowing of the wide nasal tip. J Otolaryngol 1984;13(1):55–7.
11. Daniel RK. Rhinoplasty: an atlas of surgical techniques. New York: Springer-Verlag; 2002.
12. Powell N, Humphrey B. Proportions of the aesthetic face. New York: Thieme-Stratton; 1984.
13. Byrd HS, Hobar PC. Rhinoplasty: a practical guide for surgical planning. Plast Reconstr Surg 1993; 91(4):642–54.
14. Crumley RL, Lanser M. Quantitative analysis of nasal tip projection. Laryngoscope 1988;98:202–8.
15. Anderson JR. The dynamics of rhinoplasty. In: Proceedings of the Ninth International Congress in otorhinolaryngology. Excerpta Medica, International Congress Series 206. Amsterdam; 1969.
16. Boahene KD, Orten SS, Hilger PA. Facial analysis of the rhinoplasty patient. In: Papel ID, Frodel JL, Holt GR, et al, editors. Facial plastic and reconstructive surgery. New York: Thieme Medical Publishers; 2009. p. 477–87.
17. Tardy ME. Rhinoplasty tip ptosis: etiology and prevention. Laryngoscope 1973;83:923–9.

Surgical Anatomy of the Nose

Robert M. Oneal, MD, Richard J. Beil, MD*

KEYWORDS

• Nasal anatomy • Rhinoplasty • Anatomic nasal analysis

Assessing the external nose requires an understanding of the anatomic components that contribute to its normal topographic features. Structures that influence the external appearance include the skin, which varies in thickness, and the underlying bony/cartilaginous skeletal framework. Because skin thickness is greatest at areas of skeletal narrowness, the external appearance of the nose from the frontal view is one of a soft, gentle curve emanating from the medial brows and extending to the tip-defining points (dorsal esthetic line) (**Fig. 1**). The lobule can be defined as an area including the tip of the nose and bounded by a line connecting the upper edge of the nostrils, the supratip breakpoint, and the anterior half of the lateral alar wall. The lobule is subdivided into the tip, supratip, and infratip lobule. On lateral view, one should be aware of the marked differences in the thickness of the soft tissue (**Fig. 2**).

The internal structure most frequently responsible for the prominence of the lateral tip-defining point or pronasalae is the cephalic edge of the domal segment of the middle crus. On lateral view, the tip of the nose is the apex of the lobule and ideally the most defined element on the profile.[1–3] In non-Caucasian, however, the tip tends to lack definition.[4] The infratip lobule is between the tip and the apex of the nostrils. The configuration of the infratip lobule depends on the shape, size, and angulation of the medial and middle crura of the alar cartilage (see **Fig. 2**). The supratip lobule lies between the pronasalae and the supratip breakpoint. The nasolabial angle is defined as the angle formed by a line drawn from the anterior to the posterior nostril apices and intersects with the vertical facial plane. It determines the amount of cephalic rotation of the tip.

In an esthetically pleasing nose, the columella projects as a gentle curve below the alar margin as seen on lateral view. In the non-Caucasian nose, however, a common variation is for the ala to overhang the columella posteriorly.[4] The columella and infratip lobule projection are influenced by the configuration of the medial and middle crura. Because of the thin, adherent skin, asymmetries or prominences in these structures are easily visible in external configuration. In addition, projections of the caudal edge of the septum can produce a prominence of the columella also.

On base view (**Fig. 3**), the flaring of the caudal edges of the medial and middle crura is noted. The degree of flare plus the lateral curve of the medial crural footplates determine the width of the columella and infratip lobule. Columellar deviations and asymmetries are frequently caused by deflections in the caudal septum. Medially, the relationship should be noted of the anterior nasal spine to the depressor septi muscle, which is paired and inserts into the medial crural foot plates. Laterally, the alar part of the nasalis muscle should be noted.

SOFT-TISSUE COVERING OF THE NOSE

Skin

Skin thickness is one of the most important features to assess preoperatively in planning rhinoplasty. The skin tends to be thinner and more mobile in the upper half of the nose and

This article is adapted from Oneal RM, Beil Jr RJ, Schlesinger J. Surgical anatomy of the nose. Clin Plast Surg 1996;23(2):195–222.

Department of Surgery, University of Michigan, Center for Plastic and Reconstructive Surgery, St Joseph Mercy Hospital, 5333 McAuley Drive, Suite 5001, PO Box 994, Ann Arbor, Michigan, MI 48106, USA
* Corresponding author.
E-mail address: rjbeil@earthlink.net (R.J. Beil).

Clin Plastic Surg 37 (2010) 191–211
doi:10.1016/j.cps.2009.12.011
0094-1298/10/$ – see front matter

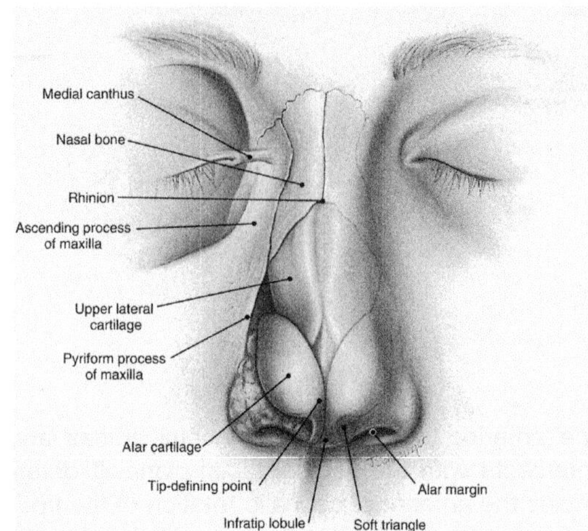

Fig. 1. Frontal view of nose. (*Courtesy of* Jaye Schlesinger, Ann Arbor, MI.)

thicker and more adherent distally. In dissections reported by Lessard and Daniel,[5] average skin thickness was noted to be greatest at the nasofrontal groove (1.25 mm) and least at the rhinion (0.6 mm). There are usually more sebaceous glands in the lower half of the nose, causing an oiliness and thickness in the skin that may limit topographic definition, sometimes obscuring entirely the underlying framework and the natural esthetic lines normally visible, particularly in the non-Caucasian nose, which may have a larger subcutaneous dense fibrofatty layer than the Caucasian nose.[4] Some of the nasal changes seen with aging (ie, tip droop, nasal lengthening) may be caused by changes in skin character.[6] The skin is usually thinner along the alar margin and in the columella, where the configuration of the alar cartilages may be visualized through a thin skin cover. The skin-to-skin approximations in the soft triangle area at the nostril apex makes it extremely vulnerable to notching and irregularities due to scarring when intranasal incisions violate this delicate area.

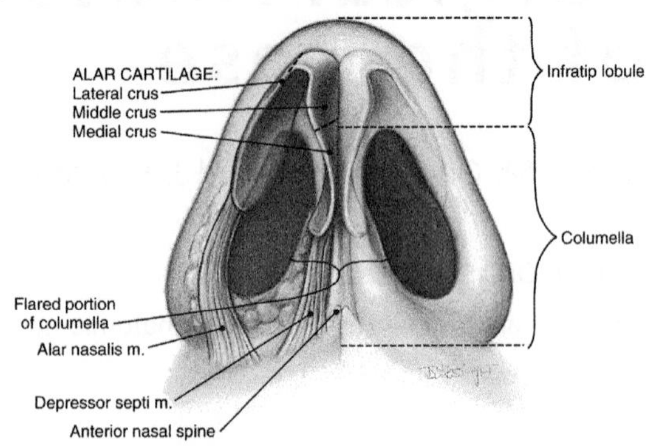

Fig. 3. Basal view of nose. (*Courtesy of* Jaye Schlesinger, Ann Arbor, MI.)

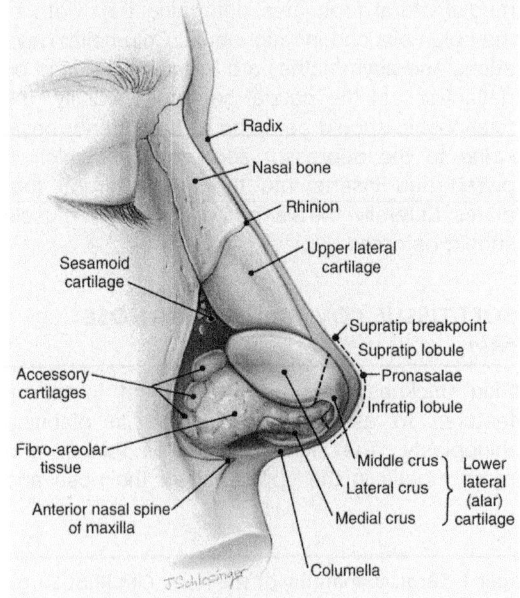

Fig. 2. Right lateral view of nose. Note the distance of the lateral crus from the skin edge of the nostril. (*Data from* Daniel RK. Discussion of Constantian, MB. Two essential elements for planning tip surg. Plast Reconstr Surg 2004;114:1582. *Courtesy of* Jaye Schlesinger, Ann Arbor, MI.)

Subcutaneous Layer

The soft tissue intervening between the skin and the osteocartilaginous skeleton is made up of four layers.[5] They are the *superficial fatty panniculus*, the *fibromuscular layer*, the *deep fatty layer* and the *periosteum* or *perichondrium*. The fibromuscular layer includes the nasal subcutaneous muscular aponeurotic system (SMAS). The nasal SMAS is a continuation of the superficial muscular aponeurotic system, which covers the entire face, interconnecting the facial musculature, the galeal-frontalis layer, and the platysma. Ignorance of the importance of this level or inadvertent surgical or traumatic division of the superficial muscular aponeurotic system (SMAS) leads to its bilateral retraction. This retraction exposes the deeper skeletal components to possible adherence through scar tissue to the superficial fatty layer, which is directly connected to the dermis.[7,8] The major superficial blood vessels and motor nerves run within the deep fatty layer.[9] Just beneath it and superficial to the periosteum and perichondrium is the proper plane of dissection, similar to the areolar layer beneath the galea aponeurotica in the scalp.

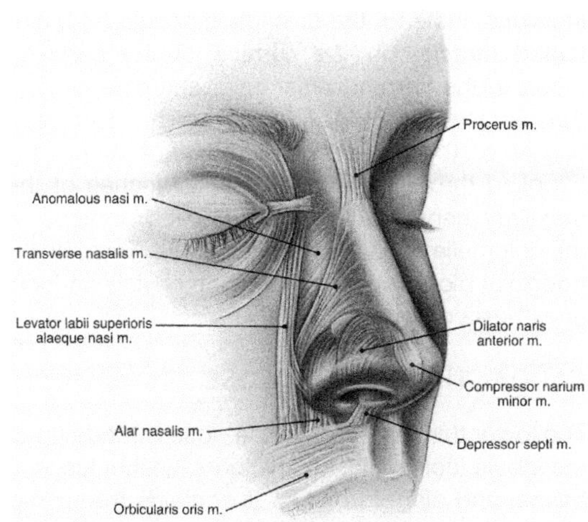

Fig. 4. Nasal muscles of facial expression. (*Courtesy of* Jaye Schlesinger, Ann Arbor, MI.)

Muscles

Griesman[10,11] subdivided the nasal muscles into four groups. Letourneau and Daniel[9] substantiated these findings in 30 fresh cadaver dissections (**Fig. 4**). The *elevator* muscles, which shorten the nose and dilate the nostrils, include (1) the procerus, (2) the levator labii superioris alaeque nasi, and (3) the anomalous nasi. The *depressor* muscles, which lengthen the nose and dilate the nostrils, include (4) the alar portion of the nasalis muscle (dilator naris posterior) and (5) the depressor septi. The *minor dilator* muscle is the (6) dilator naris anterior. The *compressor* muscles, which lengthen the nose and narrow the nostrils, include (7) the transverse portion of the nasalis and (8) the compressor narium minor. An in-depth discussion of these muscles can be found in articles by Griesman[10] and Letourneau and Danie1.[9] All the muscles are innervated by the zygomaticotemporal division of the facial nerve.

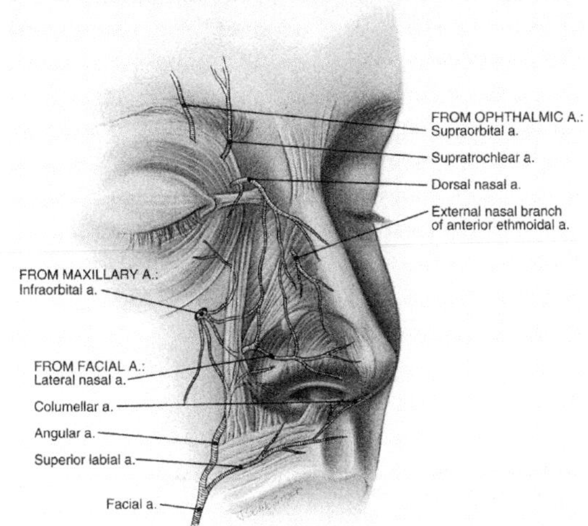

Fig. 5. Arterial supply of the external nose. (*Courtesy of* Jaye Schlesinger, Ann Arbor, MI.)

EXTERNAL BLOOD SUPPLY

The superficial arterial supply to the external structures of the nose is derived from the internal carotid artery (through the ophthalmic) and external carotid artery (through the facial and internal maxillary) (**Fig. 5**).[12,13] The lateral surface of the caudal nose is supplied by the lateral nasal branch from the angular artery, which is the continuation of the facial artery. This branch anastomoses with its pair from the opposite side across the dorsum of the nose. Herbert[14] referred to the angular artery as an alar branch of the superior labial artery. He noted that it passed deep in the groove between the ala and the cheek and lay buried in the levator labii superioris alaeque nasi muscle.[14] It tended to follow closely the margin of the pyriform aperture. Sequentially it gives off between 7 and 12 short branches, which perforate the enveloping muscle and enter the subdermal plexus of the nostril and cheek.[14] These branches provide a rich axial blood supply to subcutaneous based cheek and nasolabial flaps and the nasalis myocutaneous flap.[15,16]

An external branch of the ophthalmic artery, the dorsal nasal artery, perforates the orbital septum above the medial canthal ligament and runs downward on the side of the nose to anastomose with the lateral nasal branch of the angular artery. It gives off a branch to the lacrimal sac. All of these vessels, which vary in size, are supplemented by twigs laterally from branches of the infraorbital artery. The dorsal nasal artery, which also can have communications with the supratrochlear and infraorbital arteries, forms an axial arterial network for the dorsal skin as described by Marchak and Toth.[17] Injection studies quoted in their article show the rich anastomotic blood supply to the lateral skin of the nose, allowing elevation of this entire soft-tissue envelope on a narrow vascular pedicle.

Branches of the superior labial artery supply the nostril sill and the base of the columella. Consistently a substantial branch ascends in the columella just superficial to the medial crura (see **Fig. 5**). The columellar artery, which is often bifurcated, is cut with a transcolumellar incision used in the open rhinoplasty approach.[18] The branches of the external nasal branch of the anterior ethmoidal artery along with the angular artery in the ala also contribute to the arterial supply to the nasal tip.

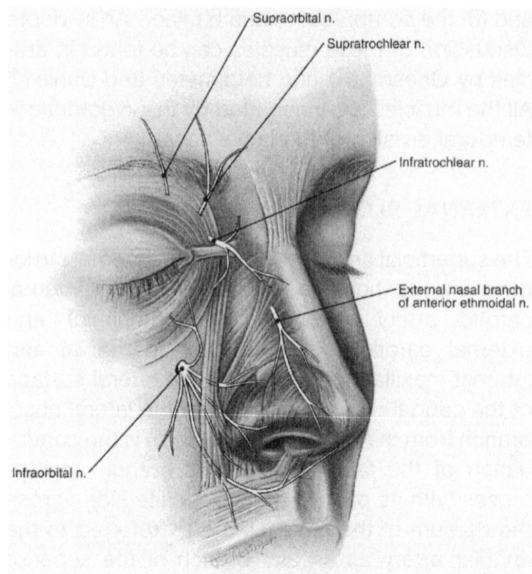

Fig. 6. Sensory nerve supply of the external nose. (*Courtesy of* Jaye Schlesinger, Ann Arbor, MI.)

The level of these vessels should be considered in open rhinoplasty to minimize compromise of the circulation to the nasal tip and columellar skin. It is also important to maintain dissection just superficial to the lateral crura of the alar cartilage to avoid injuring these lateral vessels. For the same reason, when performing open rhinoplasty, alar base excisions should always be limited to skin and superficial subcutaneous tissue.[19]

The venous drainage of the external nose has the same-named veins, which accompany the arteries. These veins drain via the facial vein and the pterygoid plexus and through the ophthalmic veins into the cavernous sinus.

EXTERNAL SENSORY NERVE SUPPLY

Sensibility to the external nose is mediated through branches of the ophthalmic and maxillary divisions of the fifth cranial nerve (**Fig. 6**). Sensibility to the skin of the nose at the radix, the rhinion, and the cephalic portion of the nasal side walls is supplied by twigs from the supratrochlear and infratrochlear branches of the ophthalmic nerve. The external nasal branch of the anterior ethmoidal nerve, which emerges between the nasal bone and the upper lateral cartilage, accompanying the same-named artery, supplies the skin over the dorsum of the distal nose down to and including the tip of the nose. Injury to this nerve explains tip numbness commonly noted after rhinoplasty, as this branch is vulnerable during intercartilage or cartilage-splitting incisions. To minimize the chance of injury to this nerve, it is best to avoid deep endonasal incisions. Instead, the dissection should be maintained directly on the surface of the cartilage (deep to the fibromuscular layer and extension of the periosteum [SMAS]).[10] Sensibility to the soft tissues on the side of the lower half of the nose is supplied through the infraorbital branches of the maxillary nerve, which also supplies portions of the columella and the lateral vestibule. Thus, an infraorbital block is important when relying on local anesthesia during rhinoplasty.

CAUDAL THIRD OF THE NOSE

The lower third, or base, of the nose is made up of the lobule, columella, nostril floors, vestibules, alar bases, and alar side walls. It contains the paired alar cartilages and accessory cartilages and fibrous fatty connective tissue (see **Figs. 1–3**).

Alar Cartilage Morphology

The traditional concept of alar cartilage morphology was that of medial and lateral crura connected by an anatomic domal segment. To clarify the understanding of the surgical anatomy of the nasal tip, Sheen and Sheen[3] introduced the concept of a *middle crus*, with its inferior limit at the columellar lobule junction and its superior limit at the junction of the medial extent of the lateral crus (**Figs. 7–9**). Daniel's[20] observations place the domal segment in the most superior aspect of the middle crus. After Sheen's original observation, the middle crus has also been referred to as the *intermediate crus*.[19,21] The concept of a distinct and independent middle or intermediate crus has been challenged by another study, in which the term *body* or *intercrural segment* was applied.[22] It is the authors' opinion, however, that this structure is more than a connecting link between the medial and lateral crura.

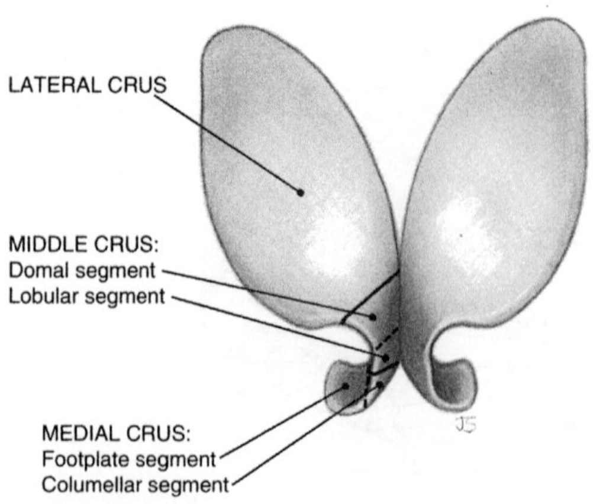

Fig. 7. Paired alar cartilages: frontal view. (*Courtesy of* Jaye Schlesinger, Ann Arbor, MI.)

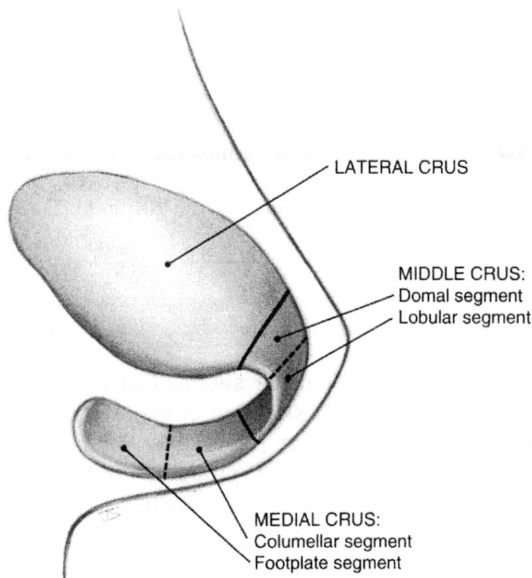

Fig. 8. Paired alar cartilages: lateral view. (*Courtesy of* Jaye Schlesinger, Ann Arbor, MI.)

Its complex and variable structure is so important to the configuration of the nasal lobule that it deserves separate description and consideration. In this discussion, each alar cartilage is divided into 3 components: the *medial*, *middle*, and *lateral crura*.

Medial crus

The medial crus consists of two components: the *footplate segment* and the *columellar segment*. In most patients, angulation occurs in 2 planes: the

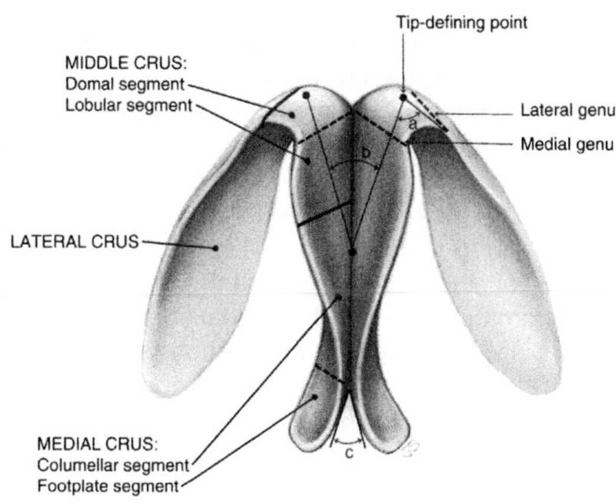

Fig. 9. Paired alar cartilages: basal view shows angles of divergence and angle of domal definition. a, angle of domal definition; b, angle of domal divergence; c, angle of footplate divergence. (*Courtesy of* Jaye Schlesinger, Ann Arbor, MI.)

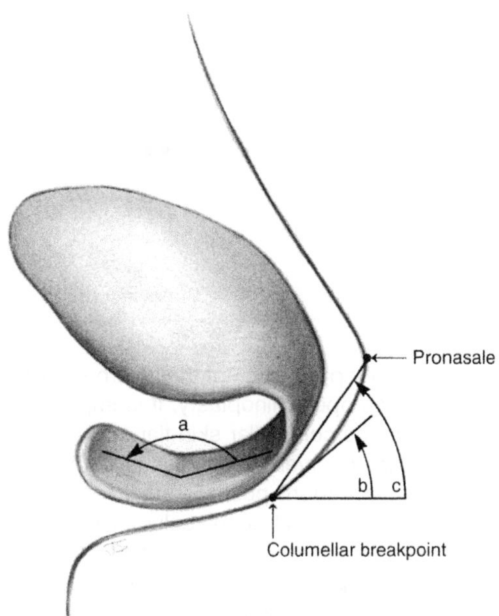

Fig. 10. Alar cartilage: right lateral view of angles of rotation. a, angle of cephalic rotation; b, columellar-lobular angle; c, angle of tip rotation. (*Courtesy of* Jaye Schlesinger, Ann Arbor, MI.)

angle of cephalic rotation, as noted on lateral view (**Fig. 10**), and the *angle of footplate divergence*, as noted on base view (see **Fig. 9**C). The effect of the configuration of the medial crus produced by these angles greatly influences the shape and prominence of the flared portion of the base of the columella (see **Fig. 3**). The footplate segment of the columella is influenced not only by its intrinsic shape but also by the posterior caudal edge of the cartilaginous septum, and by the amount of soft tissue in the base of the columella.

The *columellar segment* begins at the upper limit of the footplate segment and ends at the columellar lobule junction (columellar breakpoint), where it joins the middle crus. The length of the columellar segment varies. Elongated nostrils are due in part to vertically long columellar segments. Natvig and colleagues described three common anatomic variations of the medial crus in a cadaver study that were confirmed by others (**Fig. 11**).[5] The most common type is an asymmetric parallel (75%) (**Fig. 12**). The other two types, the flared symmetric and the straight symmetric, occur about equally (12.5%).[20] Although the skin is thin and the subcutaneous tissue is almost nonexistent laterally, the intervening soft tissue between the columellar segments of the medial crus frequently camouflages any asymmetries. In contrast, the absence of sufficient intervening soft tissue

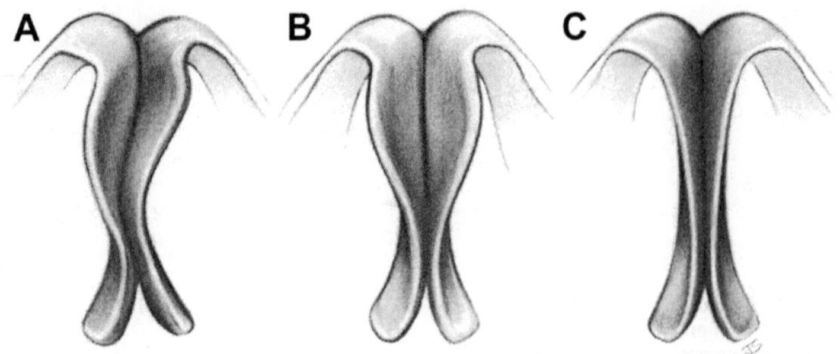

Fig. 11. Paired alar cartilages: basal view shows variations in shape of the medial crus and lobular segment of the middle crus. (*A*) Asymmetric parallel. (*B*) Flared symmetric. (*C*) Straight symmetric. (*Courtesy of* Jaye Schlesinger, Ann Arbor, MI.)

creates a bifid appearance of the columella. When performing an open rhinoplasty, it is important to elevate with the columellar skin flap at a depth to include all the intervening soft tissue. If this is not done, the inadvertent postoperative result could be an unplanned bifidity in the columella. When repositioning the columellar segments or resuturing them after separation to expose the caudal septum in open rhinoplasty, it is important to retain the natural flare of the caudal edges by placing any fixation sutures only at the cephalic borders.

From the lateral view, the most convex portion of the columellar lobular curve is termed the *columella breakpoint* (see **Fig. 10**). Its configuration is determined intrinsically by the shape of the junction of the columellar segment of the medial crus and the lobular segment of the middle crus. Acute angulations can produce an unattractive protrusion. The amount of protrusion of the columella (caudal projection) depends not only on the horizontal width of the columellar segment but also on the width of the membranous septum and the amount of protrusion of the caudal edge of the septal cartilage. Likewise, upward retraction depends on a deficiency of the same factors but most often is caused by retraction of the caudal septum because of trauma or congenital deformity or iatrogenically because of overresection of the edge of the caudal septum or failure to leave an adequate caudal septal strut during submucous resection of the septum.

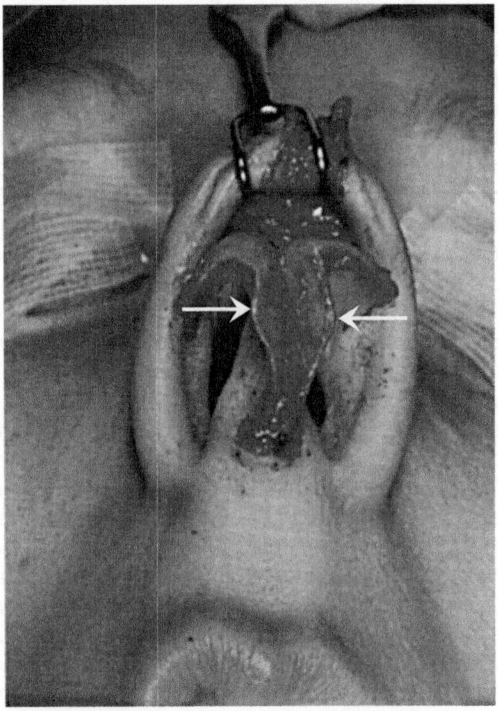

Fig. 12. Operative view of the medial and middle crura during open rhinoplasty. Note the flared symmetric configuration, the flare of caudal borders, and the domal segment.

Middle (intermediate) crus

The middle crus is made up of the *lobular segment* and the *domal segment*. The lobular segment of the middle crus tends to be the most variable and have the least correlation between the actual internal structural configuration and the external appearance. Its superficial expression is camouflaged by the thicker, overlying soft-tissue envelope.

The lobular segment tends to have the same variable configuration as described by Natvig and colleagues for the medial crus. Their description did not include the middle crus as a separate anatomic unit. Daniel and Letourneau, in describing their observations from open rhinoplasty, noted that in almost all cases the cephalic edges of the lobular segment were in close approximation but that the caudal edges diverged (**Fig. 13**). Their length, configuration, and angulation determine the shape, height, and protrusion of the infratip lobule.

The domal segment is usually short and also frequently the most thin, delicate, and narrow portion of the entire alar cartilage arch. In contrast to Sheen's earlier description, Daniel has described a medial genu at its connection with the lobular segment and a lateral genu at its junction with the lateral crus.[3,5] The domal segment

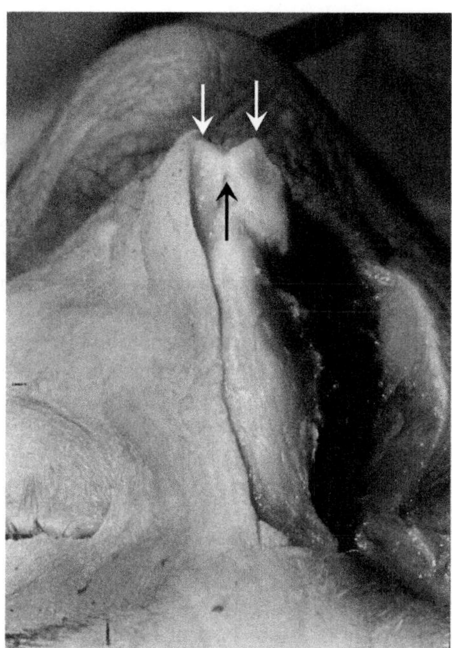

Fig. 13. Fresh cadaver dissection: a topdown view from the forehead. Note the flared caudal edges of the middle crura, the closed approximation of the cephalic edge of the middle crus, and the domal segment symmetry (*arrows*).

can vary in configuration (**Fig. 14**). It may be concave, which is the least common. With the convex medial and lateral genu, this configuration produces a double-dome effect. It also can be smooth, which gives the tip of the nose a wide, boxy configuration.[5] Varying degrees of convexity of the domal segment produce a more esthetic tip.[20,23] The concave caudal edge of the domal segment frequently has a notched configuration (the domal notch), which is largely responsible for the facet of the *soft triangle*. The soft triangle is at the apex of the nostril, where dermis is in direct contact with dermis containing no intervening subcutaneous tissue.[24] Because the caudal edge of the domal segment is so irregular and the cartilage itself is so delicate, great care must be taken in making infracartilaginous incisions to avoid injuring the cartilage edge or intruding into the soft triangle, where postoperative scarring may produce deformity in this delicate skin. The cephalic edges of the paired domal segments are frequently in close approximation or have minimal separation (**Fig. 15**).[19,20] The approximation of the domal segments also may extend to include the adjacent cephalic edge of the lateral crus. The cephalic edge usually slopes posteriorly from the high point of the domal segment in the normal esthetic nose to contribute to the supratip breakpoint (see **Fig. 15**). The paired domal defining points characteristically decrease at the most anterior projecting point along the domal segments. These defining points can be narrowed using sutures.[25]

The medial and middle crura are also tightly bound together by transverse fibrous connective tissue. The most anterior thickening is termed the *interdomal ligament* (**Fig. 16**A). These fibers fuse with the more cephalic transverse fibers between the cephalic edges of the lateral crura and to vertically oriented fibers connected to the overlying dermis, termed the *dermocartilaginous* ligament by Pitanguy (see **Fig. 16**B).[26] There is strong evidence to support the idea that the fibrous tissue connections between the full length of the medial and middle crura create a single function or unit of these paired structures (J Tebbets, personal communication, 1990).[27] Thus this paired structure can be considered one leg of a tripod, with the lateral crura (and their extensions) being the other 2 legs (**Fig. 17**).[28,29]

The external expression of the domal segment depends on 3 factors: (1) its specific angulation, (2) its position relative to the opposite domal segment as determined by the divergence of the dome-defining points, and (3) the thickness of the overlying soft tissue (**Fig. 17**). The subcutaneous fat is thickest in the supratip area, and the soft-tissue thickness over the tip of the nose varies considerably from patient to patient. A bifid tip is caused by a deficiency of intervening soft tissue between the domal segments and thin skin as much as it is caused by the amount of divergence between the dome-defining points.

The supratip breakpoint is important esthetically because it defines the cephalic limit of the nasal tip

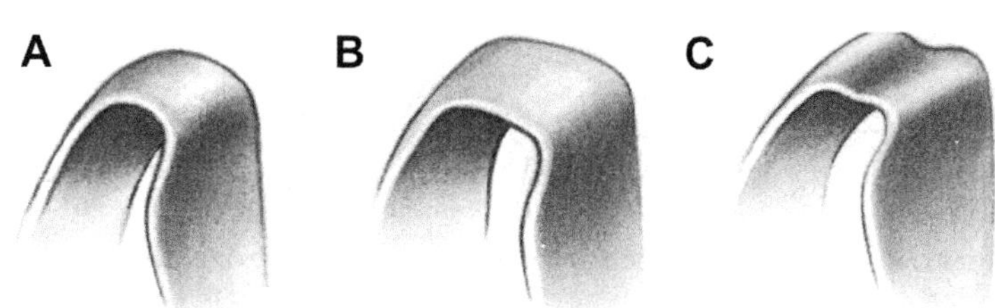

Fig. 14. Variations in domal configurations. (*A*) Convex domal segment configuration. (*B*) Boxy broad with minimal convexity. (*C*) Double-dome, concave dome segment. (*Courtesy of* Jaye Schlesinger, Ann Arbor, MI.)

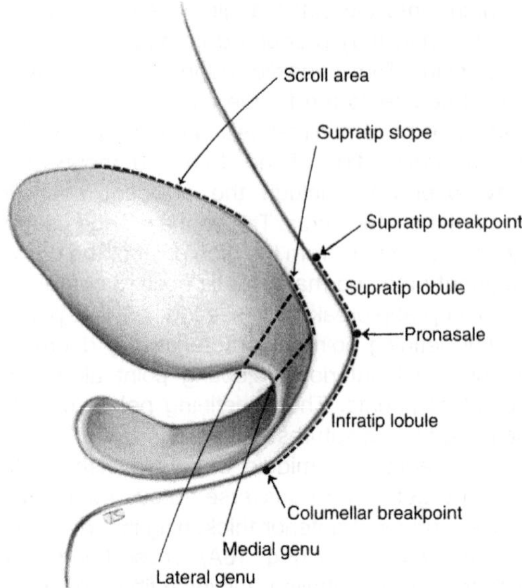

Fig. 15. Note the supratip slope of the right alar cartilage and the scroll area of the lateral crus. (*Courtesy of* Jaye Schlesinger, Ann Arbor, MI.)

and the inferior limit of the nasal dorsum. It is created in part by the difference between the projection of the dome-defining points and the height of the anterior septal angle (**Fig. 18**). Equally important is the degree of posterior slope of the lateral crus immediately adjacent to the convex domal segment of the middle crus.[20,23] The most common relationship between the anterior septal angle and the nasal tip is where the distal portion of the caudal septum does not have much influence on the position of the clinical domes; the domes are as much as 8 to 10 mm caudal to and 3 to 6 mm anterior to the anterior septal angle. The latter differential constitutes the supratip break. This distance may have to be exaggerated to 10 to 12 mm in thick-skinned noses to create an adequate supratip.

Surgical techniques to create a satisfactory supratip breakpoint have been described using suturing of the medial aspect of the lateral crura to narrow and elongate the tip of the nose, and lowering the dorsal surface of the caudal septal cartilage. This technique leaves an iatrogenic tissue void, which has a propensity to fill in with scar tissue and can be one of the causes leading to a supratip fullness or "pollybeak deformity".[25] An alternative is direct suture sculpturing, thereby emphasizing the alar cartilage projection to create an esthetically pleasing supratip break with minimal cartilage excision and potentially less "dead space" and possibly a more predictable result (J Tebbets, personal communication, 1990).[16,30]

Lateral crus

The lateral crus is the largest component of the nasal lobule and plays a major role in defining the shape of the anterior superior portion of the alar side wall. Medially the lateral crus is directly contiguous with the domal segment of the middle crus and laterally with the first of a chain of accessory cartilages that abut the pyriform process.[6,31] Caudally its free edge may be flat or it may be curved posteriorly to varying degrees. The caudal edge parallels and provides support for only the anterior one-half of the alar rim.[7,31] Thus, any excessive excision of the medial half of the lateral crus can potentially contribute to weakening of support of the anterior alar rim. As it progresses laterally the caudal edge turns cephalically away from the alar rim. Thus a marginal (infracartilaginous) incision does not follow the rim of the ala, except medially, but ascends cephalically following the edge of the cartilage.[23]

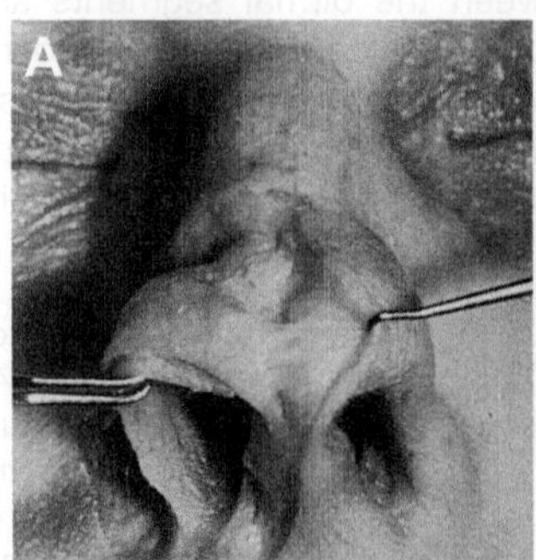

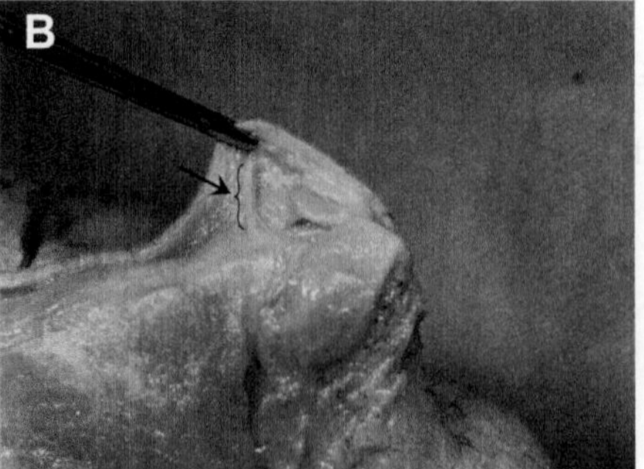

Fig. 16. Fresh cadaver dissection. (*A*) Basal view shows the interdomal condensation of fibrous connective tissue between the medial and middle crura. (*B*) Right oblique view shows the dermocartilaginous ligament (*From* the dermis to the domal segment of the middle crus).

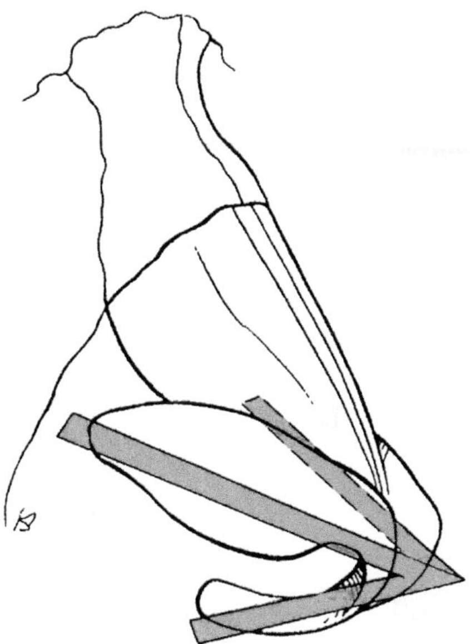

Fig. 17. Tripod concept of nasal tip cartilages. (*Courtesy of* Jaye Schlesinger, Ann Arbor, MI.)

Usually the lateral crus is at its widest just medial to where the caudal border takes its cephalic turn (S Stahl, personal communication, 1990). The longitudinal axis of the lateral crus (from dome point to lateral point) is more vertical than indicated in classic texts and may be close to 45°.[5,14] On frontal view this axis is directed toward the pupil. A more exaggerated cephalic positioning of the alar cartilage produces what Sheen describes as a malpositioned or "parenthesis" tip.[3,32,33]

Zelnick and Gingrass[34] described several variations of shape of the lateral crus in a report of preserved cadaver dissections (**Fig. 19**). In types C and D, the lateral crus adjacent to the domal segment is concave. This variation is favorable in achieving a more convex dome, possibly requiring only minimal modification of the lateral crus if combined with the creation of a more acute angle of domal definition.[20] As noted by Zelnick and Gingrass, however, because of the camouflaging effect of the overlying soft tissues, in many cases it would be impossible to appreciate these variations without direct exposure of the alar cartilages. Dion and colleagues[31] observed side-to-side asymmetry in lateral crus shape in more than half of their 31 cadaver specimens.

The junction of the cephalic edge of the lateral crus and the caudal edge of the upper lateral cartilage is known as the scroll area. An early study on the configuration of the caudal edge of the upper lateral cartilage showed some degree of lateral (downward) curling. Conversely, the slope of the adjacent cephalic edge of the lateral crus is usually a convex curve downward (**Fig. 20**). In most

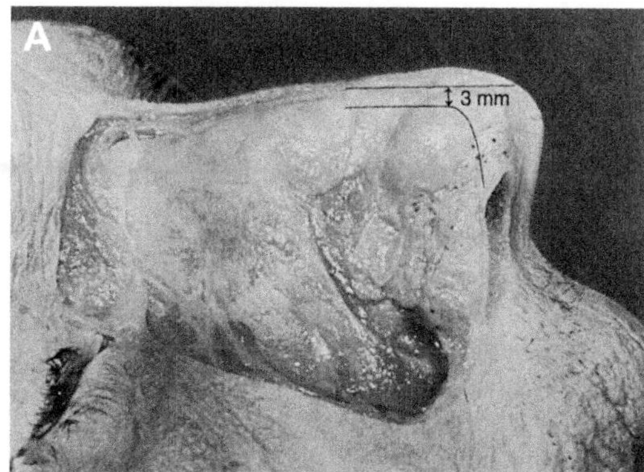

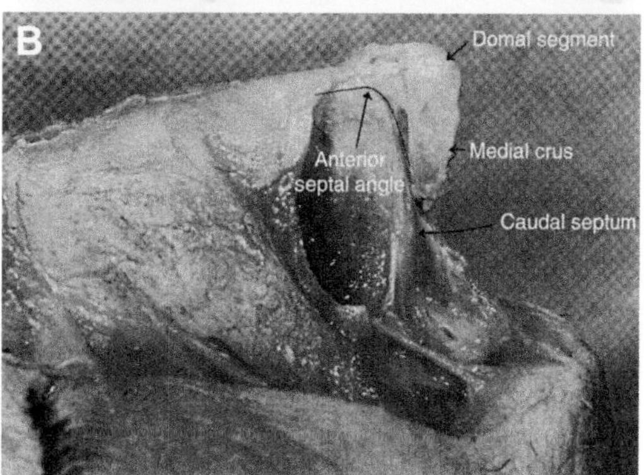

Fig. 18. Fresh cadaver dissection. (*A*) Right lateral view: the domal segment (*right alar cartilage*) projects (3 mm) above the anterior septal angle. (*B*) Right lateral view: the soft tissue and alar cartilage of the right side of the alar base (*lower one-third of the nose*) have been removed. The left-side medial and middle crura are in anatomic position. Note the relationship of the medial crus to the caudal septum and the relationship of the domal segment to the anterior septal angle.

people there is some degree of overlap of these cartilages, which may enhance the function of the internal nasal valve.[10] The degree of this curvature determines in part the flare and fullness (bulbousness) of the lateral lobule. If resection of either cartilage edge is contemplated, the underlying mucosa should be preserved carefully and the cartilage excision should be minimized to avoid unpredictable, undesirable late changes.[35]

More details of this junction were described after microscopic study. The presence of a variable number of small sesamoid cartilages was noted. The cartilage pieces were interconnected by a dense, fibrous connective tissue contiguous with the superficial and deep perichondrium of the upper lateral cartilage and the lateral crus. The configuration of this junction was likened to reptile skin or armor as it is characterized by closely inherent multiple plates of cartilage with

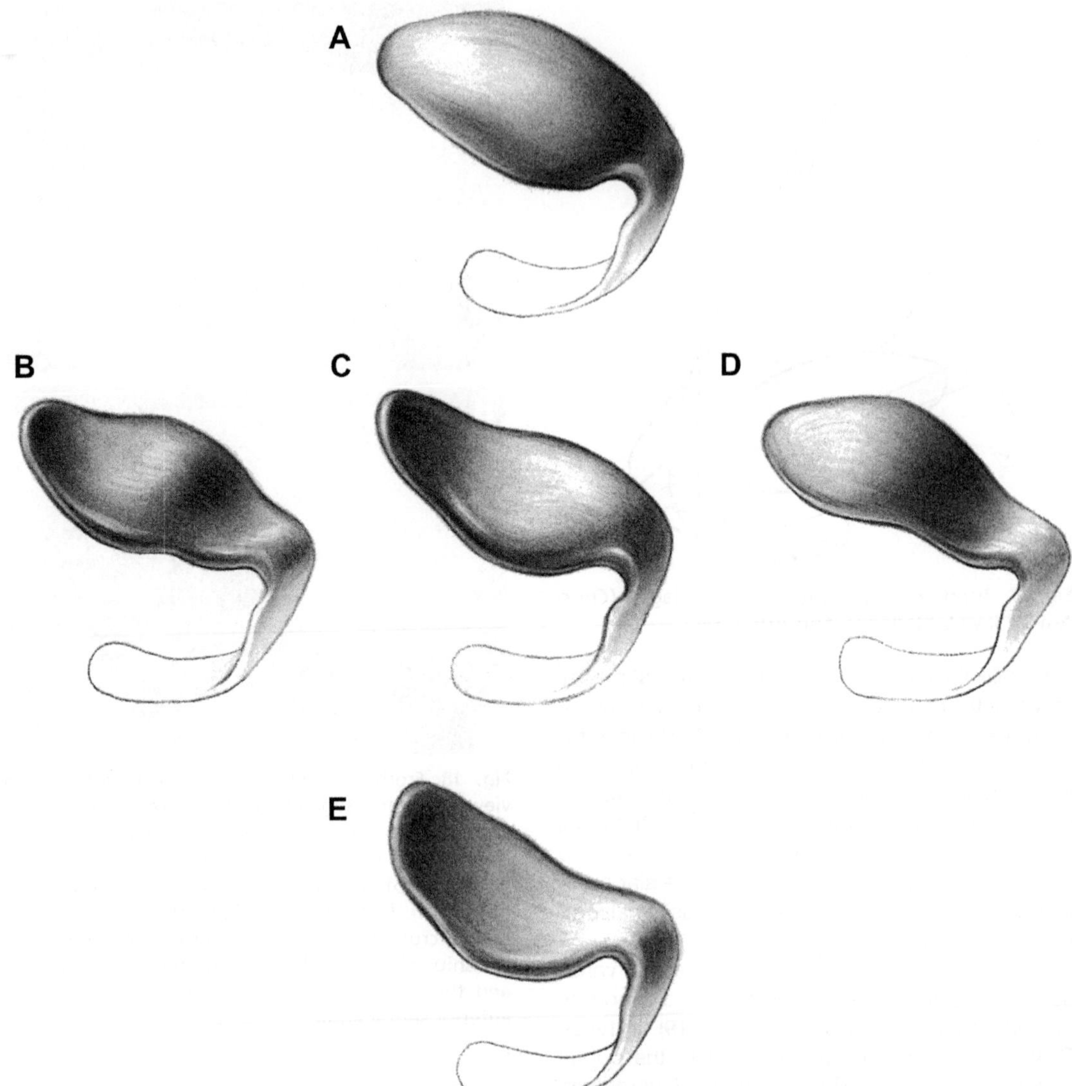

Fig. 19. Variations of form of the lateral crus of the alar cartilage. (*A*) Smooth convex. (*B*) Convex medial, concave lateral. (*C*) Concave medial, convex lateral. (*D*) Concave medial, convex central, concave lateral. (*E*) Smooth concave. (*Courtesy of* Jaye Schlesinger, Ann Arbor, MI.)

flexibility but little or no extensibility.[6] Because of the frequent overlap, the interspersed sesamoids, and the nondistensibility, the *intercartilaginous* incision is rarely that but probably almost always an *intracartilaginous* incision.[6,36,37]

The intrinsic shape and form of the alar cartilaginous arch depends entirely on its inherent form and resiliency. LePesteur and Firmin showed that the paired alar arches are also a part of 2 cartilaginous rings, one for each nostril (**Fig. 21**). Each ring consists of the following components: the medial crus embracing the caudal septum; the septum firmly set on the anterior nasal spine; the continuity of middle and lateral crus; and laterally a chain of accessory cartilages. The most posterior accessory cartilage is attached to the anterior nasal spine through fibrous connections in the nostril floor. These laterally placed cartilages contained within a distinct structural formation are accessory in contrast to the highly variable sesamoid cartilage found between the upper lateral cartilage and the lateral crus. The lateral accessory cartilage configuration may vary, from multiple to one or two larger pieces.[7,38]

In the non-Caucasian nose, the medial and lateral crura are frequently shorter and the cartilage structures comparatively weak, affording

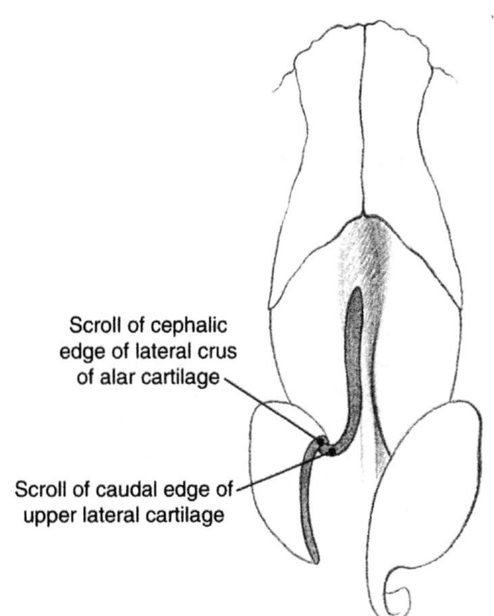

Fig. 20. Nasal skeleton: frontal view. Note the cutaway section of the right upper lateral cartilage and the lateral crus of the right alar cartilage and the scroll junction of the upper lateral cartilage and lateral crus (interlocked configuration). (*Courtesy of* Jaye Schlesinger, Ann Arbor, MI.)

less support.[4] Even in some Caucasian noses with thick skin and soft tissue, the cartilages are thin, providing less support than normal.[1]

THE NOSTRIL

The nostril is composed of the alar base and the vestibule. There is wide variation in the shape and size of the external naris.

Alar Bases

The shape and resiliency of the nostril and the posterior half of the alar side walls depend on dense fibrofatty connective tissue. Griesman[10] reported on variations in configuration and offered a classification of the junction of the alar bases with the cheek, which forms the alar cheek groove. The variations in configuration are the following (**Fig. 22**):

1. *Cheeked junction*: the alar side wall is relatively straight and the foot, or base, is only slightly curved medially.
2. *Labial junction*: the foot (base) turns medially and joins the columella in the middle of the nostril floor.
3. *Columellar junction*: the alar base turns across the nostril floor in a tubular configuration and continues across the nostril floor in a broad sweep. The size and shape of the tube vary considerably in addition to the location of its attachment to the skin of the base of the columella.

The shape of the nasal base is considered the most pleasing when it has the form of an equilateral triangle with the ratio of the columellar length to the height of the infratip lobule approximately 2:1 (see **Fig. 3**). In Caucasians, attractive nostrils normally have a teardrop shape. Nostril configurations vary considerably according to racial and ethnic types, as described by Farkas.[38–42]

Vestibule

The vestibule of the lower third of the nose is the cavity just inside the external nares bounded medially by the mobile septum and columella and laterally by the alar side wall with a protruding fold of skin with hair (vibrissae) under the lateral crus. Inferiorly, it is bordered by the skin overlying the alveolar process of the maxilla.[43] Cephalic to that is the inferior edge of the pyriform ridge, which demarcates the junction of the vestibule with the floor of the nasal cavity. The vestibule forms part

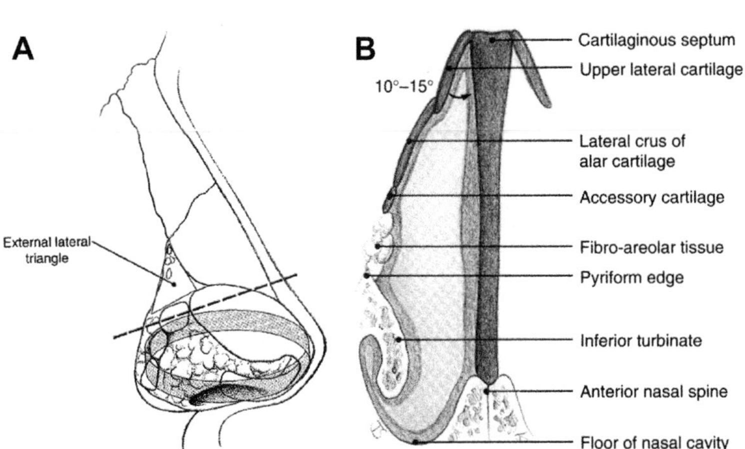

Fig. 21. (*A*) Lateral view of nose-view from right side. Note cartilage ring consisting of alar cartilage, accessory cartilages, caudal septa1 cartilage, and their fibrous interconnections. The dotted line shows the level of the cross-sectioned view. (*B*) Nasal valve area. (*Courtesy of* Jaye Schlesinger, Ann Arbor, MI.)

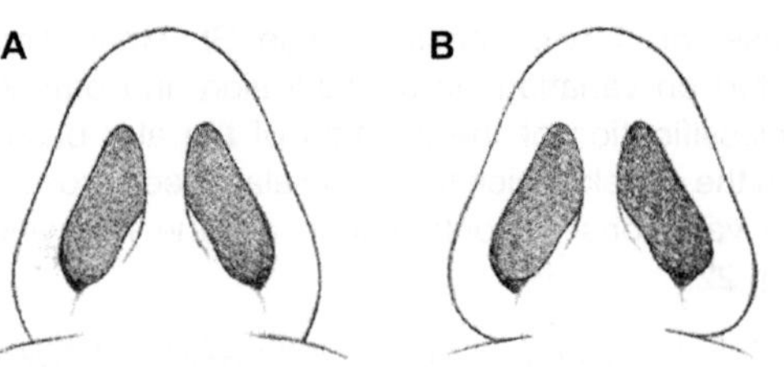
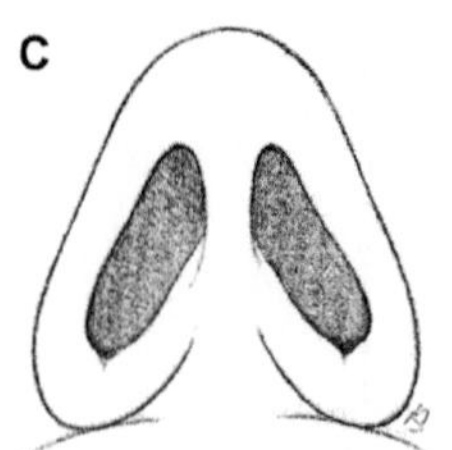

Fig. 22. Variations in alar base: nostril floor configuration. (*A*) Cheek type. (*B*) Labial type. (*C*) Tube type. (*Courtesy of* Jaye Schlesinger, Ann Arbor, MI.)

of a valve mechanism for inspired air.[44] As described by Cottle,[45–47] the vibrissae together with the vestibule provide a series of baffles, or resistors, to the stream of air, slowing down the currents of air and directing them backward into the nasal cavity for warming and moisturizing.

THE CARTILAGINOUS VAULT

The upper (cephalic) cartilaginous vault is made up of the paired upper lateral nasal cartilages and the dorsal cartilaginous septum. Early studies suggested that the cephalic one-third of the vault was a unified structure.[48] McKinney and colleagues[49] showed that actually the entire cephalic two-thirds of the vault is a single cartilaginous unit (**Fig. 23**). Inferiorly, there is gradual separation of the upper lateral cartilages from the septum to a level just above the septal angle. Embryologically, a single cartilaginous nasal capsule is present by 4 months.[48] During development, as chondrification proceeds, fibrous tissue ingrowth produces separation of the upper lateral cartilage from the pyriform process laterally and from the caudal septum. The amount of separation and flare from the septum varies, as does the amount of projection of the caudal end of the septum, which can project 1 cm beyond the caudal edge of the upper lateral cartilage (see **Fig. 20**).[50] The lateral border of the upper lateral cartilage frequently terminates at the level of the nasal bone lateral suture line. The fetal orientation of the cartilages extending beneath the piriform and the nasal bones, however, is maintained at birth, and this anatomic variation needs to be respected when performing nasal surgery in young children.[51] The lateral configuration of the upper lateral cartilage tends to be more rectangular than triangular and does not, as is commonly believed, rest on the pyriform process (see **Fig. 21**). This lateral space is termed the *external lateral triangle*. It is bordered by the lateral edge of the upper lateral cartilage, lateral prolongation of the lateral crus, and the edge of the pyriform fossa. It is lined by mucosa and covered by the transverse portion of the nasalis muscle. It also may contain one or more small sesamoid cartilages, and it functions as a bellows during

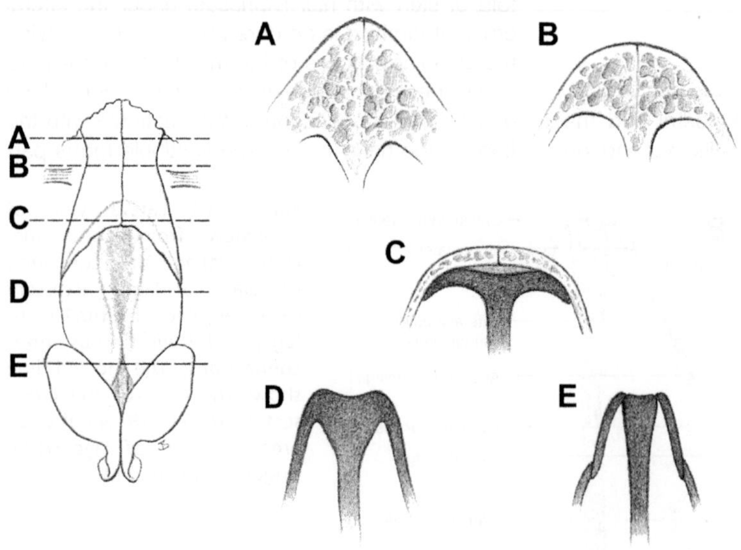

Fig. 23. Cross-sectional views of the nasal skeleton showing the osseous and upper cartilaginous vault. (*A*) Bony vault caudal to nasofrontal suture (near radix). (*B*) Bony vault, just cephalic to intercanthal line. (*C*) Junction of bony and cartilaginous vault. Note the overlap of nasal bones over the cephalic edge of the upper lateral cartilage and the T configuration of the nasal septum continuous structure with the paired upper lateral cartilages. (*D*) Middle third of upper cartilaginous vault. Note Y configuration of the nasal septum and the persistent structural continuity of the nasal septum and the upper lateral cartilage. (*E*) Caudal upper cartilaginous vault. Note that the nasal septum and the upper lateral cartilages are separate structures at this level. (*Courtesy of* Jaye Schlesinger, Ann Arbor, MI.)

respiration.[6,46] There is no lateral skeletal support for the upper lateral cartilage; its support comes only from attachments to the nasal bones and septum.

There is a common perichondrial lining on the undersurface of the upper lateral cartilages and the septum (**Fig. 24**). During traditional rhinoplasty techniques, whenever the dorsum is lowered, the apex of the cartilaginous vault is often interrupted depending on the amount of cartilage removed.[30,52] The upper lateral cartilages are thus separated from the septum through their length and totally depend on their connection with nasal bones for their support.[45,50] If the mucoperichondrial lining between the septum and the upper lateral cartilage is divided further, instability is created. By creating submucosal tunnels and performing an extra mucosal rhinoplasty, the integrity of the mucoperichondrial layer can be maintained beneath these structures (see **Fig. 24**).[9,50,53] Caudally, where the upper lateral cartilage diverges from the septum, the mucoperichondrium contains a fibrous aponeurosis that lends support to this area of the internal valve; it should be protected by gentle and judicious dissection. As it approaches its caudal end, the upper lateral cartilage ideally forms an angle of 10 to 15° with the septum (see **Fig. 21**). This is the area of the internal nasal valve, which requires flexible patency for a normal airway.[3,35,46,54]

There are many variations in configuration and position of the anterior septal angle because of

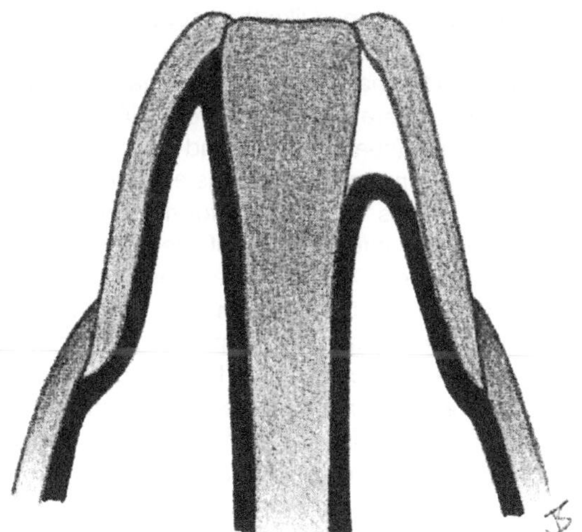

Fig. 24. Caudal upper cartilaginous vault. The dark black line on the left represents the continuous mucoperichondrial layer in its normal configuration. The submucosal tunnel on the right is the approach to the nasal skeleton. (*Courtesy of* Jaye Schlesinger, Ann Arbor, MI.)

development and racial influences.[24,50] The high angular nose with a prominent dorsum tends to have a more prominent caudal septal cartilage than the nose with a low fat dorsum.[55] Occasionally the septal border of the distal septal cartilage may be definitively felt at the anterior septal angle and may present almost subcutaneously between the caudal ends of the upper lateral cartilages and medial lateral crus. Most commonly, however, the closely approximated medial aspects of the lateral crura are superimposed.[20,56]

Lateral deviations of the caudal dorsal septum can "artificially" produce asymmetries in the position of the domal segments similar to the secondary effect of caudal deflections of the septal cartilage or the medial crus. These external influences on tip position should be carefully documented preoperatively by careful clinical examination.

THE BONY VAULT

The bony vault consists of the paired nasal bones and the paired ascending processes of the maxilla.[57] The vault is generally pyramidal in shape; however, the cephalic portion of the bones flare outwardly as they approach the nasofrontal suture (see **Fig. 23**). The most narrow part of the bony pyramid is at the intercanthal line, which connects the attachments of the medial canthal tendons at the anterior crest of the lacrimal bone (see **Fig. 1**).[10] The nasal bones are thicker and denser above the level of the medial canthus.[58] The nasofrontal suture line averages 10.7 mm cephalic to the intercanthal line.[5] The nasal bones average 25 mm in length, although there may be considerable variation. Thus, the bony vault is divided approximately in half at the intercanthal level (**Fig. 25**). One variation described by Sheen is of short nasal bones.[3] Preoperative recognition is important because standard osteotomies in such patients may lead to excessive postoperative collapse of the bony and cartilaginous vault. Nasal bones also tend to be shorter and smaller and the bony pyramid is widened in the non-Caucasian nose.[4]

At the cephalic end of the nasal dorsum, the soft-tissue nasion, or sellion, is the deepest portion of the curve between the glabella and the nasal dorsum (nasofrontal groove or curve) (see **Fig. 25**).[10] This is generally at a level approximately between the supratarsal fold and the upper lid margin with the eye open and approximately 9 to 14 mm anterior to the corneal projection.[59] This area is referred to as the radix. The thin caudal edge of these 2 bones and the adjacent thin anterior ridge of the premaxilla, continuous with the

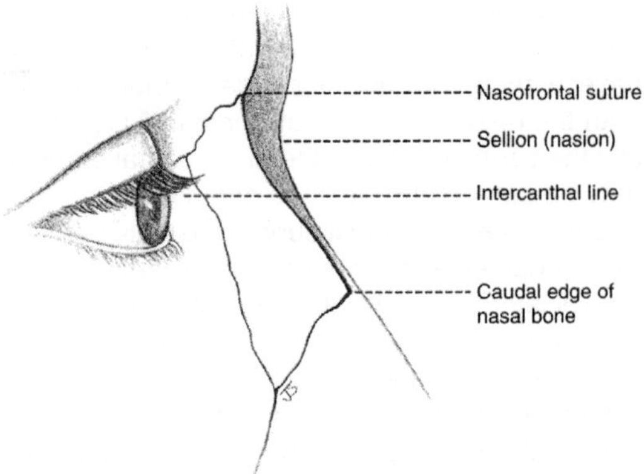

Fig. 25. Lateral view of the bony skeleton and overlying soft tissue from the right side. Note the relationship of the sellion (nasion) to the nasofrontal suture line and the level of the intercanthal line. The intercanthal line splits the dorsal (anterior) length of the nasal bone approximately in half. (*Courtesy of* Jaye Schlesinger, Ann Arbor, MI.)

anterior nasal spine, make up the pyriform aperture.

Caudal to the intercanthal line, under the midline of the fused nasal bones, there is an inward curved bony spine that articulates with the superior edge of the perpendicular plate of the ethmoid. This spine is also just cephalic to where the dense fibrous tissue connects the overlapped cephalic edges of the upper lateral cartilages. These cartilages are, in turn, fused to the cartilaginous nasal septum, which articulates solidly with the perpendicular plate of the ethmoids (**Fig. 26**). This confluent area of 4 solid structural elements is called the keystone area (**Fig. 27**).[24,36,50,] This area provides critical support for the nasal dorsum in the middle third of the nose. If the bony and cartilaginous dorsum is lowered and the side walls separated in the midline, then the integrity of both the perpendicular plate of the ethmoid and the dorsal-cartilaginous septum is essential to support the nasal dorsum once osteotomies are performed. To maintain this support, these midline bony and cartilaginous structures must be preserved, or if mobilization is required during reconstruction of the septum, they must be reconstituted carefully.

INTERNAL ANATOMY OF THE NOSE

Nasal Cavities

The normal spatial relationships of the nasal cavities with surrounding structures in the skull are illustrated by a series of coronal computed tomography (CT) scans (see **Fig. 26**). The location of these sections is depicted in relation to the sagittal view of the nasal septum lateral wall and surrounding structures, which also provide additional orientation for structures anterior and posterior to the CT scan cuts.

The nasal vestibule is lined with squamous epithelium that contains numerous thick stiff vibrissae. The limen nasi is consistently at the junction of the skin with the nasal mucosa. This mucosa has a highly specialized function in respiration and should be preserved carefully when possible. Superiorly, the lining consists of olfactory mucous membrane, which has a yellowish hue.

Bony Septum

The *perpendicular plate of the ethmoid* forms the upper third of the bony septum and is continuous above with the frontal bone and the cribriform plate. Anteriorly, it articulates with the inward projection of the nasal bones in the midline, caudally with the septal cartilage, and inferiorly with the vomer (see **Figs. 26** and **27**). The degree of contact between ethmoid and vomer depends on how much septal cartilage is interposed between them. The level of the junction of the perpendicular plate with the septal cartilage at the dorsal keystone area varies with the amount of distal nasal bone overlap of the upper lateral cartilage, but can be 1 cm or more cephalic to the caudal end of the nasal bone. Along its anterior junction with the septal cartilage, the ethmoid is sometimes grooved, making its disarticulation from the septal cartilage difficult during septoplasty. In some patients it may be easier to incise through the cartilage 2 to 3 mm anterior to this junction to separate the two structures.

The *vomer* is shaped like the keel of a boat and extends anteriorly and inferiorly from the sphenoid superiorly to the nasal crest of the palatine bones and maxilla, where it joins the premaxillary wings of the maxilla (see **Figs. 26** and **27**). Anteriorly the vomer and premaxillary wings embryologically are paired bones that fuse to form a groove for insertion of the inferior edge of the quadrilateral septal cartilage. Caudally, the most projecting part of the premaxilla is the anterior nasal spine, which is the most caudal attachment at the inferior edge of the septal cartilage. In the non-Caucasian nose, the anterior nasal spine may be undeveloped or even totally absent.[4] The bony groove that supports the septal cartilage is most prominent caudally in the premaxilla and gradually becomes more flattened as it progresses posteriorly along the vomer.

Cartilaginous Septum

The septal cartilage is a flat plate of cartilage of irregular quadrilateral shape and varying size (see

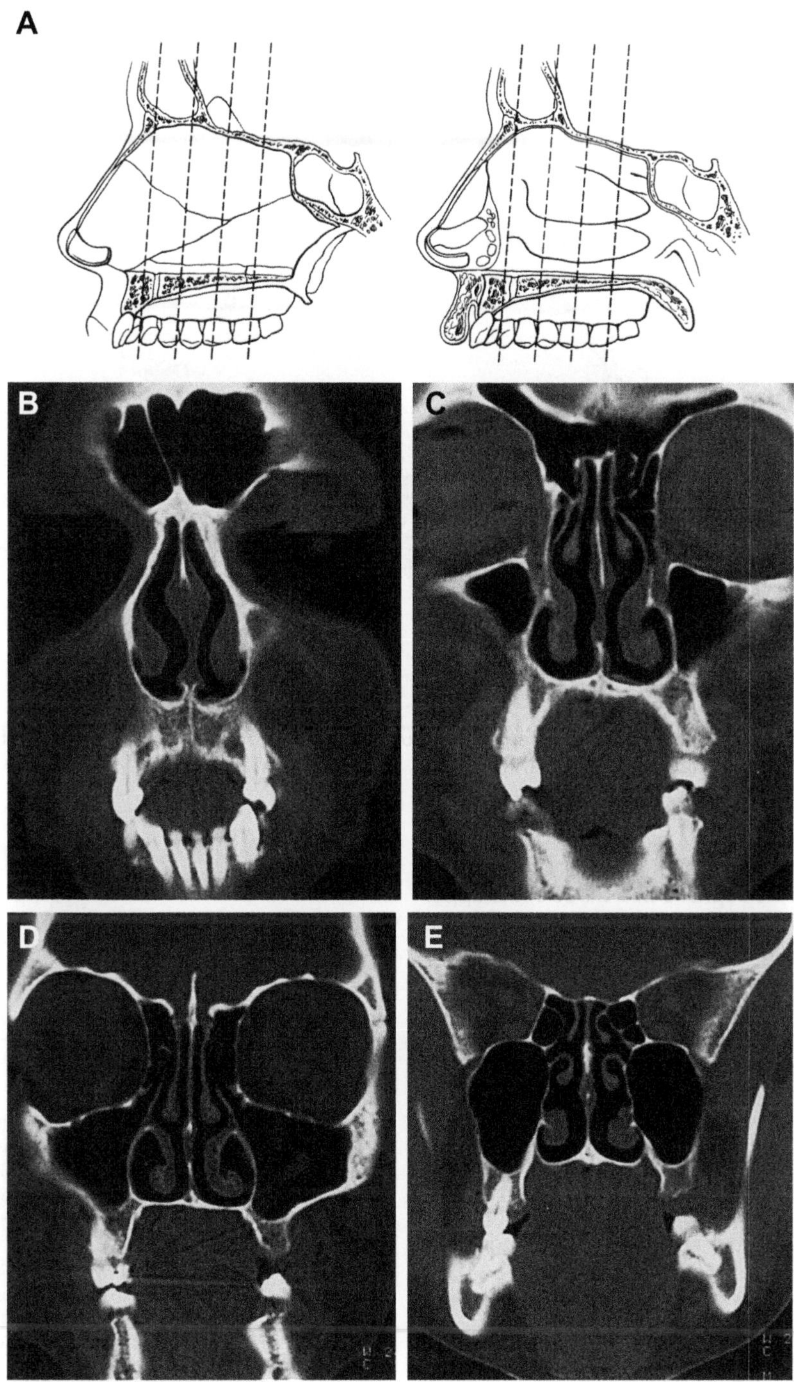

Fig. 26. (*A*) Location of coronal CT sections projected on sagittal view of the cranium. (*B*) Level of the anterior maxilla and frontal sinus. Note the groove in the premaxillary crest and the groove in the perpendicular plate of the ethmoid. (*C*) Level of the anterior aspect of the maxillary sinus and posterior frontal sinus. Note the cephalic septa1 cartilage extension between the vomer posteriorly and the perpendicular plate of the ethmoid anteriorly. (*D*) Level of the midseptum. Note the following: the crista galli above the roof of the nasal cavity; the nasal crest of the maxilla; the middle and inferior turbinates and meatuses; and the ethrnoid cells between the lateral wall of the nose and the medial wall of the orbit. (*E*) Posterior septum. Note the nasal crest of the palatine bone or floor of the nose and the superior turbinate with the lateral ethmoid interposed next to the medial orbital wall.

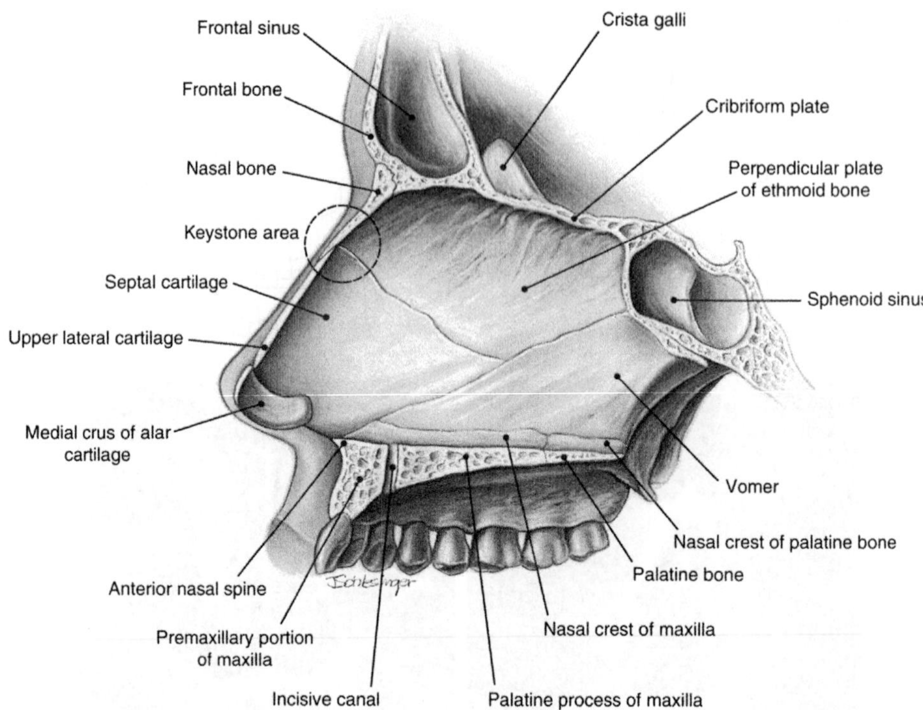

Fig. 27. Lateral view of the left side of the nasal septum. The left lateral wall of the nose has been removed. (*Courtesy of* Jaye Schlesinger, Ann Arbor, MI.)

Fig. 27). Embryologically, it develops as a single unit along with the cephalic two-thirds of the upper lateral cartilages.[48,49] It articulates with the perpendicular plate of the ethmoid and the fused portions of the vomer and premaxillary wings. Its shape depends in part on the length and angulation of the cephalic extension between the vomer and perpendicular plate of the ethmoid. The quadrilateral cartilage provides support and form of the nasal dorsum from the cartilaginous bony junction (rhinion) to just cephalic to the lobule in the supratip area. The *anterior septal angle* is at the junction of the dorsal and caudal septum. The other two caudal angles are the intermediate and posterior (**Fig. 28**).

There are some critical aspects about the tongue-and-groove articulation between the quadrilateral septal cartilage and the premaxilla and vomer (**Fig. 29**).[36] Although some periosteal fibers are continuous with the ipsilateral perichondrial fibers, many pass around the superior articulated edge of the bone to become continuous with the opposite periosteum or cross to become continuous with the opposite perichondrial fibers. The perichondrium has a similar crossed configuration around the inferior edge of the quadrilateral cartilage. There are fibrous connections within the groove that allow mobility of the cartilaginous

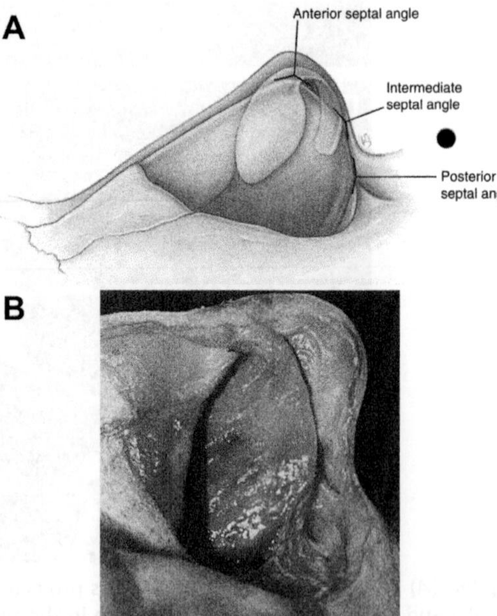

Fig. 28. (*A*) Lateral view of nose from right side. The soft tissue has been removed. Note the 3 angles of the caudal septum and the anterior nasal spine. (*B*) Fresh cadaver dissection: view from right side with right nasal wall removed. Note the 3 angles of the caudal septum, the anterior nasal spine, and the position of the left medial and middle crus. (*Courtesy of* Jaye Schlesinger, Ann Arbor, MI.)

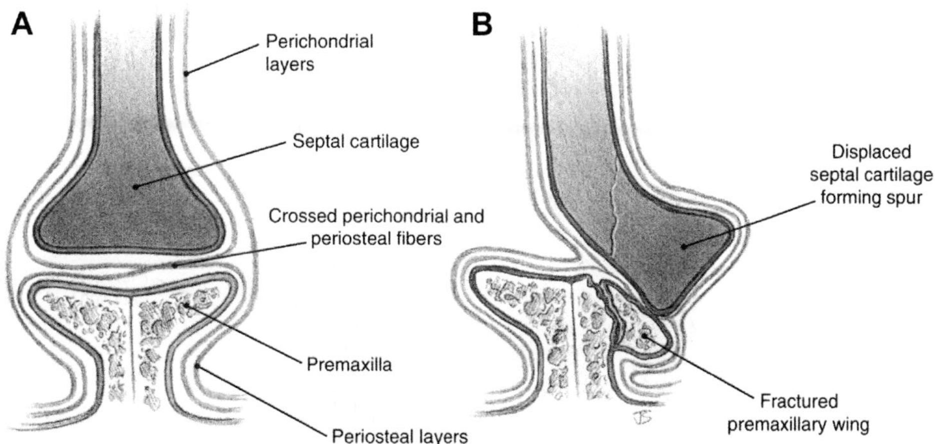

Fig. 29. (*A*) Cross-sectional diagram depicting the joint between the septal cartilage and premaxilla. (*B*) Common posttraumatic configuration of this junction. (*Courtesy of* Jaye Schlesinger, Ann Arbor, MI.)

septum in this bony groove, permitting slight rotation laterally when the cartilage is compressed, reducing the danger of fracture. The sum effect is a joint with intricate interweaving of periosteum and perichondrium that makes a continuous mucoperichondrial dissection difficult.

Lateral Wall of the Nasal Cavity

The lateral wall of the nasal cavity is a specialized area (**Fig. 30**). It contains the 3 turbinates: superior, middle, and inferior. They are scrolls of bone covered by mucosa containing a plexus of large veins, which can become markedly engorged. The turbinates can cause interference with visualization and manipulation during intranasal examination and usually require vasoconstriction to allow adequate intranasal examination preoperatively. Vasoconstriction also facilitates visualization of the posterior reaches of the nasal cavities during surgical procedures. The inferior turbinates often become compensatorily enlarged on the side opposite septal deviations. There is crucial juxtaposition of the caudal end of the inferior turbinate within the narrow flow-limiting segment of the nasal valve area (see **Fig. 21**).[60] Consequently, alterations of their size and position are required frequently during operations for nasal airway

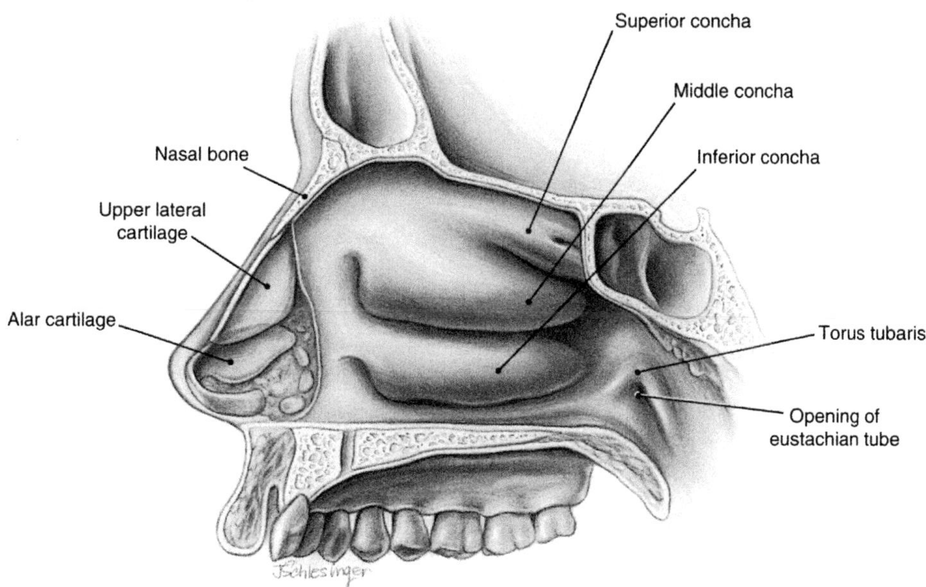

Fig. 30. Right lateral wall of the nasal cavity viewed from left side with left nasal wall and septum removed. The palate is sectioned in the midline. (*Courtesy of* Jaye Schlesinger, Ann Arbor, MI.)

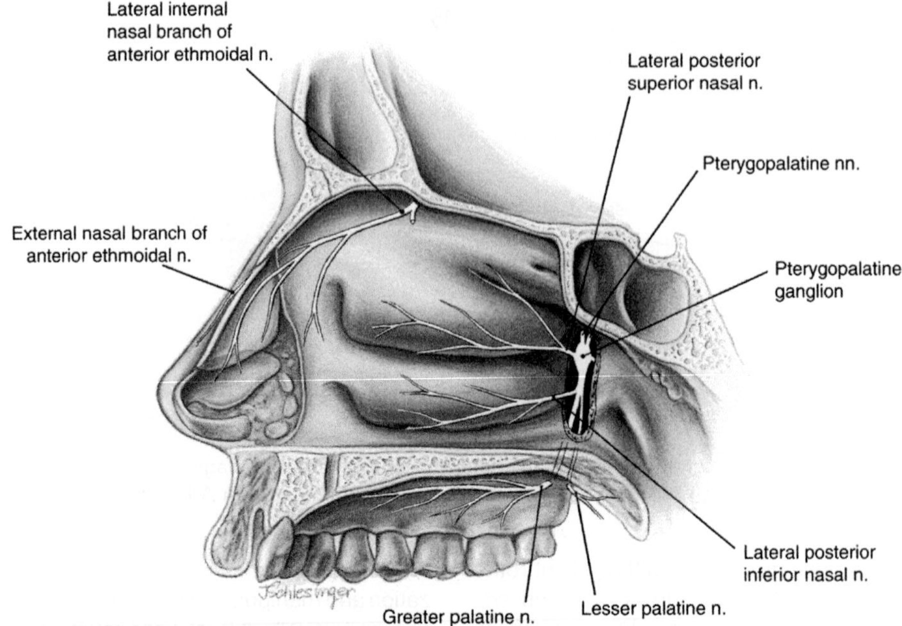

Fig. 31. Right lateral wall of the nasal cavity (same view as in **Fig. 30**), showing the sensory nerve supply of the lateral nasal wall. (*Courtesy of* Jaye Schlesinger, Ann Arbor, MI.)

obstruction. Inferior to each turbinate are the superior, middle, and inferior meatuses, respectively. Openings from the various paranasal sinuses open into these meatuses and the nasolacrimal duct, which drains into the inferior meatus approximately 1 cm behind the pyriform opening. There can be temporary interference with drainage of these adjacent structures because of intranasal swelling, which may explain the increase in tearing and sinus stuffiness seen after rhinoplasty.

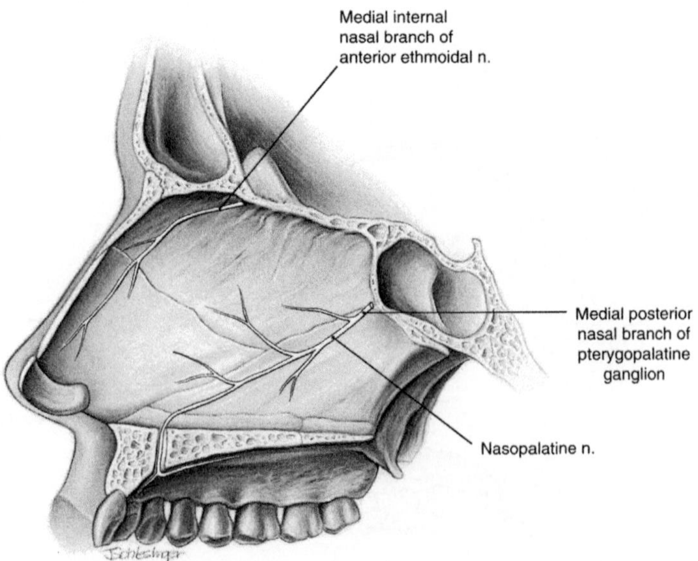

Fig. 32. Left side of the nasal septum with left lateral wall of nose removed (same view as in **Fig. 27**), showing the sensory nerve supply to the nasal septum. (*Courtesy of* Jaye Schlesinger, Ann Arbor, MI.)

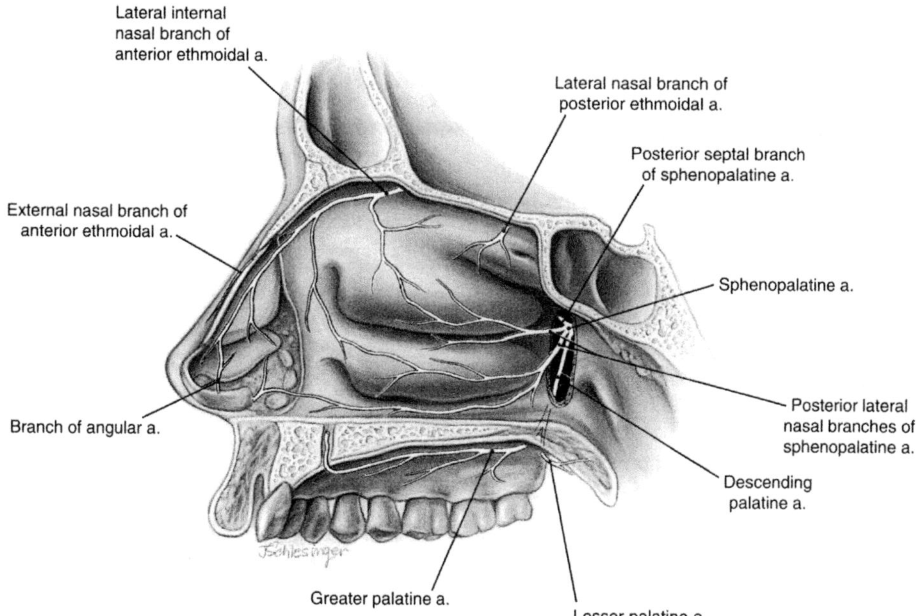

Fig. 33. Right lateral wall of the nasal cavity (same view as in **Fig. 30**), showing the arterial blood supply to the right lateral nasal wall. (*Courtesy of* Jaye Schlesinger, Ann Arbor, MI.)

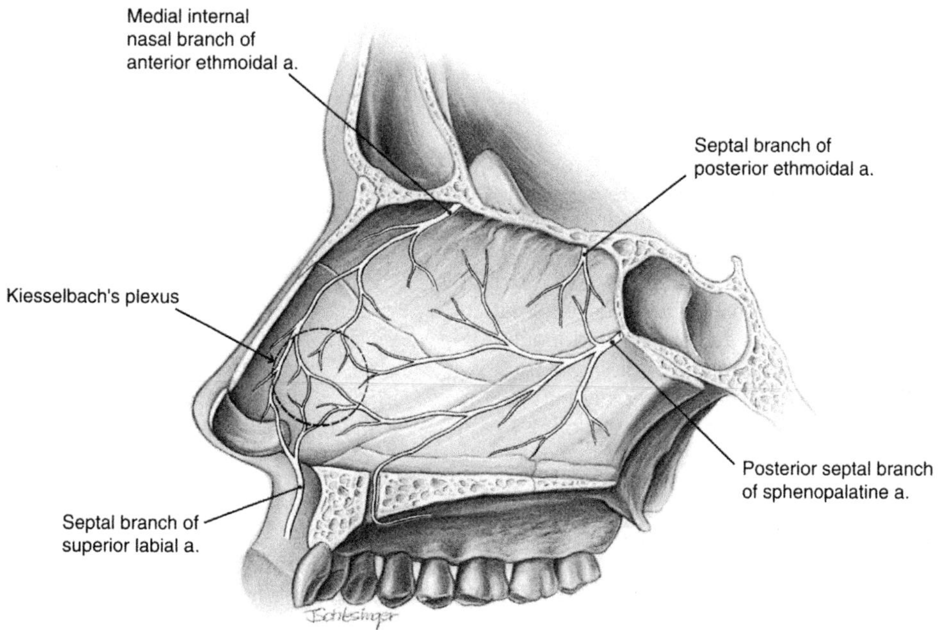

Fig. 34. Left side of the nasal septum with the left lateral wall of the nose removed (same view as in **Fig. 32**), showing the arterial blood supply to the left side of the nasal septum. Kesselbach's plexus is shown in the dotted circle. (*Courtesy of* Jaye Schlesinger, Ann Arbor, MI.)

The Nerves, Blood Supply, and Lymphatics of the Inside of the Nose

Figs. 31 to 34 clearly depict the nerves and arteries of the inner nose. They should be studied carefully. Special mention of only a few facts needs to be made. Little's area on the anterior septum is one of these (see **Fig. 34**). This is an area of vascular confluence of the superficial terminal branches of the anterior ethmoidal, sphenopalatine, and superior labial arteries.[12,29,61] This is called Kesselbach's plexus (see **Fig. 34**). Because of the rich supply of superficial blood vessels in this concentrated area, it is a common location for anterior nasal bleeding and is easily accessible for cauterization.[12,61] It is particularly relevant with anterior septal deviations.

Veins

The submucosa of the interior of the nose is composed of well-developed venous plexi, which are particularly prominent on the inferior nasal concha, the inferior meatus, and the posterior part of the septum. They function like erectile tissue. Batson,[62] in 1954, noted a rich venous plexus on his injection studies, with interlacing veins of diameters of 0.1 to 0.5 mm forming a widely intermingled valveless network.[62] This rich venous plexus forms essentially a cast of all the internal nasal structures. This venous plexus also is present in the tissues of the vestibule, but to a lesser degree.[62] Dion and colleagues[31] noted microscopic veins on the deep surface of the lateral crus and the intercartilaginous area.[31] There is some evidence from careful airflow studies that there may be some mucosal congestion in the vestibular mucosa.

These various venous plexi converge into definitive veins that correspond to the arteries on the lateral nasal wall and septum mentioned earlier. They pass through the pterygopalatine foramen into the pharyngeal plexus and via the ethmoid branches into the cavernous sinus. The external nasal vein drains into the facial vein and jugular system. Thus, injected materials or drainage from infection theoretically can spread rapidly into the cerebral, ophthalmic, and central circulation.[34]

Lymphatics

Anteriorly, the nasal lymphatics drain through the soft-tissue nares and into the lymphatics of the upper lip. Posteriorly, they are larger and more prevalent, and some drain toward the deep cervical lymph nodes. The majority, however, pass into a plexus in front of the eustachian tube, where they join the lymphatics from the upper pharynx and middle ear to pass into the retropharyngeal nodes.[12,63]

SUMMARY

Knowing the details of nasal anatomy is essential when undertaking rhinoplasty surgery. Careful study of these details makes for a more confident, prepared practitioner.

REFERENCES

1. Peck GC, Michelson LN. Anatomy of aesthetic surgery of the nose. Clin Plast Surg 1987;14:737.
2. Philippou M, Stenger GM. Cross-sectional anatomy of the nose and paranasal sinuses. Rhinology 1990;28:221.
3. Sheen JH, Sheen AP. Aesthetic rhinoplasty. 2nd edition. St. Louis (MO): CV Mosby; 1987. p. 1506.
4. Zmgaro EA, Falees E. Aesthetic anatomy of the non-caucasian nose. Clin Plast Surg 1987;14:749.
5. Lessard M, Daniel RK. Surgical anatomy of septorhinoplasty. Arch Otolaryngol Head Neck Surg 1985;111:25.
6. Jost G, Meresse B, Torossan F. Studies of junction between lateral cartilages and the nose. Ann Chir Plast Esthet 1973;18:175.
7. Gunter JP. Anatomic observations of the lower lateral cartilages. Arch Otolaryngol Head Neck Surg 1969; 89:599.
8. Gunter JP, Rohrich RJ, Adams WP. Dallas rhinoplasty: nasal surgery by the masters. 2nd edition. St. Louis (MO): Quality Medical Publishing; 2007. p. 1500.
9. Letourneau A, Daniel RK. Superficial musculoaponeurotic system of the nose. Plast Reconstr Surg 1988;82:48.
10. Griesman BL. Muscles and cartilages of the nose from the standpoint of typical rhinoplasty. Arch Otolaryngol Head Neck Surg 1944;39:334.
11. Gruber R, Freeman M, Hsu C, et al. Nasal base reduction by alar release: a laboratory evaluation. Plast Reconstr Surg 2009;123(2):709–15.
12. Hollingshead WH. Anatomy for surgeons: volume I. Head and neck. 3rd edition. Philadelphia: Harper and Row; 1982.
13. Johnson CM, Toriumi DM. Open structure rhinoplasty. Philadelphia: WB Saunders; 1990. p. 516.
14. Herbert DC. A subcutaneous pedicled cheek flap for reconstruction of alar deficits. Br J Plast Surg 1978;31:78.
15. Rybka FJ. Reconstruction of nasal tip using nasalis myocutaneous sliding flaps. Plast Reconstr Surg 1983;71:40.
16. Wee SS, Hruza GJ, Mustoe TA. Refinements of nasalis myocutaneous flap. Ann Plast Surg 1990;25:271.
17. Marchak D, Toth B. The axial fronto nasal flap revisited. Plast Reconstr Surg 1985;76:686.
18. Rohrich RJ, Gunter JP. Vascular basis for external approach to rhinoplasty. Surg Forum 1990;13:240.

19. Tebbets J. Primary rhinoplasty. Philadelphia: Mosby; 1998. p. 708.
20. Daniel RK. The nasal tip: anatomy and aesthetics. Plast Reconstr Surg 1992;89:216.
21. Tardy ME, Brown RJ. Surgical anatomy of the nose. New York: Raven; 1990.
22. Pollack RA. Greater alar cartilage anatomy and biomechanics of the nasal tripod. Presented at the Seventh Annual Meeting of the American Association of Clinical Anatomists, Saskatoon, Canada, 1990.
23. Bernstein L. Surgical anatomy in rhinoplasty. Otolaryngol Clin North Am 1975;8:549.
24. Converse JM. The cartilaginous structures of the nose. Ann Otol Rhinol Laryngol 1955;64:220.
25. Tardy ME, Cheng E. Transdomal refinement of the nasal tip. Facial Plast Surg 1987;4:317.
26. Pitanguy I. Surgical importance of a dermocartilaginous ligament in bulbous noses. Plast Reconstr Surg 1965;36:247.
27. Bachman W, Legler U. Studies on the structure and function of the anterior section of the nose by means of luminal impressions. Acta Otolaryngol 1972;73:433.
28. Anderson JR. A new approach to rhinoplasty: a five year appraisal. Arch Otolaryngol Head Neck Surg 1971,93:284.
29. Burgett G, Menica FJ. Nasal support and lining: the marriage of beauty and blood supply. Plast Reconstr Surg 1989;84:189.
30. McKinney P, Cunningham B. Avoiding secondary rhinoplasty. Operat Tech Plast Reconstr Surg 1995;2:31.
31. Dion MD, Jefek BW, Tobin CE. The anatomy of the nose. Arch Otolaryngol Head Neck Surg 1978;104:145.
32. Daniel RK. Discussion of Constantian, MB. Two essential elements for planning tip surg. Plast Reconstr Surg 2004;114:1582.
33. Dingman RO, Natvig P. Surgical anatomy in aesthetic and corrective rhinoplasty. Clin Plast Surg 1977;4:111.
34. Zelnik J, Gingrass RP. Anatomy of the alar cartilage. Plast Reconstr Surg 1979;64:650.
35. Toriumi DM. Management of middle nasal vault in rhinoplasty. Operat Tech Plast Reconstr Surg 1995;2:16.
36. Drumheller GW. Topology of the lateral nasal cartilages. Anat Rec 1973;176:321.
37. Enlow DH. The human face: an account of post nasal growth and development of the craniofacial skeleton. New York: Hober; 1968.
38. Farkas LG, Hreczko TA, Deutsch CK. Objective assessment of standard nostril types–a morphological study. Ann Plast Surg 1983;11:381.
39. Farkas LG, Kolar JC, Munro IR. Geography of the nose: a morphologic study. Aesthetic Plast Surg 1986;10:191.
40. Firmin F. Discussion on Letourneau A, Daniel RK: the superficial musculoaponeurotic system of the nose. Plast Reconstr Surg 1988;82:56.
41. Gray VD. Physiologic returning of the upper lateral cartilage. Rhinology 1970;8:56.
42. Griesman BL. Base of nose anatomy and plastic repair. Arch Otolaryngol Head Neck Surg 1950;51:541.
43. Bridger CP. Physiology of the nasal valve. Arch Otolaryngol Head Neck Surg 1970;92:543.
44. Mann DG, Sasaki CT, Fukuda H, et al. Dilator nares muscle. Ann Otol Rhinol Laryngol 1977;86:362.
45. Cottle MH. Nasal roof repair and hump removal. Arch Otolaryngol Head Neck Surg 1954;60:408.
46. Cottle MH. Structures and function of the nasal vestibule. Arch Otolaryngol Head Neck Surg 1955;62:173.
47. Cottle MH, Loring RM, Fischer GG, et al. The "maxilla-premaxillary" approach to extensive nasal septum surgery. Arch Otolaryngol Head Neck Surg 1958;68:301.
48. Straatsma BR, Straatsma CR. The anatomical relationship of the lateral nasal cartilage to the nasal bone and the cartilaginous nasal septum. Plast Reconstr Surg 1951;8:443.
49. McKinney P, Johnson P, Walloch J. Anatomy of the nasal hump. Plast Reconstr Surg 1986;77:404.
50. Converse JM. Corrective surgery of nasal deviations. Arch Otolaryngol Head Neck Surg 1950;52:671.
51. Poublon RM, Verwoerd CD, Verwoerd-Verhoef HL. Anatomy of the upper lateral cartilages in the human newborn. Rhinology 1990;28:41.
52. Bernstein L. Submucous operation on the nasal septum. Otolaryngol Clin North Am 1975;6:549.
53. Robin JL. Extra mucosal method in rhinoplasty. Aesthetic Plast Surg 1979;3:171.
54. Kern EB. Surgery of the valve. In: Sisson GA, Tardy ME Jr, editors, Plastic and reconstructive surgery of the face and neck: proceedings of the second international symposium, vol. 2. New York: Grune and Stratton; 1977. p. 501–54.
55. Parell GJ, Becker GD. The tension nose. Facial Plast Surg 1984;1:81.
56. Daniel RK. Rhinoplasty: creating an aesthetic tip. Plast Reconstr Surg 1987;80:775.
57. Wright WK. Study on hump removal in rhinoplasty. Laryngoscope 1967;77:508.
58. Wright WK. Surgery of the bony and cartilaginous dorsum. Otolaryngol Clin North Am 1975;8:575.
59. Byrd HS, Andochick S, Copit S, et al. Septal extension grafts: a method of controlling tip projection, rotation and shape. Plast Reconstr Surg 1997;100:999.
60. Haight JS, Cole P. Site and function of the nasal valve. Laryngoscope 1983;93:49.
61. Ritter FN. Vasculature of the nose. Ann Otol Rhinol Laryngol 1970;79:468.
62. Batson OV. The venous networks of the nasal mucosa. Ann Otol Rhinol Laryngol 1954;63:571.
63. Robison M. Lymphangitis of the retro pharyngeal lymphatic system. Arch Otolaryngol Head Neck Surg 1944;105:333.

Principles of Photography in Rhinoplasty for the Digital Photographer

Ravi S. Swamy, MD, MPH[a], Jonathan M. Sykes, MD[b,*], Sam P. Most, MD[a]

KEYWORDS

- Digital single-lens reflex camera • Depth of field
- Field of view • Charged coupled devices

The art and technology of photography can be overwhelming to the facial plastic surgeon. A basic understanding and appreciation of this vital tool is invaluable in surgical practice, especially in rhinoplasty. Photographic documentation of patients undergoing rhinoplasty is essential for patient consultation, perioperative planning, and postsurgical evaluation.[1] Developing a technique to ensure standardized, high-quality images requires an understanding of the basic principles of photography as well as an understanding of the equipment used, proper lighting, and patient positioning. This article reviews the basic principles of photography and discusses their application to facial plastic surgery practice, and rhinoplasty in particular.

EQUIPMENT/CAMERA

With the advent of the digital single-lens reflex (SLR) photography, 35-mm film SLR cameras are no longer the gold standard.[2] Digital cameras offer many new advantages, such as instantaneous pictures, ability to crop and adjust on a computer, and images that can be easily stored and filed. Although point-and-shoot cameras are less expensive, the resolution of these models is lesser than the digital SLR cameras. Digital SLR cameras also afford the ability to change lenses and adjust settings that control aperture size, shutter speed, and exposure. An understanding of the correct manipulation and use of these settings is critical to obtain consistent, high-quality images.

Focus/focal Point

The goal of photography in rhinoplasty is to attain sharp, clear images, which emphasize the fine details of nasal anatomy.[3] Depth of field (DOF) in a photograph is the distance range in which all included portions of an image are in sharp focus. The DOF should be sufficient to allow focus of the entire face, and the focal point, which is the point in the photograph that appears to be the sharpest, should be the nose.[4] Digital SLR cameras allow the photographer to change the DOF through manipulation of the focal length of the lens, distance from photographer to subject, and aperture size. These 3 factors are critical to get the best DOF for photographing patients undergoing rhinoplasty.

The DOF varies inversely with the focal length of the lens used. Point-and-shoot cameras have lenses with short focal lengths that help to keep everything in focus (large DOF). Digital SLR cameras allow for interchanging lenses with different focal lengths. However, as discussed later in this article, distortion can occur with

[a] Division of Facial Plastic and Reconstructive Surgery, Stanford University School of Medicine, 801 Welch Road, Stanford, CA 94305, USA
[b] Department of Otolaryngology-Head and Neck Surgery, 2521 Stockton, Boulevard Suite 6206, Sacramento, CA 95817, USA
* Corresponding author.
E-mail address: jonathan.sykes@ucdmc.ucdavis.edu (J.M. Sykes).

Clin Plastic Surg 37 (2010) 213–221
doi:10.1016/j.cps.2009.12.003
0094-1298/10/$ – see front matter

change of focal lengths. Thus, changing focal length to optimize DOF is less than ideal in facial plastic surgery.

The DOF varies directly with the distance between the photographer and the subject. Objects that are photographed at long distances will be seen with greater DOF for any given aperture or focal length of the lens. Given the space constraints, the distance between the photographer and the subject cannot be easily manipulated to increase DOF in the photography studio.

Controlling the aperture size is the best way to increase the DOF because aperture size can be manipulated without the distorting effects of changing focal length and the manipulation does not require a large room. The aperture size varies inversely with the DOF. Thus, a camera with an infinitely small aperture size would have an infinite DOF. This is most closely demonstrated in pinhole film cameras, which have a near-infinite DOF. Aperture size is measured in f-stops, the value for which is a calculation based on the ratio of the focal length of the lens to aperture diameter in millimeters. An f-stop of f/2 is therefore a much larger aperture size than an f-stop of f/8. An f-stop of f/8 provides greater DOF than an f-stop of f/2. This can be appreciated in **Table 1**, which gives the corresponding aperture area for different f-stops of a 50-mm lens; with each stepwise increase in f-stop, the aperture area is roughly halved. The effect of aperture size on DOF is illustrated in **Fig. 1**. In this figure, the DOF increases dramatically as the f-stop is increased from f/2.8 to f/32.

While attempting to improve DOF by changing aperture size, it is important to realize that changing the aperture size will affect the exposure. Increasing the f-stop, and thus increasing DOF, results in less light entering the camera. Two factors may be manipulated to maintain proper photographic exposure when the f-stop is increased. The first factor is the sensitivity of the medium used to light. In film cameras, this was measured with the American Standards Association (ASA) or International Organization for Standardization (ISO) scale. The higher the ISO the greater the sensitivity of the medium to light. Digital SLRs have the capability to change the ISO value. The effect of decreasing the aperture size can also be counter-balanced by decreasing the shutter speed to prevent underexposure. Typical shutter speeds include a range from 1/60 to 1/1000 of a second. Therefore, if an increase in the DOF is achieved by increasing the f-stop, it is important to decrease the shutter speed as well.

Although these settings can be completed manually, most digital SLR cameras now have multiple modes that take the guessing out of determining the correct shutter speed for a particular aperture size for each lens. These automated options include the aperture priority mode (A mode), in which setting the photographer manually adjusts the aperture size and the camera adjusts the remaining settings, and the shutter priority mode (S mode), in which the photographer controls shutter speed and the camera automatically adjusts the rest. There is also a programmed mode, in which the camera automatically adjusts all of the settings. It is the author's experience that using the aperture priority mode will ensure the best DOF, while the camera adjusts other parameters to ensure optimal exposure.

Table 1
F-stop nomenclature and its relationship to aperture area

F-stop	Aperture Size (mm) (50 mm/f-stop)	Aperture Radius (mm) (Diameter/2)	Aperture Area (mm^2)
f/1	50	25	1963
f/1.4	35.7	17.9	1002
f/2.0	25	12.5	491
f/2.8	17.9	8.9	250
f/4	12.5	6.3	123
f/5.6	8.9	4.5	63
f/8	6.3	3.1	31
f/11	4.5	2.3	16
f/16	3.1	1.6	8
f/22	2.3	1.1	4

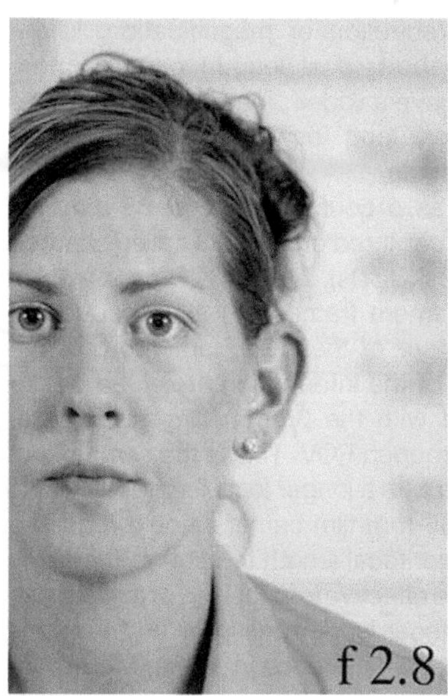

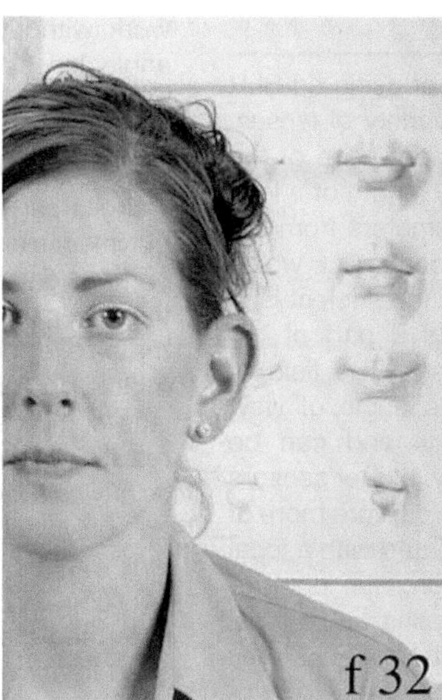

Fig. 1. Effect of aperture on DOF. In this set of photos, there is a limited DOF in the left figure. The plane of focus is limited to the nasal tip and facial plane; the ears and hair are out of focus. In the second photograph, the aperture is reduced significantly (with concomitant decrease in shutter speed and increase in ISO to maintain appropriate exposure). In this photograph, the patient's nasal tip, face, ears, and hair are all in focus. The line drawings, located 2 ft behind the patient, are also in focus.

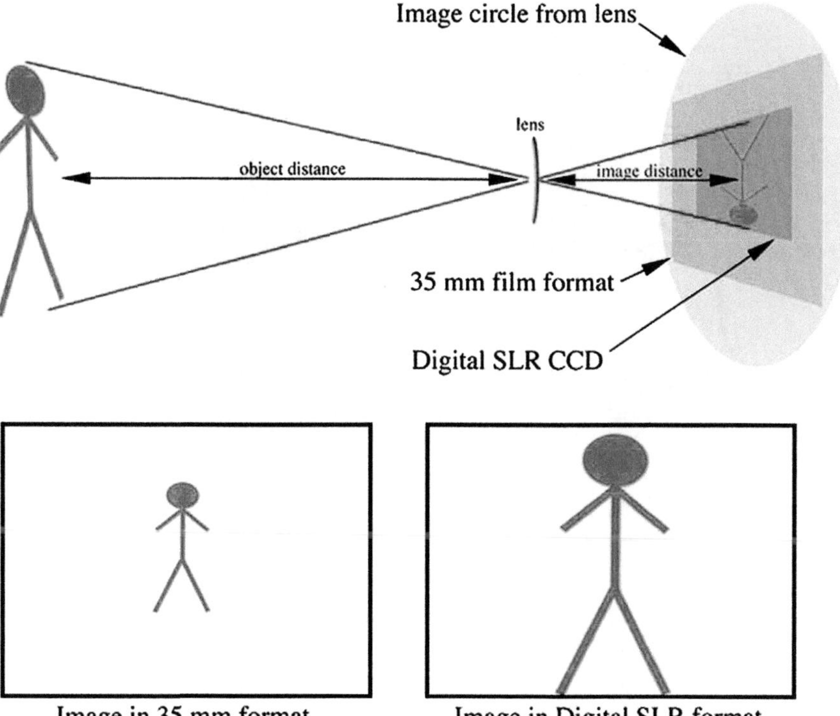

Fig. 2. Focal length multiplier (FLM) effect. The FLM is calculated by dividing the diagonal of 35-mm film by the diagonal of the CCD used by the digital SLR camera. This multiplier gives us the effective increase in focal length engendered by use of the digital SLR. This varies with the manufacturer. In the case of Nikon (used for taking the photos in this article), the multiplier is 1.5. The image in the case of the digital SLR appears larger, which is effectively the same as using a lens with a longer focal length.

Lenses

Although one of the advantages of using an SLR camera is the choice of a wide variety of lenses, it is crucial to understand the importance of the focal length of the lens. The focal length of a lens is defined as the distance in millimeters from the optical center of the lens to the focal point, which is located on the sensor or film if the subject is in focus. The camera lens projects a part of the scene onto the film or the sensor. The field of view (FOV) is determined by the angle of view from the lens out to the scene and can be measured horizontally or vertically. Larger sensors or films have wider FOVs and can capture more of the scene. The FOV that is associated with a focal length is usually based on 35-mm film photography. In 35-mm photography, lenses with a focal length of 50 mm are called normal because they work without reduction or magnification. Wide-angle lenses (short focal length) capture more because they have a wider picture angle, whereas telephoto lenses (long focal length) have a narrower picture angle.

Digital cameras, of course, do not use 35-mm film, but images are captured on sensors called charged coupled devices (CCDs). These CCDs are smaller than 35-mm camera frames. As a consequence, the smaller sensor of the CCD captures only the middle portion of the information projected by the lens compared with the 35-mm film frame area, resulting in a cropped FOV. This is the same effect as having a lens with a longer focal length. Similarly, an equivalent 35-mm film camera would require a lens with a longer focal length to achieve the same FOV (**Fig. 2**). The effective lengthening of focal length is termed the focal length multiplier (FLM) and is used to correct the difference in size of the sensor

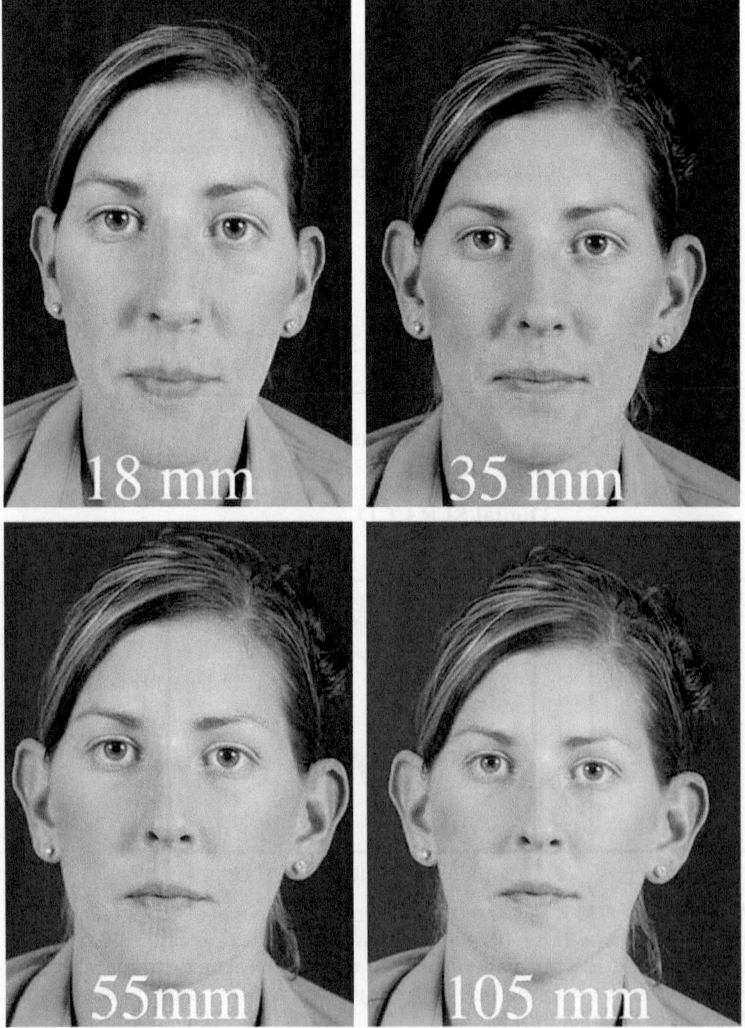

Fig. 3. Effect of lens focal length on facial proportions. The subject was photographed in the same sitting with a Nikon D70 digital SLR camera, using a dual-flash studio. Only focal length was changed, as indicated on each photograph. A visible distortion to the nasal tip and facial shape is noted on using the 18-mm lens. More realistic facial proportions are achieved with 55-mm or 105-mm lenses. The conversion for digital CCD is not included in the figure (1.5x for Nikon digital SLR, see text).

to the traditional 35-mm window. The FLM is equal to the diagonal of 35-mm film (43.3 mm) divided by the diagonal of the sensor. For example, for Nikon digital SLR cameras (Nikon Corp, Tokyo, Japan) the FLM is 1.5. Therefore a lens with a focal length of 60 mm would be equivalent to a 90-mm SLR lens when fitted on a digital Nikon SLR. By convention, the focal lengths on lenses are listed as calculated for a 35-mm film camera.

In photodocumentation of the patient undergoing rhinoplasty, it is important to use a lens that produces the least distortion and provides the largest DOF to ensure that the whole face is in focus.[5] Lenses between 90 and 105 mm in focal length meet these criteria. Although lenses with shorter focal lengths provide better DOF, the distortion of facial anatomy becomes obvious. This is depicted in **Fig. 3**.

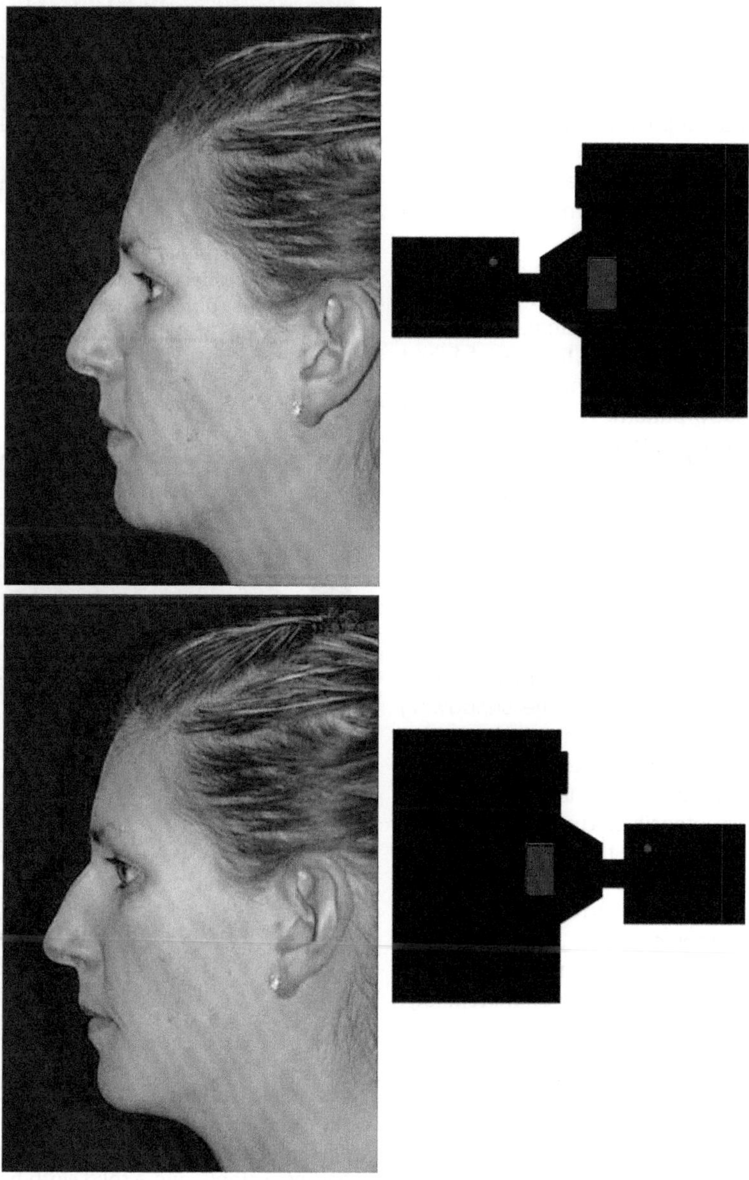

Fig. 4. Appropriate orientation of single on-camera flash. When using a single, camera-mounted flash, the orientation of the flash should be toward the patient's nasal tip, as in the top photograph and diagrammatic representation of the camera's orientation. When the opposite orientation is used, a significant shadow effect of the patient's profile ensues (*bottom photograph*).

Lighting

Lighting is the most critical component and the most studied area in photography of patients undergoing rhinoplasty. Use of different lighting arrangements, light sources, or even light positions can have a dramatic effect on the final photographic product. The most inexpensive form of lighting is to use a single mounted camera flash. However, this will produce harsh shadows and uneven lighting.[6] **Fig. 4** illustrates the sharp difference of flash position using a single mount flash. When a single-flash camera is used, the flash should be oriented toward the nose of the subject to avoid the shadow effect (see **Fig. 4**). The twin camera-mounted flash (not pictured) will help to improve the problem of uneven lighting but is unwieldy and does not provide adequate separation (horizontal angle of incidence, see later discussion). The most effective way to avoid harsh shadows would be to use a formal photo studio with lighting system.

Two major studio light systems have been described: the key light system and the quarter light system.[7,8] The key light system, developed for portrait photography involves the use of 1 light (the key light) as the major light source, which produces the shadow pattern. The key light is first moved around the camera in a horizontal plane until the nose and the cheek shadows merge and then in a vertical plane until the shadow of the nose touches the corner of the mouth. A fill light, which is less intense with a softer and a more diffuse quality, is then positioned to light or fill in the area of the shadow on the face produced by the key light. Two backlights are used simultaneously to separate the subject from the background. The technique minimizes the shadowing seen in using single mounted flashes and provides lighting that helps better delineate nasal anatomy.[7] The downside of this system is that the light sources are not of equal intensity and are placed asymmetrically. Unfortunately, the resultant light reflexes that are often used to define the nasal tip will also be asymmetrical and may even appear deviated. To overcome these limitations the quarter light system was specifically designed for medical photography, especially for rhinoplasty. The quarter light system consists of 2 lights of equal intensity, positioned at 45° from the subject-camera axis, and overcomes the limitations of other lighting systems (**Fig. 5**). Although this system is ideal, the downsides are cost and large space requirements. The author has used a modified version of this system, and it is illustrated in **Fig. 6**. This system works well in small spaces, and the backlights are not necessary. A

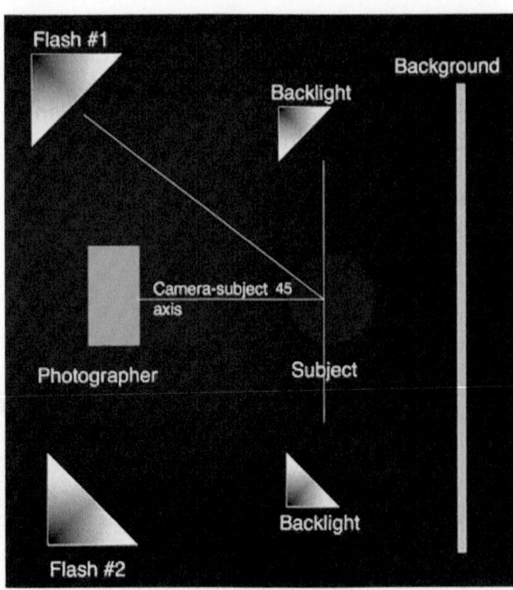

Fig. 5. The ideal key light photography setup for facial plastic surgery. The flashes are set up at 45° to the camera-subject axis. Backlighting and the distance between the subject and background provide separation from the background.

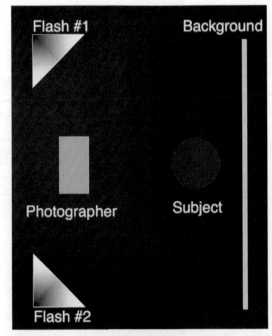

Fig. 6. The practical photography setup for facial plastic surgeons. It requires only 2 synchronized studio flashes, 2 stools, and a solid cloth background. In this scenario, with which most of the author's photographs are taken, consistent, well-balanced photographs can be taken for facial plastic surgery.

distance of 12 to 18 in is maintained between the subject and the background to minimize shadow effects of the subject on the background.

The distance between the main lights can have a profound effect on the appearance of the nasal tip anatomy and can simulate the postoperative appearance of tip rhinoplasty without surgery. The horizontal angle of incidence is the angle between the subject-camera axis and the flash (see **Fig. 5**). The ideal angle is 45°. When the angle is increased, the tip-defining points (and light reflexes in the eyes) appear wider apart and vice versa (**Fig. 7**). The term "photographic tip rhinoplasty" was coined to refer to this variance in nasal appearance with change in horizontal angle of incidence.[7]

Patient Views

The standardized views for photographing the patient undergoing rhinoplasty are well known and have been described in detail.[9] However, correct execution of these 6 standard views is imperative to critically evaluate the nasal anatomy. These standard views include the anteroposterior (AP) view, lateral view from right and left, the

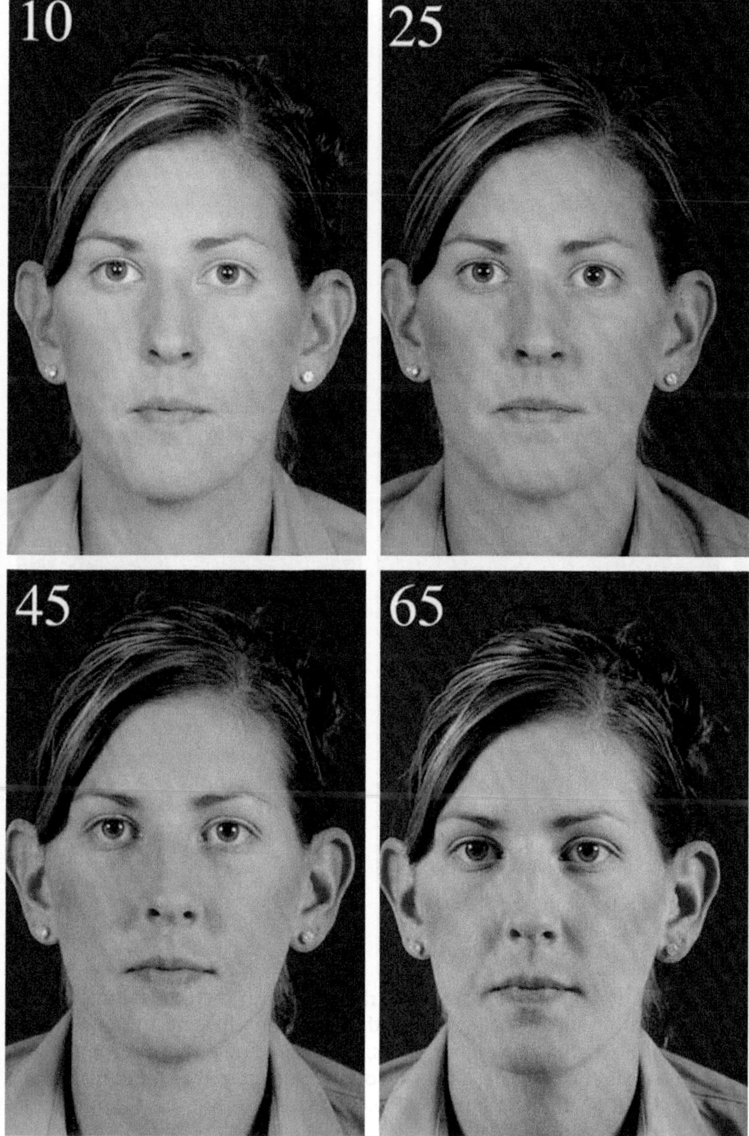

Fig. 7. The effect of angle of incidence on photography in rhinoplasty. The width of the tip-defining points is affected by the angle of incidence (angle between the flash and the camera-subject axis). At 10°, the dual-flash becomes nearly equivalent to a single light source. The tip-defining points are at close proximity. At 25°, increased separation of the tip-defining points ensues. At 45°, (ideal) appropriate and realistic separation is noted. At 65°, the tip-defining points have migrated to the lateral nasal tip. The light reflexes indicate flash separation in the subject's eyes.

oblique view from right and left, and the basal view. It may also be beneficial to obtain a cephalic view to evaluate the nasal dorsum and a smiling lateral view to capture dynamic changes to the nasal tip.

Patient Positioning

It is critical to maintain standardization between the different views. A brief review of standard patient positions in photography in rhinoplasty is listed herein, and as a detailed description listed in the article by Henderson and colleagues.[9] Photographs should be taken with a solid background, such as medium blue, because this provides contrast but does not obscure facial features. Pictures should be taken at the patient's eye level, and the patient should be exactly 90° from the lens. The Frankfort horizontal line, an imaginary line from the top of the tragus to the infraorbital rim, is used as a guide, and the patient should be positioned with this line parallel to the

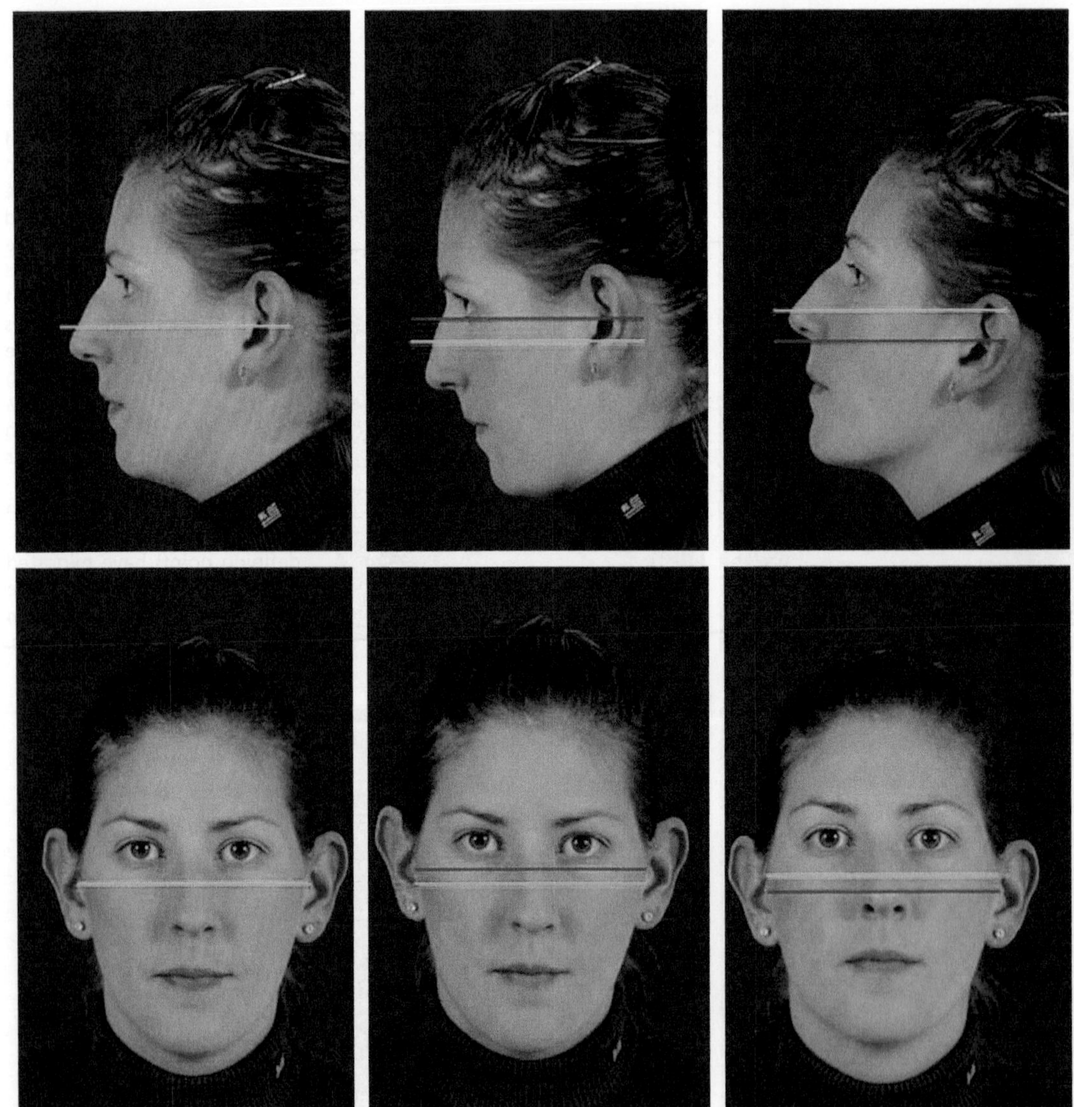

Fig. 8. The Frankfort horizontal plane and positioning in photography in rhinoplasty. In each row of photos, the left photograph demonstrates the proper position of the patient, with the green line passing through the infraorbital rim and external auditory canal. In the middle and right photos, the green line passes through the infraorbital rim and parallel to the floor, whereas the red line passes through the external auditory canal and parallel to the floor. There are changes in apparent tip rotation on AP view (*bottom row*) with slight changes in Frankfort plane.

ground. Examples of correct position in relation to the Frankfort line are pictured in **Fig. 8**. In the AP view, the patient should be at eye level and looking directly into the lens (see **Fig. 8**). This view is useful to evaluate the root and base of the nose for any deviations, asymmetries, and curvatures. The other essential views for rhinoplasty are the paired oblique views, the basal view, and lateral smiling view. In some cases, a cephalic view is useful for evaluation of the nasal dorsum as well.

COMPUTER IMAGING IN RHINOPLASTY

The use of computer imaging to enhance communication between patients and surgeons has grown in popularity for rhinoplasty surgeons and their patients. Patients request computer simulation as a preoperative display of anticipated results. Surgeons use this tool as an effective means to show the expected surgical outcomes and to evaluate patient acceptance of these outcomes.

When used appropriately, computer imaging to display rhinoplasty results facilitates communication between the patients and surgeons. The surgeon should not try to oversell the outcome and should represent with the imaging programs a realistic surgical outcome. The patient should listen to and understand the limitations of the surgery and not be overwhelmed by the presented image.

The advantages of computer imaging in rhinoplasty include the ability to show patients changes that are difficult to express verbally (eg, lip shortening or top rotation). This is particularly important when displaying profile changes, such as chin augmentation or reduction. The patient is able to visualize the effect of rhinoplasty alone versus the result of rhinoplasty and chin augmentation. It is clear that lateral, or profile, changes are much more effectively and accurately shown than are AP, or frontal, changes.

It is important that the surgeon does not guarantee a result by using computer technology. The patient often sees the computerized result as their photographic result. For this reason, it is important that the surgeon does not give the patient any hard copy of the computerized image. This will avoid the patient staring at the image and expecting results similar to the computerized image. Also, if the patient is given the simulated result, they will compare the actual result with the computerized result.

If used intelligently and effectively, computerized imaging can enhance communication between the rhinoplasty patient and surgeon. It becomes an effective tool for communication, planning, and even marketing of adjunctive procedures.

SUMMARY

It is critical for the facial plastic surgeon to obtain high-quality standardized photographs for all patients undergoing rhinoplasty. These photographs, when implemented correctly, are invaluable for presurgical planning, patient education, record keeping, and presentations to demonstrate surgical outcomes. Possession of a basic understanding of photographic principles, technique, and equipment as well as consideration to consistency of patient positioning is essential for producing the best photographic results.

REFERENCES

1. Karlan MS. Photographic documentation techniques. Ear Nose Throat J 1979;58(6):246–51.
2. Persichetti P, Simone P, Langella M, et al. Digital photography in plastic surgery: how to achieve reasonable standardization outside a photographic studio. Aesthetic Plast Surg 2007;31(2):194–200.
3. Beekhuis GJ, Rosenbaum JM. Office photography for facial cosmetic surgery. Laryngoscope 1979;89(4): 677–81.
4. Staffel JG. Photo documentation in rhinoplasty. Facial Plast Surg 1997;13(4):317–32.
5. Becker DG, Tardy ME Jr. Standardized photography in facial plastic surgery: pearls and pitfalls. Facial Plast Surg 1999;15(2):93–9.
6. Schwartz MS, Tardy ME Jr. Standardized photodocumentation in facial plastic surgery. Facial Plast Surg 1990;7(1):1–12.
7. Daniel RK, Hodgson J, Lambros VS. Rhinoplasty: the light reflexes. Plast Reconstr Surg 1990;85(6):859–66 [discussion: 867–8].
8. Galdino GM, DaSilva D, Gunter JP. Digital photography for rhinoplasty. Plast Reconstr Surg 2002; 109(4):1421–34.
9. Henderson JL, Larrabee WF Jr, Krieger BD. Photographic standards for facial plastic surgery. Arch Facial Plast Surg 2005;7(5):331–3.

Diagnosis and Correction of Alar Rim Deformities in Rhinoplasty

Fred L. Hackney, MD, DDS

KEYWORDS

• Retracted ala • Hangng ala • Concave ala
• Convex ala • Alar rim deformities • Rhinoplasty

Recognition of alar rim deformities is an important component of the preoperative analysis of the nose. Correction of these deformities improves the esthetic balance of the nose and has the added benefit, in some patients, of improving the function of the external nasal valve.

In recent years classification systems have been proposed, which enable surgeons to more accurately diagnose alar deformities.[1,2] These classification systems help guide surgeons as to the appropriate surgical procedure to correct the problem. The purpose of this article is to review the proposed classification systems for alar rim deformities and review the specific surgical techniques that have been proposed for each of the deformities.

CLASSIFICATIONS OF ALAR RIM DEFORMITIES

Gunter and colleagues[1] proposed a classification for alar-columellar discrepancies, which defines the normal alar columellar relationship based on a line drawn through the most anterior and posterior points of the nostril on the lateral view (**Fig. 1**). The nostril represents an oval in which the alar rim forms the upper border of the nostril and the columellar rim, at the junction of the external skin with the vestibular skin, forms the lower border of the nostril. This oval is occasionally interrupted by flaring of the feet of the medial cura, but this should be disregarded when analyzing the relationship. In a normal alar-columellar relationship, the greatest distance from the long axis of the nostril to the alar rim or the columellar rim should be 1 to 2 mm.

A hanging ala results in decreased columellar show with the distance between the long axis of the nostril and the alar rim being less that 1 to 2 mm. A retracted ala is characterized by an alar rim to nostril long axis distance of more than 2 mm. The true "hanging columella" occurs when the distance between the long axis of the nostril and the columellar rim is greater than 2 mm and the distance from the long axis to the superior nostril rim is the normal distance of 1 to 2 mm. It is important not to misdiagnose a hanging columella as a retracted ala. A retracted columella is characterized by the distance between the columellar rim and the long axis of the nostril less than 1 to 2 mm.[1]

Of the four basic deformities (defined previously), retracted ala, hanging ala, retracted columella, and hanging columella, only the retracted ala and the hanging ala represent true alar rim deformities. Of these two, the retracted ala is the deformity that has generated the most interest from surgeons attempting to correct it.

Guyuron subsequently expanded the classification of alar rim deformities to include an analysis from the perspective of the alar basilar view, in contrast to Gunter's classification, which focused on the alar columellar relationships in the lateral (profile) view. In the ideal basal view, the alar rim anatomy forms an equilateral triangle. The ala forms a straight line, which constitutes two sides of the triangle, with the alar base width forming the third side. Guyuron recognized two distinct alar abnormalities, the concave and the convex ala. The concave ala is defined as the lateral border of the ala being medial to the line of the

8315 Walnut Hill Lane, Suite 225, Dallas, TX, USA
E-mail address: fred@drhackney.net

Clin Plastic Surg 37 (2010) 223–229
doi:10.1016/j.cps.2009.12.007

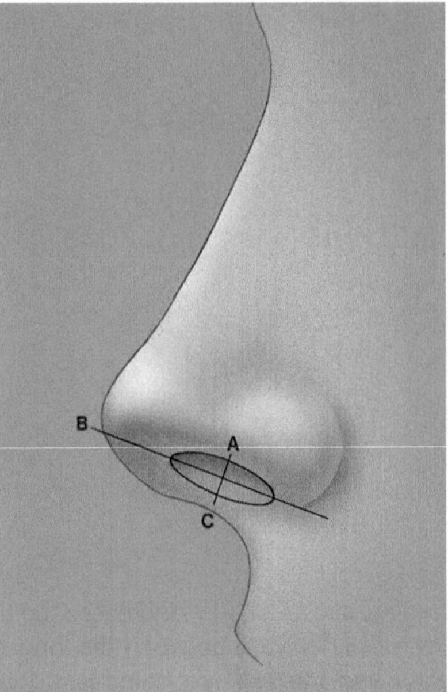

Fig. 1. The normal alar columellar relationship is based on a line drawn through the most anterior and posterior points of the nostril on the lateral view. In a normal relationship, the distance from the long axis of the nostril (line B) to the alar rim (point A) or the columellar rim (point C) is 1–2 mm. (*From* Gunter JP, Rohrich RJ, Friedman, RM. Classification and correction of alar-columellar-discrepancies in Rhinoplasty. Plast Reconstr Surg 1996;97(3):643–8; with permission.)

equilateral triangle. The convex ala is defined as the lateral border of the ala extending lateral to the line of the equilateral triangle.[2]

TREATMENT OF ALAR RIM DEFORMITIES

For the purposes of this discussion, the treatment of alar deformities is divided into deformities seen in the lateral (profile)[1] and those seen in the basilar view.[2]

Lateral View Alar Deformities

The hanging ala

The most common technique to correct a hanging ala is to excise an ellipse of vestibular skin. The ellipse should be horizontal and parallel to the alar rim. The width of the ellipse should be slightly more than the planned elevation of the alar rim (**Fig. 2**). Care should be taken not to excise too much to avoid a rolled in appearance of the alar rim, so the excision should not exceed 3 mm.[1] Other options for raising the ala include excision of skin of the nose, trimming of the cephalic or caudal border of the lateral crus and excision of nasal lining.[3] Direct excision of skin at the alar rim is best performed in patients with thick sebaceous skin but may lead to visible scarring. This is rarely used because of the scar. McKinney and Stalnecker found resection of the caudal border of the lateral crus to be useful in thin-skinned patients and has resected up to 2 mm. The trimming of the caudal border must be accurate and

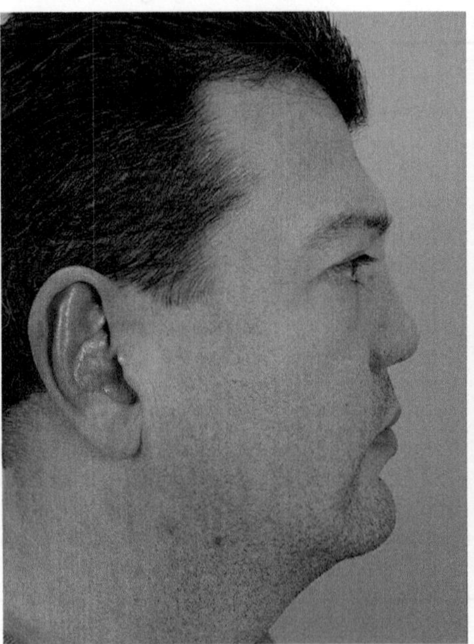

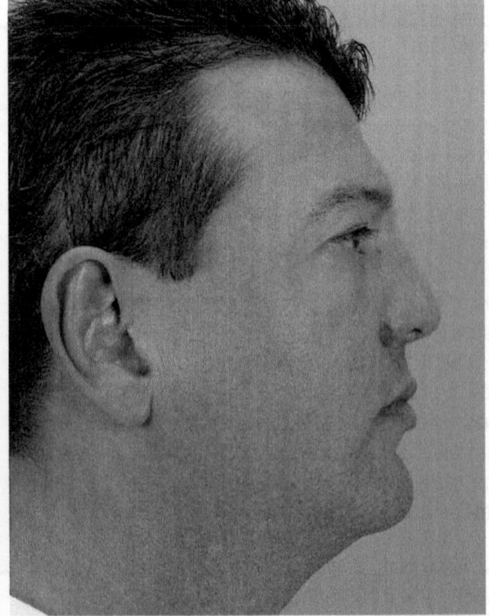

Fig. 2. Lateral view of a patient before (*left*) and after (*right*) correction of a hanging ala with excision of an ellipse of vestibular skin parallel to the alar rim.

smooth to prevent any irregularity or notching of the alar rim. This technique does not work well in thick-skinned patients because the skin is not pliable enough to conform to the new position of the cartilage. Excision of the nasal lining in the area of the cephalic border of the alar cartilage is effective in thick-skinned patients. Caution is advised, however, because the resection must be caudal to the internal nasal valve and in general over-resection of lining should be avoided.[3]

Another option for raising the alar rim is direct excision of the ala.[4] This can be done by excising the skin and mucosa and then undermining the skin edge and advancing it to close it to the mucosa. Millard[5] had also proposed alar margin sculpturing in a thick hanging ala. Irregularities and scarring of the alar rim may result so direct excision is used less often than other techniques.

The retracted ala

The correction of a retracted ala depends on the severity of the retraction. If only a small amount of lowering is desirable, an alar base resection provides some lowering of the alar rim.[6] If the retraction is mild, the deformity can be corrected by separating the lateral curs from the accessory cartilage and moving the cartilage caudally. This is only effective if there are no associated tissue deficiencies.[1]

For moderate alar retractions, cartilage grafting may be more appropriate. Rohrich and colleagues[7] have described the alar contour graft for correction of alar rim deformities. This technique is done with an open approach. Using the medial end of the infracartilaginous incision, a pocket is undermined cephalic and parallel to the alar rim. A cartilage graft of approximately 5 mm by 25 mm is used, or at least long enough to span the retracted area. The graft is placed in the pocket and stabilized to the nasal lining medially with one 5-0 plain gut suture. Septal cartilage is the first choice for grafting, but auricular cartilage is an acceptable second choice. This technique can also be used with a closed approach.[8] An incision is made in the posterior vestibule perpendicular to the rim, and a tunnel is developed along the rim and the graft is inserted.

An alternative to the alar rim graft when using an open approach is to place a cartilage graft caudal to the existing lateral curs. To facilitate this, the vestibular incision is made caudal to the caudal rim of the lateral curs, thus leaving a cuff of vestibular skin below the lateral curs. The graft is placed in a pocket under this cuff of vestibular skin.[9]

For more severe alar retraction, a lateral crural strut graft may be indicated (**Fig. 3**). This is a versatile technique, which can be used to treat other alar deformities, such as alar rim collapse, and concave lateral crura, in addition to correction of alar retraction. This is also done with an open rhinoplasty technique. The vestibular skin is dissected from the cephalic border of the crura

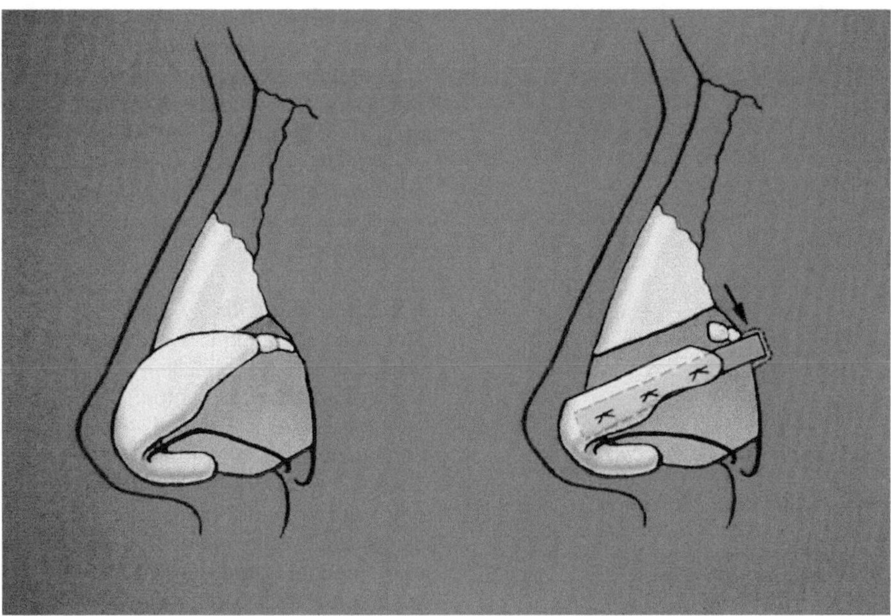

Fig. 3. A severe retracted ala can be corrected with a lateral crural strut graft. The graft is sutured to the lateral curs and repositioned more caudally to lower the alar rim. (*From* Gunter JP, Friedman RM. Lateral crural strut graft: technique and clinical applications in rhinoplasty. Plast Reconstr Surg 1997;99(4):943–52; with permission.)

toward the caudal border. The vestibular skin is left attached to the caudal border. The lateral crura are separated from the accessory cartilages. A cartilage graft measuring 3 to 4 mm in width and 15 to 25 mm in length is fashioned from septal cartilage, but auricular or rib cartilage can also be used. A longer strut is indicated for the correction of alar retraction. The pocket is made in the soft tissue below the alar groove, and the lateral end of the strut is placed in the pocket, thus positioning the lateral crura more caudally.[10] This is technically more demanding than the alar contour graft and is indicated for more severe cases of alar retraction or secondary cases.

A modification of the lateral crural strut is the intercartilaginous graft for moderate to severe alar retraction as described by Gruber and colleagues (**Fig. 4**). The graft is placed between the upper lateral cartilage and the lateral crus or the remnant of the lateral curs. This lengthens the lateral nasal sidewall. Key to this procedure is soft tissue release between the lateral crus remnant and the upper lateral cartilages. Scissors are used the spread between the two, while attempting to preserve the vestibular mucosa. A gap of 4 mm and up to 8 mm may be made with the soft tissue

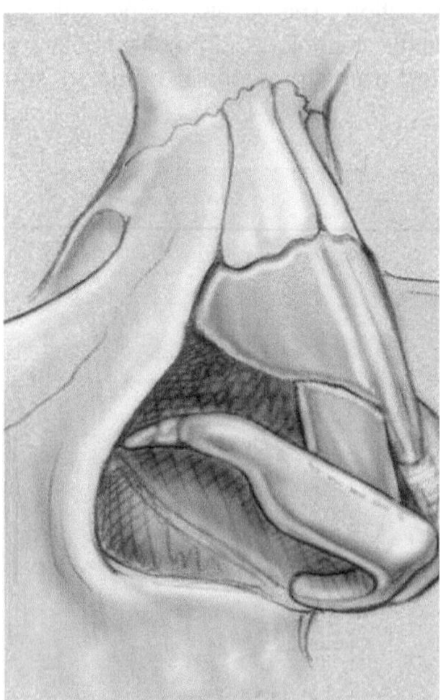

Fig. 4. The intercartilaginous septal graft is placed in the dissected space between the caudal edge of the upper lateral cartilage and the cephalic edge of the lateral crus. The graft is stabilized with sutures. (*From* Gruber RP, Kyyger G, Chang DM. The intercartilaginous graft for actual and potential alar retraction. Plast Reconstr Surg 2008;121(5):288e–96e; with permission.)

release. The release often results in some undermining of the vestibular skin of the lateral crus. The septal graft is placed between the upper lateral cartilage and the lateral curs and is sutured to the upper lateral cartilage and under the upper edge of the lateral curs.[11]

The traditional treatment for severe alar retraction in patients with scarring or lining deficiencies is composite grafting, usually with septal cartilage and mucosa or auricular cartilage and skin (**Fig. 5**). A vestibular incision is made parallel to the rim with inferior mobilization of the rim by releasing the soft tissue with scissors. The composite graft is placed in the resulting defect.[1] The graft is sutured to the defect and may be stabilized with a bolster dressing for 1 week.

An alternative to composite grafting is internal V-Y advancement flap, which has been described by Guyuron. This technique can be used with an open approach, in which the design of the V-Y flap is incorporated into the intranasal incisions. The technique can also be done as an isolated procedure for revisions. The base of the V flap is at the alar rim and the apex of the V extends to the intercartilaginous line. The flap is then elevated caudally to the alar rim. If the exposed lower lateral cartilage is missing or transected, it can be reconstructed with septal or auricular grafts. After completion of the rhinoplasty and as the incisions are closed, the V-Y advancement is performed to lower the alar rim. A bolster dressing is applied for 5 to 7 days and stabilized with a through and through suture, but caution is advised not to tighten the suture excessively as necrosis of the alar rim may occur. This technique has been used successfully for alar retractions up to 5 mm.[2] This technique may have advantages over the traditional composite graft because the composite graft is susceptible to scar contraction as the graft heals, which may lead to partial recurrence of the alar rim deformity.

Hanging columella

The hanging columella is treated based on the anatomy of the specific columellar deformity. Most often a variable amount of the membranous septum is resected and reapproximated. The cartilaginous nasal septum can also be trimmed. These maneuvers move the columella superiorly.[12] If the medial crura have increased width in a cephalic caudal orientation, then direct trimming of the caudal border help correct the deformity.[13] In some patients the intermediate crura is vertically oriented and displaces the medial crura caudally. Transverse division, overlapping and stabilizing with suture decrease the vertical length of the

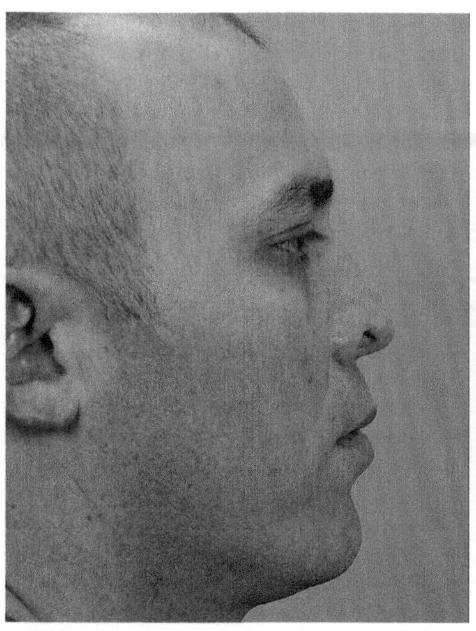
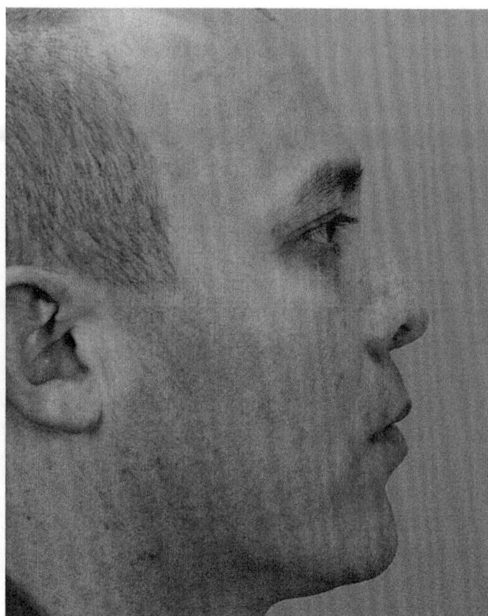

Fig. 5. Lateral view of a patient before (*left*) and after (*right*) correction of a retracted ala with auricular composite graft.

intermediate crura and allow the medial crura to move more cephalically.[1]

Retracted columella

Recognition of a retracted columella is important because this can be misdiagnosed as a hanging ala. The treatment of retracted columella is placement of a cartilage graft (**Fig. 6**). This columellar strut is shaped so its widest part corresponds to the area of greatest retraction of the columella. The strut is placed between the medial crura and caudal to the septum so the columellar skin is pushed caudally to correct the retraction.[1]

Basilar View Alar Deformities

Concave ala

The concave ala is defined as the lateral border of the ala being medial to the line of the equilateral

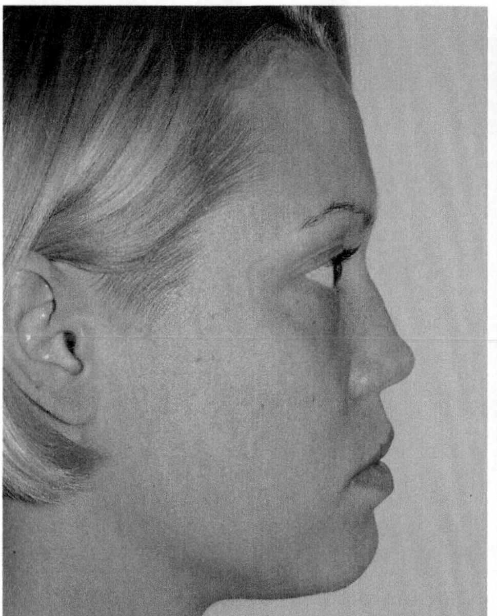
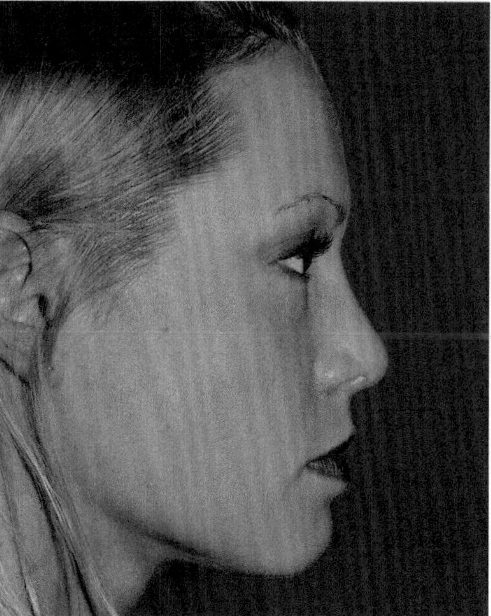

Fig. 6. Lateral view of a secondary rhinoplasty patient before (*left*) and after (*right*) correction of a retracted columella with placement of a columellar strut fashioned from rib cartilage.

triangle, which is formed by the nose from the basilar perspective. The etiology of this deformity is often inappropriate division or resection of the lower lateral cartilage. A tip graft that extends lateral to the existing dome also produces the appearance of a concave ala. Treat of a concave ala depends on the severity of the deformity. For a mild amount of concavity, Guyuron uses an alar rim graft. The graft is placed in a subcutaneous tunnel along the alar rim. Septal, auricular, or rib cartilage may be used. The edges of the graft are thinned and beveled so as not to be visible. The grafts must be of appropriate length and width to provide support to the rim and correct the deformity.[2] This is similar to the alar contour graft as described by Rohrich and colleagues.[7] Another option for a more severe or secondary rhinoplasty is a lateral crura strut graft as described by Gunter and Friedman (**Fig. 7**).[10] Options for correction of a concave ala and a retracted ala are often the same, and the two deformities often coexist.

Convex ala

If the ala is lateral to the equilateral triangle as seen in the basilar view, the ala is convex. This may be the result of a convex shape and bulging of lateral crus or thickened soft tissues of the ala. If the deformity is a result of convex shaped lateral curs, the treatment is directed to reshaping the cartilage. The options include transection and overlapping of the lateral crura posteriorly or placement of lateral crura spanning sutures or transdomal sutures.[2] When considering these options, surgeons should consider the effects these maneuvers may have on tip rotation and tip projection. For instance, transection and overlapping of the lateral crura may result in a loss of tip projection or increased tip rotation.

When the convex ala is a result of increased thickness of the alar soft tissue, there are two options for correction. If alar base resections are planned, then the alar thickness is reduced through the alar base incision, removing the excess tissue between the external skin and the vestibular skin. After debulking of the alar subunit, the width of the ala consists of the two skin surfaces in opposition to each other.[14] If no alar base resections are planned, then direct excision of the alar rim can used to reduce the thickness. A fusiform incision is made as close to the medial

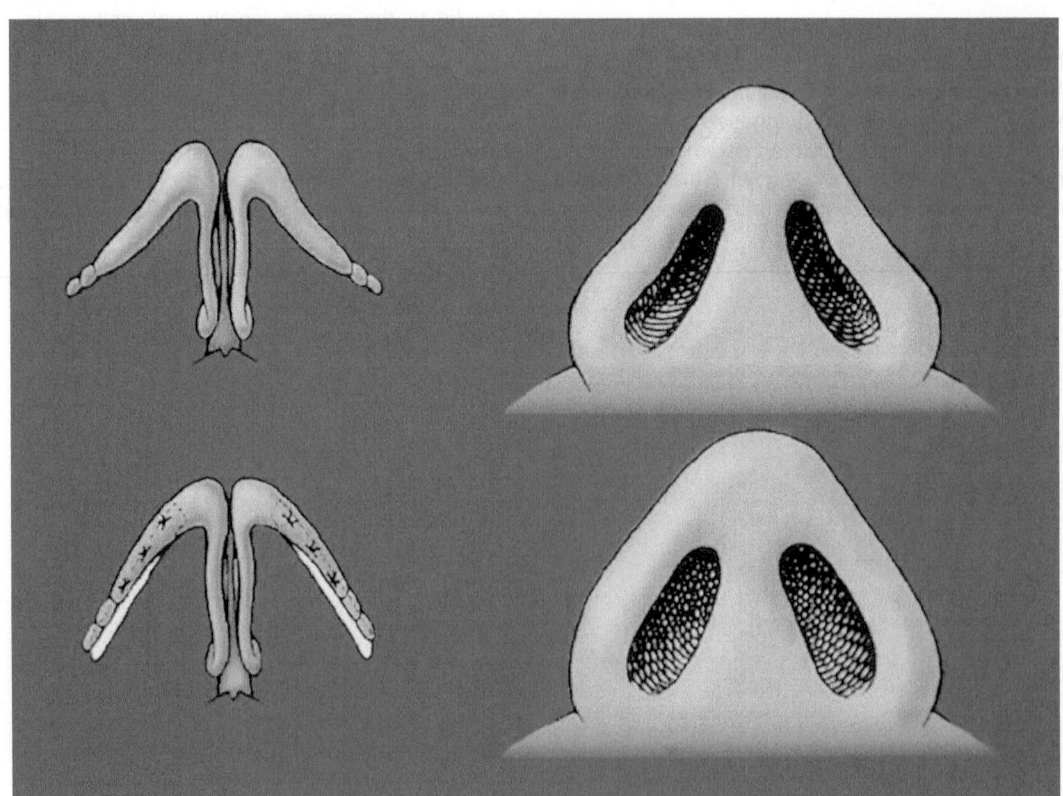

Fig. 7. A concave ala as shown above is a cosmetic deformity and can cause an incompetence of the external nasal valve. A lateral crural strut is one of several techniques that can reshape the concave ala as shown below. (*From* Gunter JP, Friedman RM. Lateral Crural Strut Graft: Technique and clinical applications in rhinoplasty. Plast Reconstr Surg 1997;99(4):943–52; with permission.)

aspect of the nostril as possible, and a combination of skin and subcutaneous tissue is removed. The incision is closed in one layer with plain gut.[2]

SUMMARY

Alar base deformities are common in rhinoplasty patients. Careful and detailed analysis of a patient's deformities leads to improved outcomes. The alar rim should be evaluated in the lateral view and the basilar view. The lateral view reveals retracted ala, hanging ala, retracted columella, hanging columella, or combinations of these. Analysis in the basilar view allows diagnosis of concave or convex ala. Treatment of each deformity varies and because combinations of deformities can exist, an accurate analysis is paramount to appropriate treatment. Treatment options for each deformity are presented for consideration.

REFERENCES

1. Gunter JP, Rohrich RJ, Friedman RM. Classification and correction of alar-columellar-discrepancies in Rhinoplasty. Plast Reconstr Surg 1996;97(3):643–8.
2. Guyuron B. Alar rim deformities. Plast Reconstr Surg 2001;107(3):866–7.
3. McKinney P, Stalnecker ML. The hanging ala. Plast Reconstr Surg 1984;73(3):427–30.
4. Ellenbogen R, Blome DW. Alar rim raising. Plast Reconstr Surg 1992;90(1):28–37.
5. Millard DM. Alar margin sculpturing. Plast Reconstr Surg 1967;40(4):337–42.
6. Guyuron B. Dynamics of rhinoplasty. Plast Reconstr Surg 1991;88(6):970–8.
7. Rohrich RJ, Raniere J, Ha R. The alar contour graft: correction and prevention of alar rim deformities. Plast Reconstr Surg 2002;109(7):2495–502.
8. Gruber RP, Rohrich RJ, Raniere J, et al. The alar contour graft: correction and prevention of alar rim deformities. Plast Reconstr Surg 2002;109(7): 2506–8 [discussion].
9. Toriumi E, Josen J, Weinbergem M, et al. The use of the alar batten grafts for correction of nasal valve collapse. Arch Otolarynogol Head Neck Surg 1997;123:802–5.
10. Gunter JP, Friedman RM. Lateral crural strut graft: technique and clinical applications in rhinoplasty. Plast Reconstr Surg 1997;99(4):943–52.
11. Gruber RP, Kyyger G, Chang DM. The intercartilaginous graft for actual and potential alar retraction. Plast Reconstr Surg 2008;121(5):288e–96e.
12. Adamson PA, Tropper GA, McGraw BL. The hanging columella. J Otolaryngol 1990;19:319–23.
13. Randall P. The direct approach to the hanging columella. Plast Reconstr Surg 1974;53(5):544–7.
14. Matarasso A. Alar rim excision: a method of thinning bulky nostrils. Plast Reconstr Surg 1996; 97(4):828–34.

Suture Techniques in Rhinoplasty

Ronald P. Gruber, MD[a,b,*], Edward Chang, MD[b], Edward Buchanan, MD[b]

KEYWORDS

- Rhinoplasty • Four-suture algorithm
- Universal horizontal mattress suture • Tipplasty

Controlling the shape of the nose in large part involves controlling the shape of the cartilages. Much of this control is obtained by excisional and grafting techniques. Scoring techniques are used less and less frequently, and in recent years and have been relegated to straightening crooked septal cartilages. It is clearly preferable to retain natural cartilage and make it conform to the desired shape, and also clearly better to minimize damage to the cartilage, which would even allow for the possibility of reversibility. Therefore, suture techniques to shape the nose have witnessed a dramatic increase since the early 1980s.[1–17] In this article on suture techniques, 2 major aspects are discussed: (1) techniques that totally and unambiguously control tip shape, and (2) a general technique that is applicable to all cartilages in the nose when one wants to eliminate undesirable convexities or concavities.

TIPPLASTY

Before undertaking nasal tip shaping with suture techniques, 3 surgical tenets should be followed to obtain consistent and reproducible results: (1) use a model, (2) preserve a 6-mm strip of lateral crus, and (3) recognize the delayed effects of suture on cartilage.

There are numerous angles and dimensions of the nose and its underlying framework to memorize. A surgeon can memorize several of them, but for the average plastic surgeon who performs the operation potentially only once a month, to become adept with all of them is a Herculean task. It is much easier to sculpt by using a model, which is a concept familiar to many commercial artists. A model is available (**Fig. 1**) that is a reasonable prototype of what the normal sculpted tip should resemble if one expects the nose to look good when the skin is redraped. The model demonstrates that the tip is usually about 6 mm above the dorsum and that there is an angle of divergence formed by the middle crurae. It also demonstrates that there is (following most all tipplasties) an axis to the dome and that the axes of the domes separate to form an angle close to 90°.

By preserving 6 mm of lateral crus after the cephalic trim, one has a substantial piece of cartilage that is not likely to buckle or collapse (**Fig. 2**), which also responds best to suture techniques. There is no need to remove more lateral crus when attempting to make the tip smaller or narrower.

Harris and colleagues[18] demonstrated that the effect of a particular suture technique may change over time. This change may not occur until half an hour after the suture is placed. This effect is a subtle but real one, caused by the entire cartilaginous framework adjusting to the new tension provided by the suture. It is best at the end of the rhinoplasty procedure to have a final look at what the sutures have done and to make any minor adjustments as necessary.

Current rhinoplasty literature contains confusing nomenclature regarding the various suture techniques. The names used in this article represent

[a] Division of Plastic & Reconstructive Surgery, Stanford University, Oakland, CA, USA
[b] Divisions of Plastic & Reconstructive Surgery, University of California (SF), 3318 Elm Street, Oakland, CA 94609, USA
* Corresponding author. Divisions of Plastic & Reconstructive Surgery, University of California (SF), 3318 Elm Street, Oakland, CA 94609.
E-mail address: rgrubermd@hotmail.com (R.P. Gruber).

Clin Plastic Surg 37 (2010) 231–243
doi:10.1016/j.cps.2009.12.010

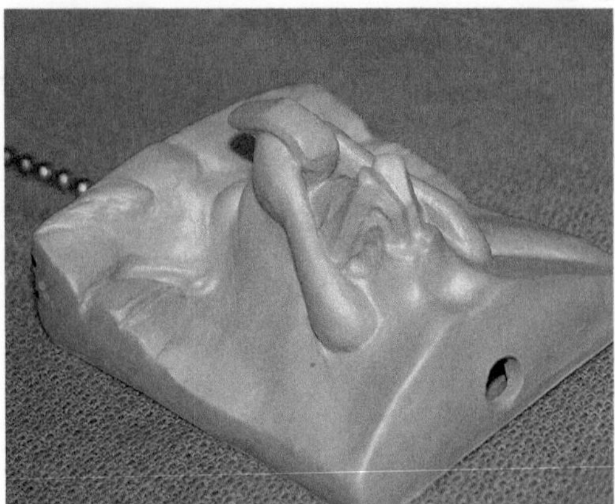

Fig. 1. A model of a prototype of the ideal sculpted nasal framework makes it easier to perform biologic sculpting of the tip. This way one does not have to memorize angles and distances. This model acts as a nasal retractor and is autoclavable. It is available from Miltex, and also Padgett Instruments. Any royalties from this product are sent to the PSEF.

the terms most commonly used by rhinoplasty surgeons. As for particular suture type, the authors tend to favor polydioxanone (PDS) whenever there is a question regarding soft tissue coverage. However, if coverage is not an issue, nylon is used. Although the study by Iamphongsai and colleagues[19] indicated little difference between nylon and PDS in maintaining the curvature of cartilage in animals at 3 months, several surgeons are concerned that when PDS is absorbed, the cartilage may return to its original state.

There are a few algorithms for suture tipplasty. One of the best and most complete analyses is that by Guyuron and colleagues[20,21] Daniel[22,23] has also developed an outstanding algorithm that will serve any plastic surgeon well. Here, the authors present an abridged version that addresses the most common issues that the average plastic surgeon will encounter in practice, namely the 4-suture algorithm.[23] However, not

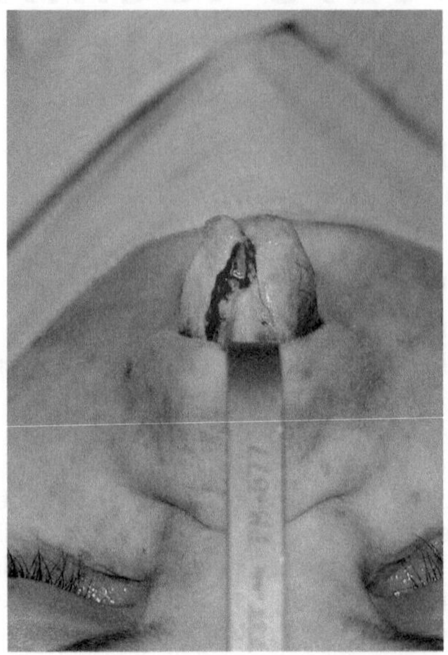

Fig. 2. In a primary rhinoplasty, a trim of the cephalic component of the lateral crus is almost always necessary before beginning suture tipplasty. Suture techniques work best on a strip of lateral crus as opposed to the entire unadulterated lateral crus.

all 4 of the techniques are necessary in every patient.

Hemi-Transdomal Suture

Perhaps the most important suture for the tip is that which controls the dome. The hemi-transdomal suture is a variation of the transdomal suture introduced by Tardy and colleagues[1] for the closed approach and by Daniel[22,23] for the open approach. The soft tissue deep to the dome is hyperinfiltrated with local anesthesia to prevent the suture from penetrating the vestibular skin. A 5-0 nylon or PDS is placed at the cephalic end of the dome (**Figs 3** and **4**). The effect of this suture is to (a) narrow the dome, (b) evert the caudal border of the lateral crus, and (c)

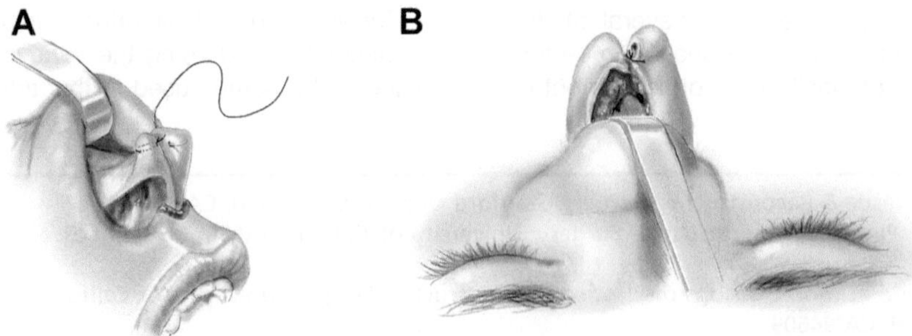

Fig. 3. (*A, B*) The hemi-transdomal suture is a new variation of the traditional transdomal suture. A 5-0 PDS or nylon that pinches the cephalic part of the dome so that the caudal border of the lateral crus is everted.

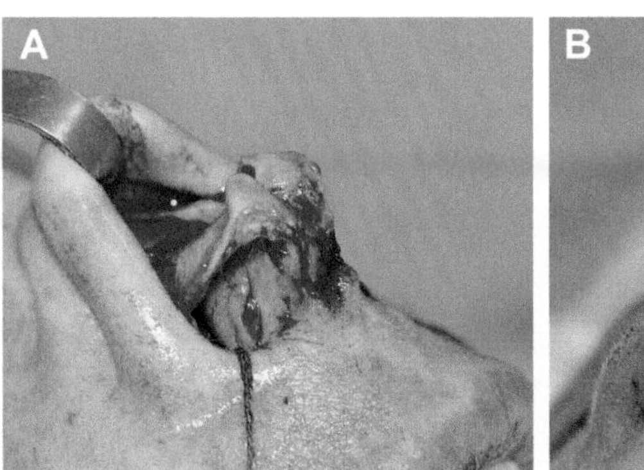

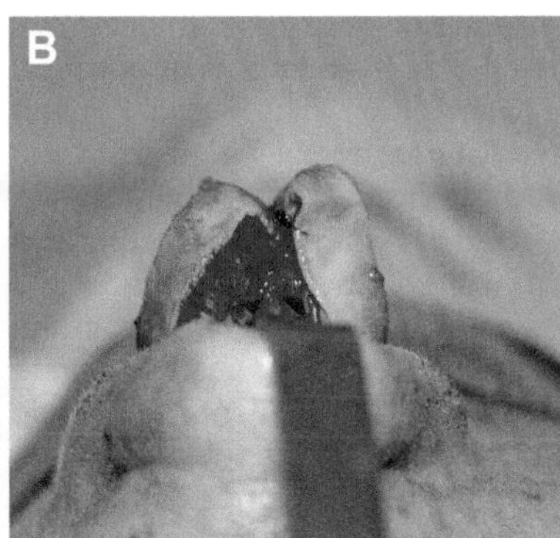

Fig. 4. (*A, B*) This intraoperative view demonstrates the effect of the hemi-transdomal suture. Note that the caudal border of the lateral crus is everted slightly as a result of that suture.

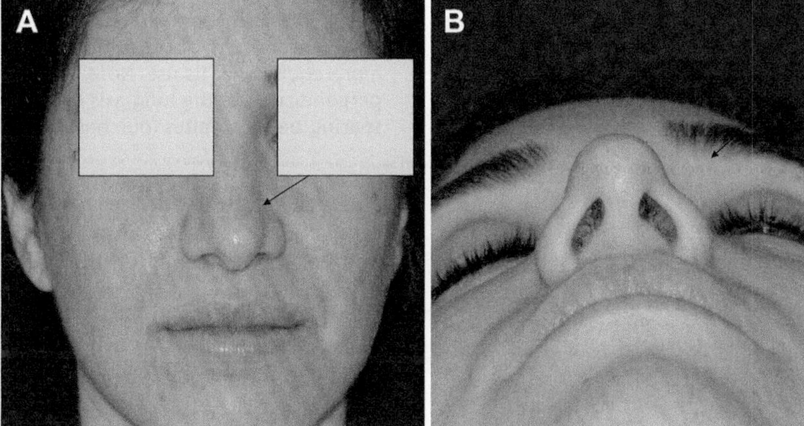

Fig. 5. (*A, B*) This patient demonstrates what may happen if a conventional transdomal suture causes inversion of the lateral crus. The result is a concavity of the alar rim.

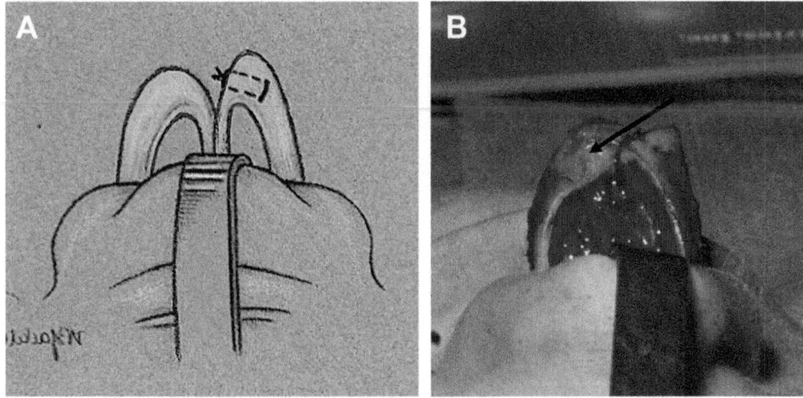

Fig. 6. (*A, B*) The traditional transdomal suture narrows the tip and on occasion is added to the hemi-transdomal suture if additional narrowing of the dome is needed.

straighten the lateral crus (remove its convexity). Everting the lateral crus is an important concept. Without it the lateral crus may actually invert when a conventional transdomal suture is placed. The result (**Fig. 5**) of inversion is a potential alar concavity that may then require a rim graft. In a few cases it will be necessary to add the conventional transdomal suture (**Fig. 6**) if the actual dome width has not been reduced substantially. These fine adjustments are made after reflecting the skin flap in the open approach to see what the suture technique has done to the dome.

Interdomal Suture

The interdomal is a 5-0 PDS suture that brings together the 2 middle crura. The suture is placed approximately 3 mm posterior to the dome on the cephalic side of the middle crus (**Fig. 7**). An interdomal suture keeps the domes together, enhances symmetry, and also provides strength to the overall tip complex. If one is attempting to create a major change in the symmetry or if the tips are very weak, it would be wiser to use a columellar strut.

Lateral Crural Mattress Suture

The lateral crus is often convex and often weak. The lateral crural mattress (**Figs. 8** and **9**) suture addresses both deficiencies by correcting the convexity and strengthening the lateral crus.[24] The suture is a 5-0 PDS or nylon applied at the apex of the convexity. After grasping the lateral crus at the apex of the convexity with a Brown Adson forceps, the needle is applied perpendicular to the long axis of the lateral crus as a bite is taken on one side of the forceps. The second bite is taken on the other side of the forceps (about 6 mm away from the first bite). The knot

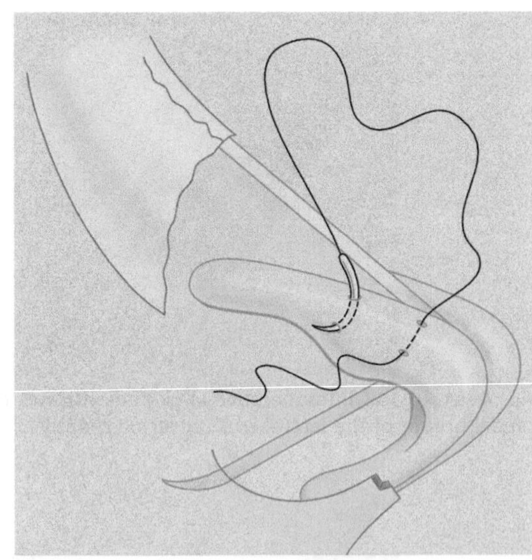

Fig. 8. The lateral crural mattress suture removes any residual convexity of the lateral crus. Cephalic trim is a prerequisite for its use. Note that the needle enters perpendicular to the long axis of the lateral crus. The spacing between bites (purchases) is about 6 mm.

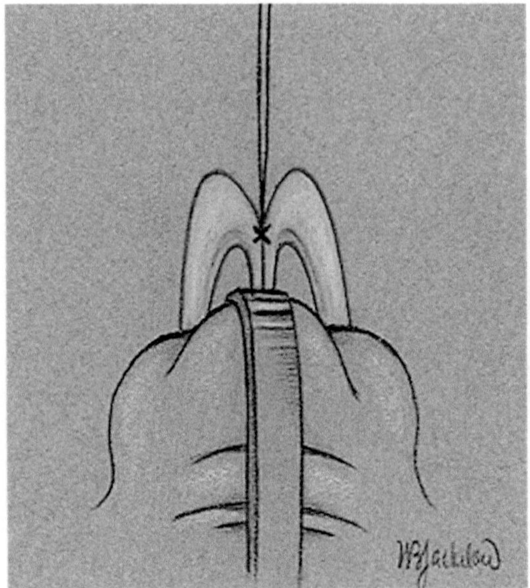

Fig. 7. The interdomal suture brings the dome together, provides symmetry and strength.

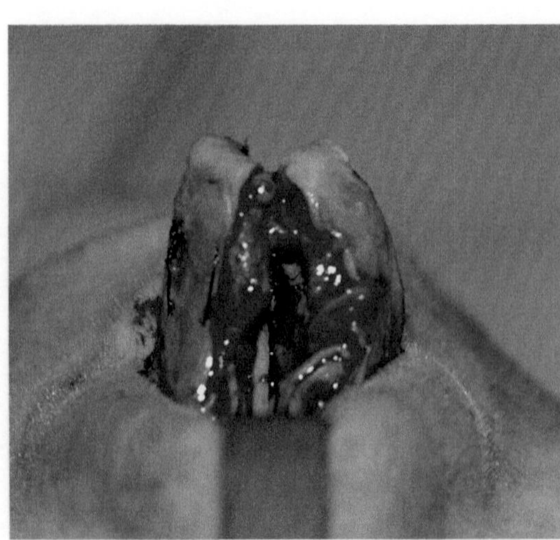

Fig. 9. This intraoperative view shows how the lateral crural mattress suture removes unwanted convexity. Often a second and third lateral crural mattress suture is needed if the convexity is large.

is not tied tightly, just tight enough to straighten the lateral crus. One also wants the lateral crus to remain straight when the weight of the skin flap is draped over it. To tell if the lateral crus is sufficiently stiff and will remain straight, it is helpful to apply an index finger to the dome and push down (in a posterior direction) and observe if a bulge (convexity) develops in the lateral crus. If a bulge develops, one or more lateral crural mattress sutures should be applied. It is often necessary to apply 2 or 3 lateral crural sutures to achieve the desired result. Of note, each suture supplies more strength to the lateral crus, and the effect is additive. **Fig. 10** exemplifies the effectiveness and power of the hemi-transdomal and lateral crural mattress sutures.

Columellar-Septal Suture

This suture (a 4-0 PDS) secures the tip complex to the caudal septum, and provides a slight amount of projection if needed. The suture is not intended to substitute for the columellar strut when there is tip deficiency; it is effective for minor adjustments of the tip complex. After determining the optimal tip location with respect to the dorsal septum (about 6 mm anterior to it), a 4-0 PDS suture with a large needle is passed

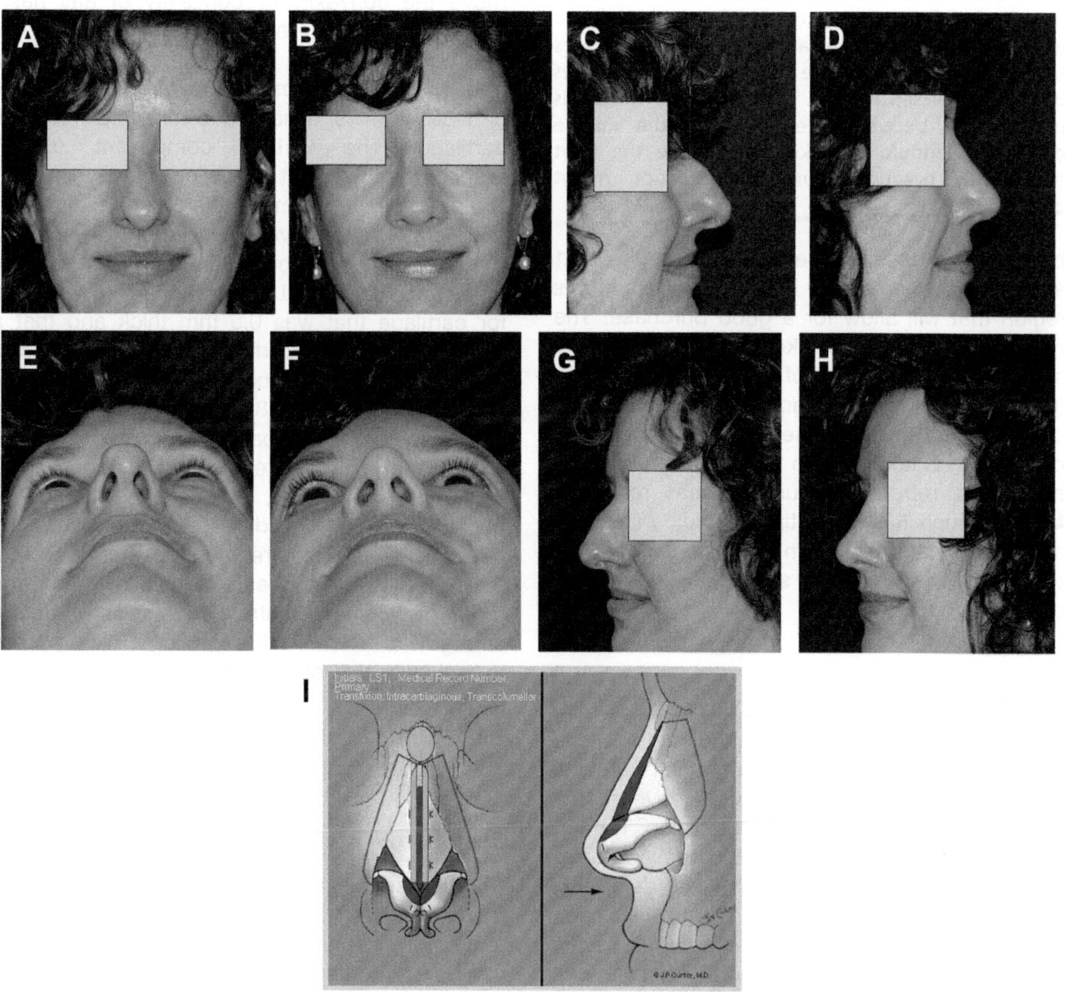

Fig. 10. This patient underwent tipplasty including cephalic trim, hemi-transdomal suture, and lateral crural mattress sutures by the open approach. (*A, B*) Front view pre/post surgery. (*C, D*) Side view pre/post surgery. (*E, F*) Basal view pre/post surgery. (*G, H*) Oblique view pre/post surgery. At 17 months after surgery, the tip is narrower but it is not pinched. On basal view the rims are straight and there was no need for rim (alar contour) grafts. The Gunter diagram (*I*) demonstrates all the other maneuvers including radix grafting, humpectomy and spreader flaps.

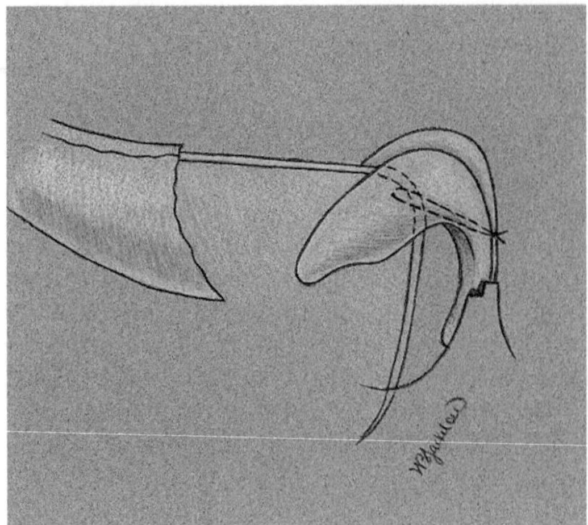

Fig. 11. The columellar-septal suture secures the tip complex to the caudal septum and provides a small amount of projection. A large-needle 4-0 PDS goes between the leaves of the middle crura. Two bites of the caudal septum are taken and the needle is passed back between the leaves of the middle crura. Care should be taken not to tie the knot too tightly because columellar retraction might occur.

between the leaves of the middle crura (**Figs. 11** and **12**). There are many intercrural fibers in this region that will allow for a good purchase. The needle is then used to take a bite of the caudal septum. A second bite of the septum is taken (to avoid a pull-through) and then the large needle is passed between the leaves of the middle crura. Care is taken not to tie the knot too tightly because a retracted columellar may result. In fact, although the entire tip complex will be up against the caudal septum it should be possible to pull it away from the septum (with forceps) by 1 to 2 mm.

Closed Approach

Some patients are not good candidates for the open approach. Patients with very thick skin who need reduction tend to get postoperative edema that is often replaced with fibrous tissue. The net result may be a thicker skinned, ill-defined nose that might even be worse than initial deformity. The wishes of those patients who request a closed approach may have to be respected. Fortunately, the 4-suture algorithm described earlier can work almost as effectively in the closed approach. It will be necessary to completely deliver the tip cartilages using marginal, intercartilaginous, and transfixion incisions (**Figs. 13** and **14**). The patient in **Fig. 15** specifically requested a closed approach because she was fearful of a columellar scar.

Secondary Rhinoplasty

The 4-suture algorithm is also effective during secondary rhinoplasties. Depending on the patient's pathology, not all of the techniques need to be used to achieve the desired outcomes. In addition, if the tip shape is not acceptable after the 4-suture algorithm, tip grafts and columellar struts may need to be used. The suture techniques will serve to stabilize the tip complex, providing symmetry and structure for future grafts.

THE UNIVERSAL HORIZONTAL MATTRESS SUTURE

Not long ago[25,26] it was realized that a horizontal mattress suture could be used to effectively remove the convexity or concavity of any nasal cartilage provided that the cartilage is in the form of a strip that is no more than 6 to 10 mm wide. For example, the lateral crus after cephalic trim is usually a 6-mm wide strip of cartilage. The vertical component of an L-shaped septal strut (following central resection) is essentially a 10-mm wide strip of cartilage. Laboratory studies were performed to ascertain the ideal spacing between suture bites. The studies indicated that a 6-mm spacing was ideal for cartilage that was 0.5 mm thick and that a 5-0 size suture was ideal. If the cartilage was 1 to 1.5 mm thick (as occurs in the septum), the ideal spacing was 8 to 10 mm using a 4-0 size suture. If the spacing was less than ideal,- no change in curvature resulted. If the spacing was more than ideal, the cartilage tended to buckle (**Figs. 16** and **17**). Furthermore, the increase in tensile strength (biplanar modulus) that resulted from these sutures was on the order of 35%, in contrast to a loss of tensile strength of 48% if the cartilage was scored to achieve the same degree of straightening (**Fig. 18**).

Examples are given here of virtually every situation in rhinoplasty whereby a horizontal mattress suture will straighten cartilage.

Septal Straightening

Creating an L-shaped strut is perhaps the commonest way to straighten the crooked septum and nose. The horizontal component of the L-strut can be scored and the vertical component grafted to correct a crooked septum. However, one or more horizontal mattress sutures to the vertical component is an effective way to stiffen and straighten the L-strut, thus avoiding the need to graft the vertical component (**Fig. 19**). After several years of using suture techniques for the vertical

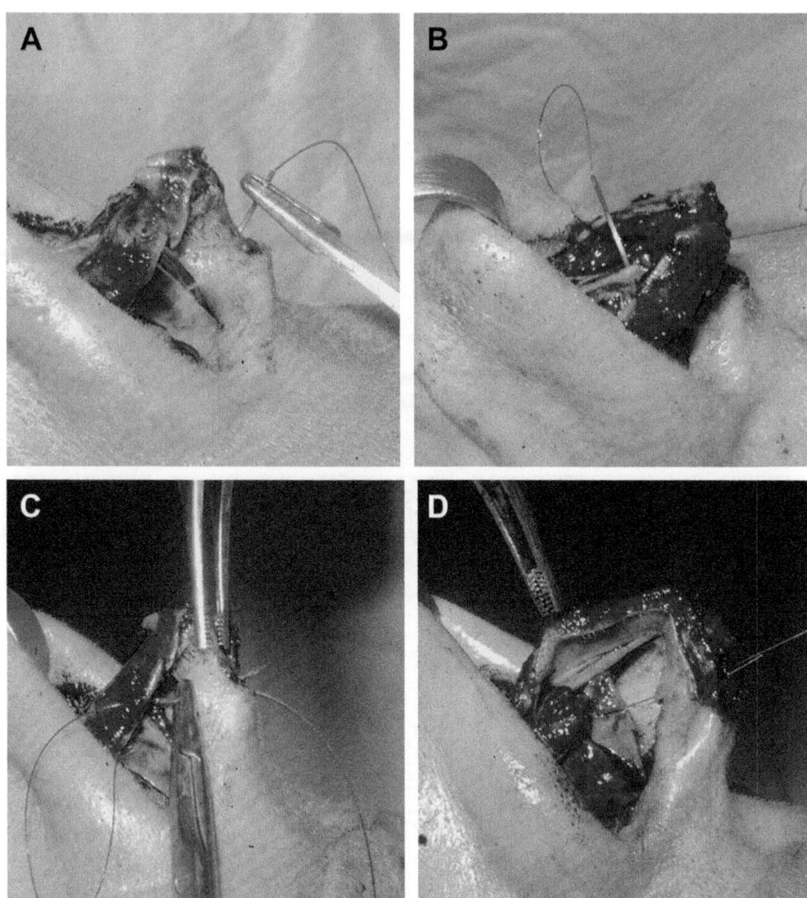

Fig. 12. (*A*) Intraoperative view of needle passing between the leaves of the middle crura. (*B*) Intraoperative view of needle passing through caudal septum near the septal angle. (*C*) Needle passing back between the leaves of the middle crurae. (*D*) Intraoperative view showing how the tip complex can be brought to the caudal septum with a columellar-septal suture.

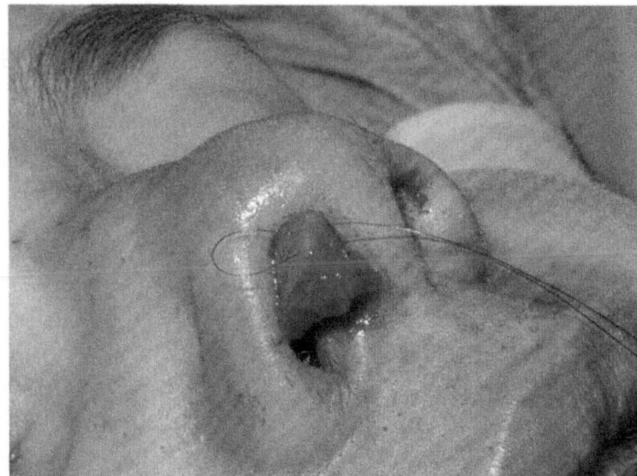

Fig. 13. The transdomal is being applied in the closed approach by delivering the tip complex through the nostril with intercartilaginous, marginal, and transfixion incisions. The hemi-transdomal suture can be done this way too.

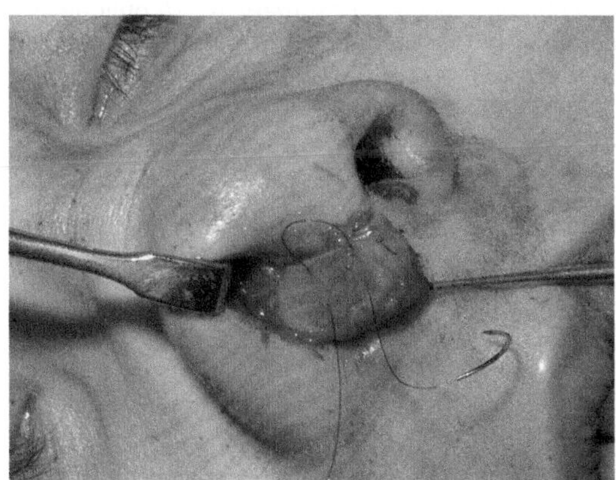

Fig. 14. The lateral crural mattress suture can also be applied in the closed approach.

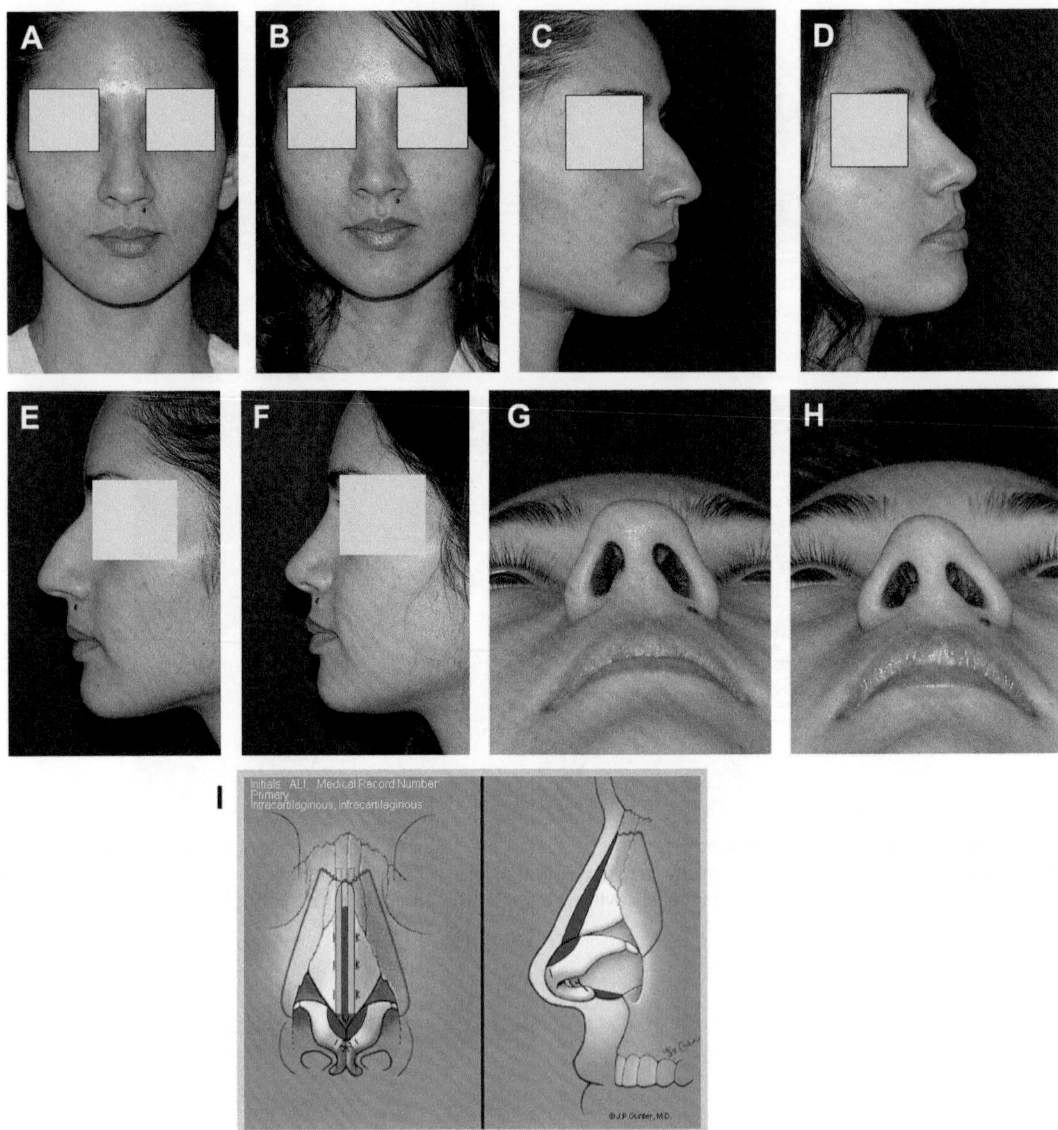

Fig. 15. This patient underwent tipplasty including cephalic trim, hemi-transdomal suture, and lateral crural mattress sutures by the closed approach. (*A, B*) front view pre/post surgery; (*C, D*) side view pre/post surgery; (*E, F*) basal view pre/post surgery; (*G, H*) oblique view pre/post surgery. At 14 months postoperatively the tip is narrower but in addition is not pinched. On basal view, the rims are straight and there was no need for rim (alar contour) grafts. The Gunter diagram (*I*) demonstrates all the other maneuvers including caudal shortening, humpectomy, and spreader flaps.

component, the authors learned that horizontal mattress sutures can just as easily be used for the horizontal component if scoring fails to achieve the desired result, and especially if for some reason the horizontal component is floppy or weak after scoring (**Fig. 20**).

Collapsed Lateral Crus (External Valve)

Not uncommonly, patients complain that they can feel a piece of cartilage in their nostril with the examining finger, which not only bothers them but may obstruct their airway. Inspection reveals a collapse of the posterior (lateral) aspect of the lateral crus. A simple method to correct this nuisance problem is to deliver the lateral crus using a U-shaped incision. In effect one creates a medially based composite flap, allowing excellent exposure to apply 1 or 2 horizontal mattress sutures on the convex side of the flap before returning it to its bed (**Figs. 21** and **22**).

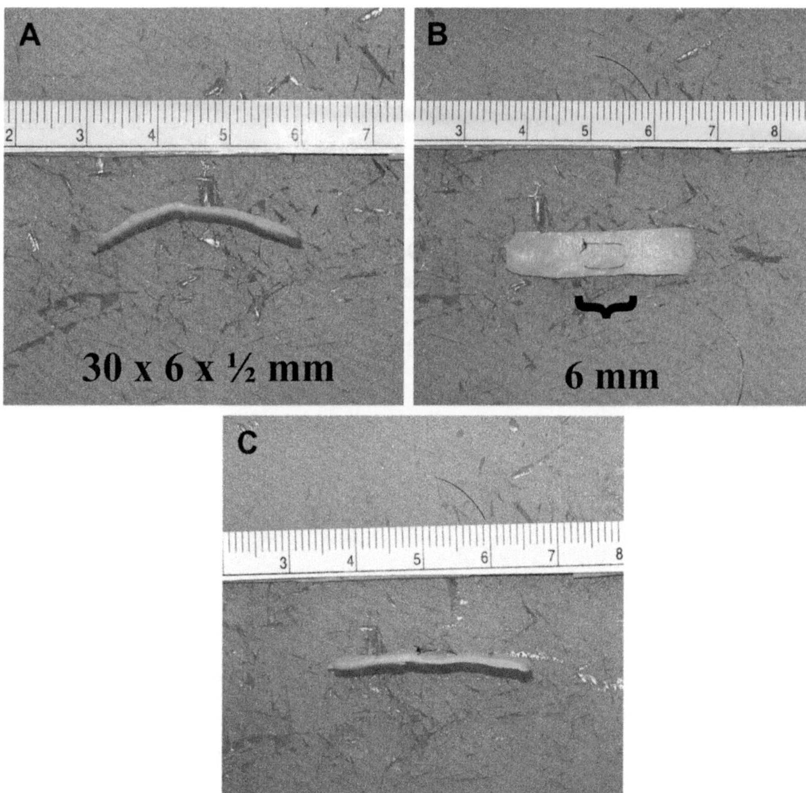

Fig. 16. When a convex piece of cartilage 6 mm wide, 0.5 mm thick (*A*) receives a horizontal mattress suture with a spacing of 6 mm (*B*), most of the convexity is removed (*C*).

Collapsed Upper Lateral Cartilages (Internal Valve)

The treatment of collapsed upper lateral cartilages (internal valves) has become a matter of routine with the advent of spreader grafts and spreader flaps. However, there are occasions when more expansion of the middle vault (internal valve) is necessary. Such is the case when prior spreader grafts have failed. Several surgeons[27–29] have described this technique in which a horizontal mattress suture is applied to the surface of both upper cartilages such that when the knot is tied, the hyperconvexity of the upper lateral cartilage

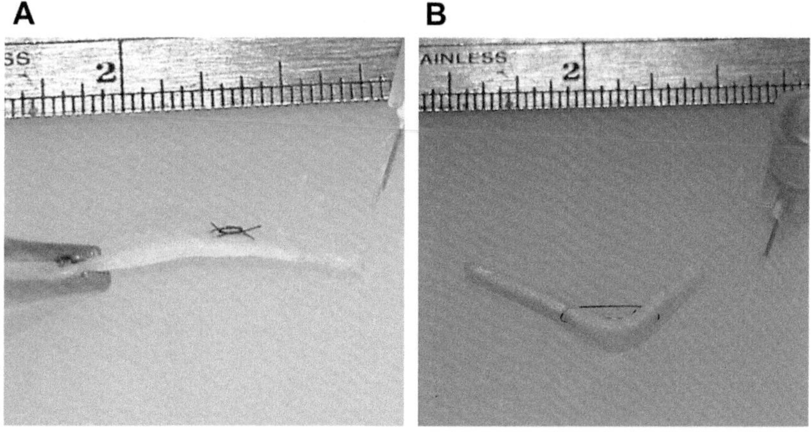

Fig. 17. If the spacing between purchases (bites) of the horizontal mattress suture is too narrow (*A*), no effect is seen. When the space is too large, buckling may occur (*B*).

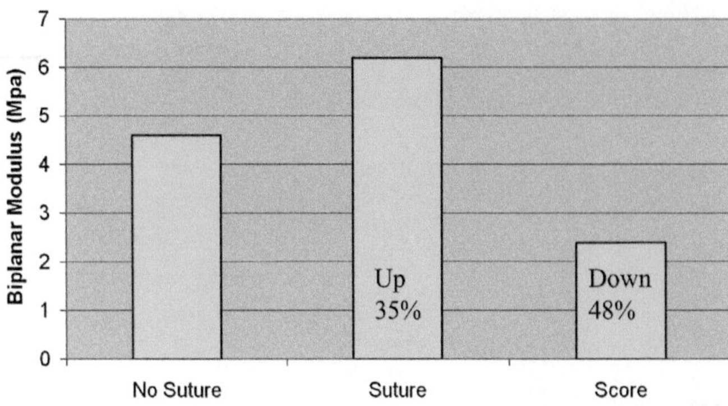

Fig. 18. Cartilage strength (biplanar modulus) is increased by approximately 35% by a single horizontal mattress suture that removes its convexity. Conversely it is decreased by approximately 48% if scoring is used to rid the convexity.

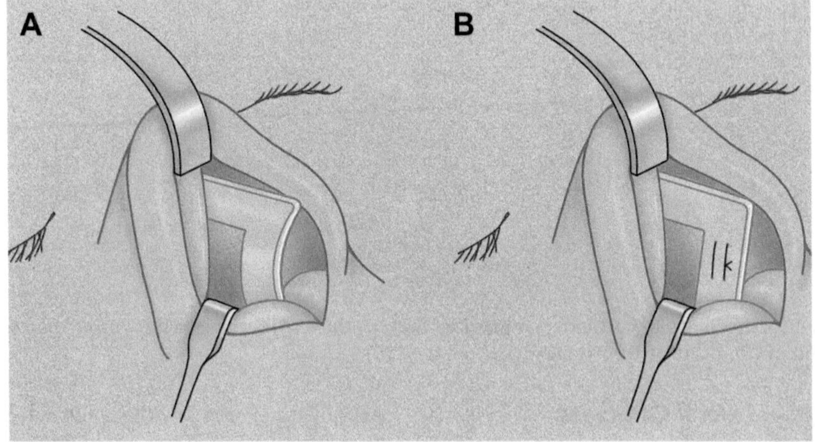

Fig. 19. (*A, B*) A 4-0 PDS horizontal mattress suture is an effective way to remove the convexity of the vertical component of an L-shaped septal strut. The suture should be applied on the convex side of the strut. More than one horizontal mattress suture may be necessary to achieve maximum straightness.

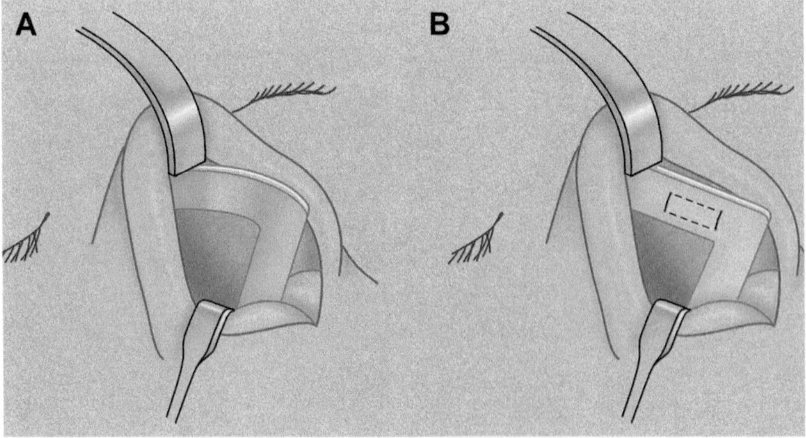

Fig. 20. (*A, B*) If scoring the horizontal component of an L-shaped septal strut is ineffective or if the strut is weak, a horizontal mattress suture (4-0 PDS) can be applied to the convex side to provide straightness and strength.

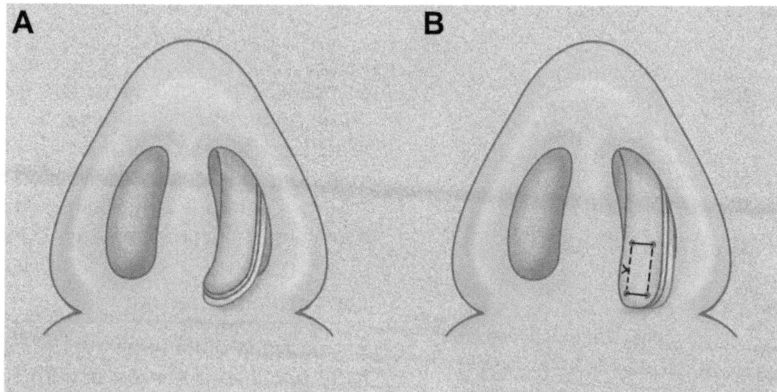

Fig. 21. (*A, B*) If the posterior (lateral) aspect of the lateral crus is collapsed and partially obstructing the vestibule, the entire lateral crus can be delivered from the nostril by making a U-shaped incision to deliver the flap. A horizontal mattress suture is placed on the convex side to straighten the flap before returning it to its bed.

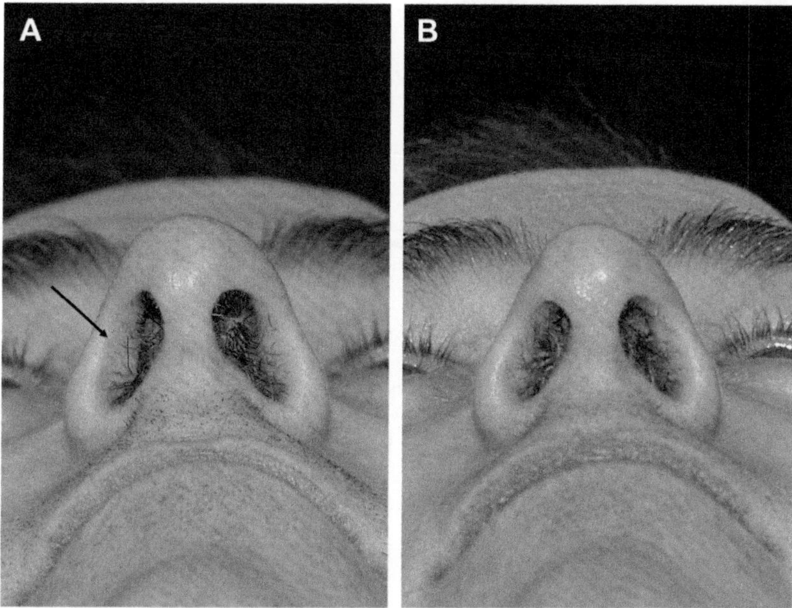

Fig. 22. (*A*) This patient had a collapse of the posterior (lateral) aspect of the lateral crus into the vestibule with obstructive symptoms. The lateral crus was delivered into the vestibule and 2 horizontal mattress sutures were applied before it was returned. Postoperatively (*B*), the vestibule is free of the obstruction.

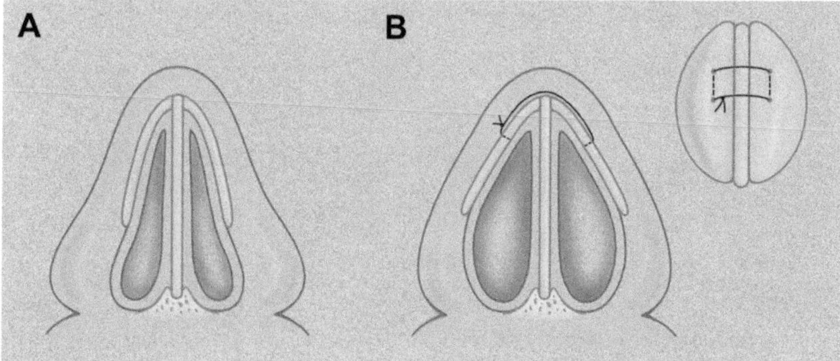

Fig. 23. (*A, B*) Despite spreader grafts or flaps, the upper lateral cartilages may fail to open properly for inspiration. These cartilages are essentially in a hyperconvex position. By applying a strong 4-0 PDS horizontal mattress suture to the surface of these cartilages, much of the hyperconvexity can be removed. This action will open the internal nasal valve.

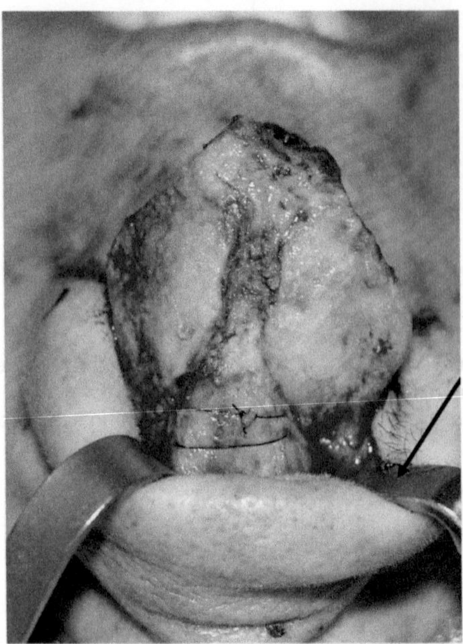

Fig. 24. Intraoperative view from the head of the bed demonstrating that a 4-0 PDS horizontal mattress suture spans the entire internal valve from one side to another. As the knot is tied, the hyperconvexity of the internal nasal valve is reduced. The "wings" of the internal nasal valve open up.

complex is reduced (to a less convex surface) (**Figs. 23** and **24**). In this specific situation one is reducing only some of the undesired convexity. Therefore, this unique application of a horizontal mattress suture is consistent with the concept of a universal horizontal mattress suture.

Ear Cartilage Grafting

Ear cartilage grafting has not gained wide popularity because it can be abnormally shaped and be too weak to provide reliable structural support. Today it is mainly used as an onlay graft. With the help of the universal horizontal mattress suture, the authors have found that the strength and shape of ear cartilage grafts can be greatly enhanced for the benefit of the rhinoplasty surgeon. Although septal cartilage is the preferred donor for most grafts due to its reliable shape and strength, if it is unavailable, ear cartilage can be used with confidence. To take full advantage of ear cartilage, the concha cymba and cavum are removed via the retroauricular approach. From this approach the cymba/cavum have a kidney-shaped appearance. With practice they are easily removed after hyperinfiltrating the anterior skin to minimize the risk of perforations.

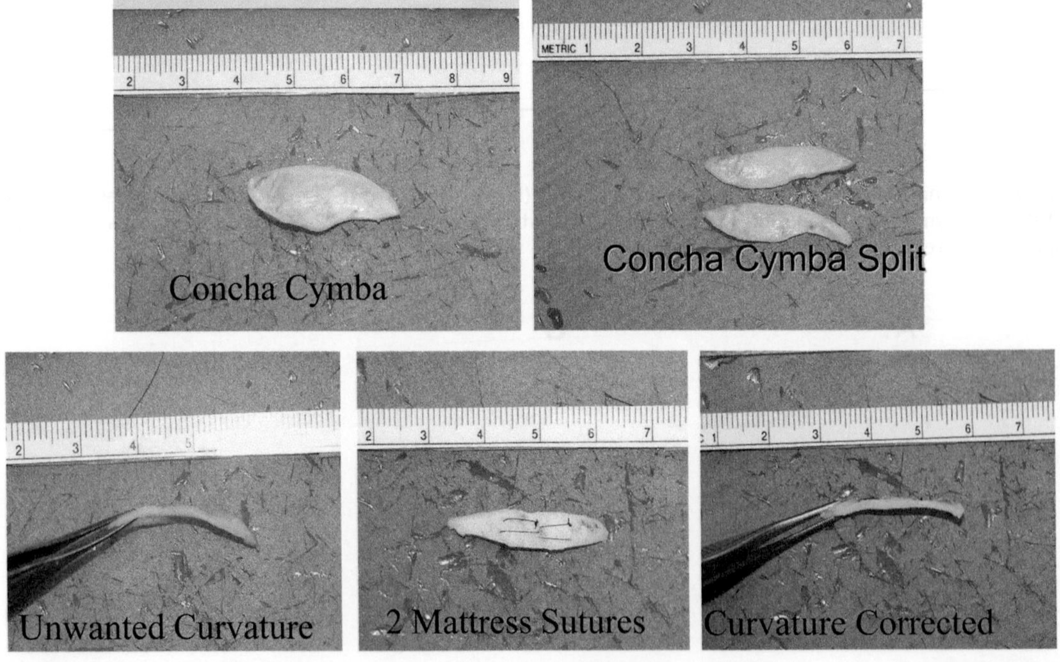

Fig. 25. The concha cymba of the ear can produce reasonably strong and straight grafts. The canoe-shaped cymba is split down the middle to make 2 grafts. A pair of 5-0 PDS horizontal mattress sutures is placed on the convex side, one at each end of the graft. The end result is a unit of graft material that is good for many purposes including columellar struts.

It is best to work with cartilage on a silicone block using needles to stabilize the cartilage grafts. The cymba is invariably separated from the cavum, and usually looks like a canoe. The cymba is split down the middle (**Fig. 25**). At this point in time it is curved and has little stability. However, it is pinned to the block and a pair of 5-0 PDS sutures are applied (to the convex surface), one at either end. No attempt is made to overtighten the knot. The sutures will give the graft strength, much like rebar does for concrete. The result will be a unit of ear cartilage that is suitable for many purposes: it can act as a columellar strut and is usually even large enough to replace the entire lateral crus, while it is certainly usable as a spreader graft.

REFERENCES

1. Tardy ME Jr, Patt BS, Walter MA. Transdomal suture refinement of the nasal tip: long-term outcomes. Facial Plast Surg 1993;9:275–84.
2. Tebbetts JB. Shaping and positioning the nasal tip without structural disruption: a new, systematic approach. Plast Reconstr Surg 1994;94:61–77.
3. Rohrich RJ, Adams WP Jr. The boxy nasal tip: classification and management based on alar cartilage suturing techniques. Plast Reconstr Surg 2001;107: 1849–63.
4. Toriumi DM. New concepts in nasal tip contouring. Arch Facial Plast Surg 2006;8:156.
5. Neu BR. Suture correction of nasal tip cartilage concavities. Plast Reconstr Surg 1996;98:971–9.
6. Baker SR. Suture contouring of the nasal tip. Arch Facial Plast Surg 2000;2:34–42.
7. Roofe SB, Most SP. Placement of a lateral nasal suspension suture via an external rhinoplasty approach. Arch Facial Plast Surg 2007;9:214–6.
8. Papel ID. Interlocked transdomal suture technique for the wide interdomal space in rhinoplasty. Arch Facial Plast Surg 2005;7:414–7.
9. Leach JL, Athre RS. Four suture tip rhinoplasty: a powerful tool for controlling tip dynamics. Otolaryngol Head Neck Surg 2006;135:227–31.
10. Tezel E, Numanoglu A. Septocolumellar suture in closed rhinoplasty. Ann Plast Surg 2007;59:268–72.
11. Perkins S, Patel A. Endonasal suture techniques in tip rhinoplasty. Facial Plast Surg Clin North Am 2009;17:41–54.
12. Corrado A, Bloom JD, Becker DG. Domal stabilization suture in tip rhinoplasty. Arch Facial Plast Surg 2009;11:194–7.
13. Cardenas JC, Carvajal J, Ruiz A. Securing nasal tip rotation through suspension suture technique. Plast Reconstr Surg 2006;117:1750–5.
14. Kuran I, Tumerdem B, Tosun U, et al. Evaluation of the effects of tip-binding sutures and cartilaginous grafts on tip projection and rotation. Plast Reconstr Surg 2005;116:282–8.
15. Lee KC, Kwon YS, Park JM, et al. Nasal tipplasty using various technique3s in rhinoplasty. Aesthetic Plast Surg 2004;28:445–55.
16. Lo S, Rowe-Jones J. Suture techniques in nasal tip sculpture: current concepts. J Laryngol Otol 2007; 121:e10.
17. Menger DJ. Lateral crus pull-up: a method for collapse of the external nasal valve. Arch Facial Plast Surg 2006;8:333–7.
18. Harris S, Pan Y, Peterson R, et al. Cartilage warping: an experimental model. Plast Reconstr Surg 1993; 92:912–5.
19. Iamphongsai S, Eshraghi Y, Totonchi A, et al. Effect of different suture materials on cartilage reshaping. Aesthet Surg J 2009;29:93–7.
20. Guyuron B, Behmand RA. Nasal tip sutures part II: the interplays. Plast Reconstr Surg 2003;112: 1130–45.
21. Behmand RA, Ghavami A, Guyuron B. Nasal tip sutures Part I: the evolution. Plast Reconstr Surg 2003;112:1125–9.
22. Daniel RK. Creating an aesthetic tip. Plast Reconstr Surg 1987;80:775.
23. Daniel RK. Rhinoplasty: a simplified three-stitch, open tip suture technique. Part I: primary rhinoplasty. Plast Reconstr Surg 1999;103:1491–502.
24. Gruber RP, Friedman GD. Suture algorithm for the broad or bulbous nose. Plast Reconstr Surg 2002; 110:1752–64.
25. Gruber RP, Nahai F, Bogdan MA, et al. Changing the convexity and concavity of nasal cartilages and cartilage grafts with horizontal mattress sutures: part I experimental results. Plast Reconstr Surg 2005;115: 589–94.
26. Gruber RP, Nahai F, Bogdan MA, et al. Changing the convexity and concavity of nasal cartilages and cartilage grafts with horizontal mattress sutures: part II clinical results. Plast Reconstr Surg 2005;115:595–606.
27. Park SS. The flaring suture to augment the repair of the dysfunctional nasal valve. Plast Reconstr Surg 1998;101:1120–2.
28. Schlosser RJ, Park SS. Functional nasal surgery. Otolaryngol Clin North Am 1999;32:37–51.
29. Ozturan O, Miman MC, Kizilay A. Bending of the upper lateral cartilages for nasal valve collapse. Arch Facial Plast Surg 2002;4:258–61.

Alar Base Disharmonies

Diana Ponsky, MD[a,*], Bahman Guyuron, MD[b]

KEYWORDS

• Alar base • Nasal base • Rhinoplasty • Nostril size
• Nostril shape • Alar cinch

Disharmony of the alar base structure with the rest of the nose is the most common imperfection encountered in secondary rhinoplasty in the senior author's (BG) practice. The deformity is often seen in the original structure of the wide base, which was neglected during the initial nasal evaluation and surgical planning. The disharmony may also arise because of changes made to the adjacent nasal structures, such as an increase in alar flare after significant reduction of the tip projection. Reduction of the nasal base width should be undertaken when the interalar distance exceeds the intercanthal distance in the Caucasian patient.[1] Ethnic variations may be handled differently.[2–4]

Alar base surgery is an important component of the aesthetic rhinoplasty procedure. Robert Weir is credited with the first external alar wedge excision in 1892 to correct the alar flaring after reduction rhinoplasty. Others, such as Joseph and Milstein, modified the technique in 1931 in an attempt to avoid the external scar by including the internal excisions from the nostril base and vestibular floor.[5] Techniques to avoid scarring during rhinoplasty have been developed, but the Weir external alar wedge excision is still in use. Most of the current written works contain some modifications in the approach to the alar base excision.[6–8] There is also a description of the cinching sutures to approximate the alae and narrow the nasal base. The most recent technique for correcting the broad nasal base, particularly for patients with a vertically oriented alar axis, uses alar release via an incision at the ala-sill junction, release of the periosteal ligaments, and approximation of the dermis on both sides with sutures to medialize the nasal base.[9]

Improper correction of these alar base abnormalities can have unfavorable aesthetic and functional consequences. Once the tissue is removed, it is much more difficult to correct. The alar base imperfections must be properly evaluated from the onset and surgical correction performed with precision to avoid the need for secondary corrective surgery. Common alar base flaws that are correctable include flaring of the alar rims, a wide nostril sill, and a combination of the two.

ANATOMY AND NASAL ANALYSIS

An essential component of achieving a natural appearing and balanced rhinoplasty outcome is attention to the alar base. In an ideal aesthetic nose, there is a harmonious relationship between the nose and other facial features. Thorough visual analysis of the face combined with the method of soft-tissue cephalometric analysis using life-sized photographs of the face facilitates planning the aesthetic goals of the operation. The life-sized photographs allow precise measurement of the facial elements.[1]

In the horizontal plane, the distance from one lateral alar base to the opposite one is approximately 2 mm wider than the intercanthal distance (ICD), the distance from one medial canthus to the opposite one. The ICD is usually 31 to 33 mm. If the ICD is abnormal, the distance of the orbital fissure (medial to lateral canthus) can

[a] Department of Otolaryngology and Plastic Surgery, University Hospitals Case Medical Center, 11100 Euclid Avenue, Mailstop LK5045, Cleveland, OH 44106, USA
[b] Department of Plastic Surgery, University Hospitals Case Medical Center, 29017 Cedar Road, Lyndhurst, OH 44124, USA
* Corresponding author.
E-mail address: diana.ponsky@uhhospitals.org (D. Ponsky).

Clin Plastic Surg 37 (2010) 245–251
doi:10.1016/j.cps.2009.12.002

be used as the reference. The ICD is bisected (point A) and a vertical line (line V) is drawn to pass the philtrum (point B) on an otherwise symmetric face. Two parallel lines (lines L and R) can then be symmetrically drawn in relation to the vertical midline, starting at the medial canthi and passing 1 mm medial to the outer boundary of the alar base (**Fig. 1**).[2,10] This is the Caucasian ideal,[11,12] but ethnic differences and personal preference may deviate from this ideal.[2–4]

In the vertical dimension, best seen on the profile view, the caudal margins of the alar base are located approximately 2 mm cephalic to a line separating the middle two-thirds from the lower one-third of the distance from the medial canthus to the stomion. Point N (nasion) denotes the deepest portion of the ideal nasofrontal groove, or the level of the lower border of the upper lid margin on straight gaze, in those with a less-shallow or too-deep nasion. Point N is connected to point S (stomion), the junction of the upper and lower lips, by the vertical line V divided into 3 equal lengths (**Fig. 2**).

Evaluation of the base of the nose should also include the size, shape, and symmetry of the nostrils and the width and length of the columella and its relationship to the height of the lobule and the thickness and contour of the alae. The ideal nasal base resembles an equilateral triangle, with the length of the columella being twice the height of the infratip lobule (**Fig. 3**). The nostrils should be oval-shaped, and should be wider than the columella.[2,3] The long axis of the nostrils in a Caucasian should be oriented almost parallel to the vertical axis of the columella, with the anterior portion slightly narrower than the posterior portion.[2] Ethnic variations can be seen in the shape and orientation of the nostrils.[2,3] The character of the skin, either thick or thin, should also be noted

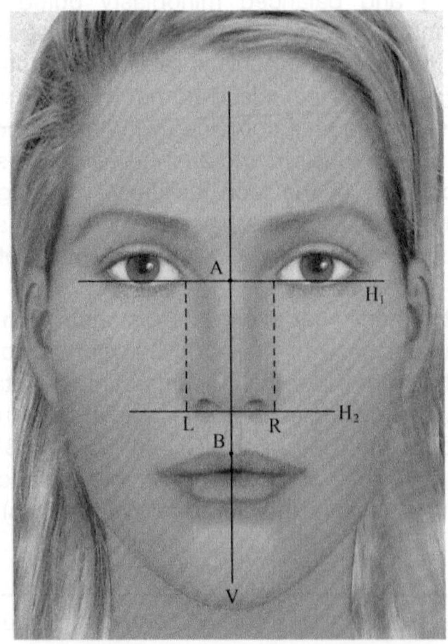

Fig. 1. Analysis of alar base position on frontal view. Point A is the bisected ICD passing through the philtrum (point B) on a symmetric face. Lines L and R are positioned in relation to the vertical midline, starting at the medial canthi and passing 1 mm medial to the outer boundary of the alar base.

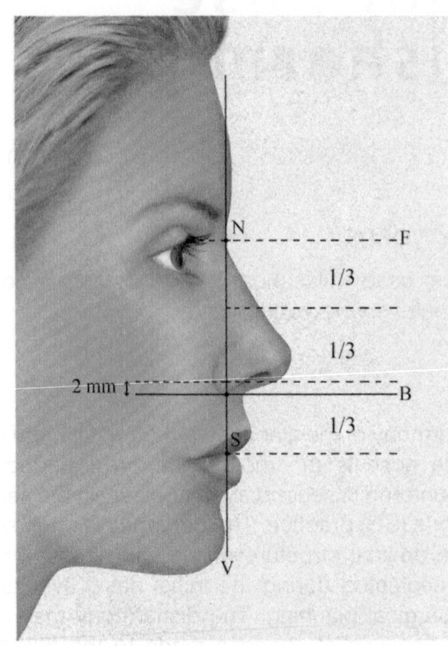

Fig. 2. Analysis of vertical alar base disharmony on the profile view. The nasion (point N) is connected to the stomion (point S) and divided into 3 equal sections. The caudal border of the alar base is located 2 mm caudal to the junction of the middle and lower thirds.

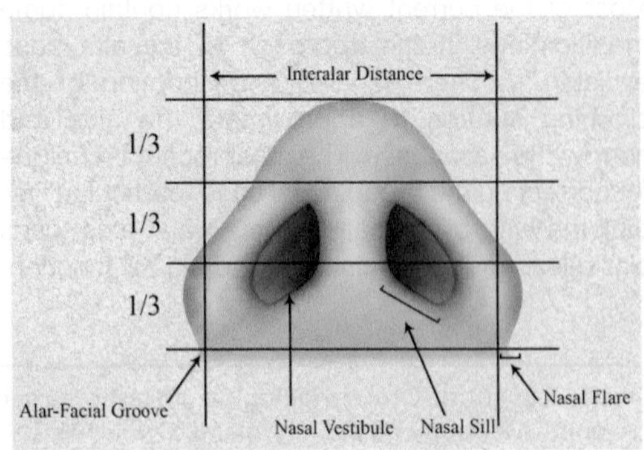

Fig. 3. Analysis of the base view of the nose, depicting the interalar distance and the horizontal one-third of the nose. The nostrils and columella occupy about two-thirds of the triangle. The nasal vestibule, nasal sill (floor), and alar-facial groove are shown.

and considered in choosing the type of alar base reduction.

VERTICAL PLANE ALAR BASE DEFORMITIES

Disharmonies of the alar base in the vertical plane result from either cephalad or caudal malposition of the alar base. These may present unilaterally or bilaterally. A cephalic malposition exposes the columella more (**Fig. 4**A), whereas a caudal malposition causes hooding of the alar base, with decreased show of columella. If the alar base is wide and cephalically malpositioned, narrowing the alar base results in medial and caudal translocation of the base. Otherwise, removal of an elliptical area of skin from the upper lip at the junction of the alar base and the lip is planned. The incision is made in the alar-facial crease and continued around the base to the nostril sill. The size of the resected skin is determined by preoperative facial analysis based on life-sized photographs. It is essential to completely release the soft tissue contained in the alar thickness so that the alar base can be advanced. Otherwise, this procedure may elevate the upper lip instead of transposing the alar base caudally. A caudally malpositioned alar base is not common and more difficult to correct (**Fig. 4**B). An incision is made in the vestibular lining just above the alar rim, and a strip of the lining is resected and repaired to reposition the alar base.

Horizontal alar base deformities are intricately interlaced with those in the vertical plane. Narrowing the wide alar base often pulls the alar rim caudally, reducing the columella-alar vertical discrepancy. For those who have retracted alae (ie, those with a cephalic malposition), this is beneficial to their nasal aesthetics. In those with caudal malposition, this medial movement of the ala during narrowing the alar base would be detrimental to the nasal harmony.[10]

HORIZONTAL PLANE ALAR BASE DEFORMITIES

Horizontal plane deformities are much more common and can present as an excess or deficiency. Alar base excess in the horizontal plane can result from a wide lateral alar base, a wide nostril sill, or a combination of the two. Rarely the base can be thick or facetted. An ostensibly excessive nasal width can result from the loss of tip projection or maxillary protrusion, which is more readily treated with correction of the underlying abnormality rather than alar base resection.

Horizontal alar base deficiency commonly results from traumatic or iatrogenic causes, making it more noticeable. Congenital deficiency of the alar base is rare. Some relative abnormalities are secondary to excess tip projection or maxillary abnormalities, usually maxillary retrusion. The correction of horizontal plane alar base disharmonies requires wedge excision of the wide nostril sill, narrowing the base laterally, reduction of the thickness of the alar base, or a combination of these techniques.

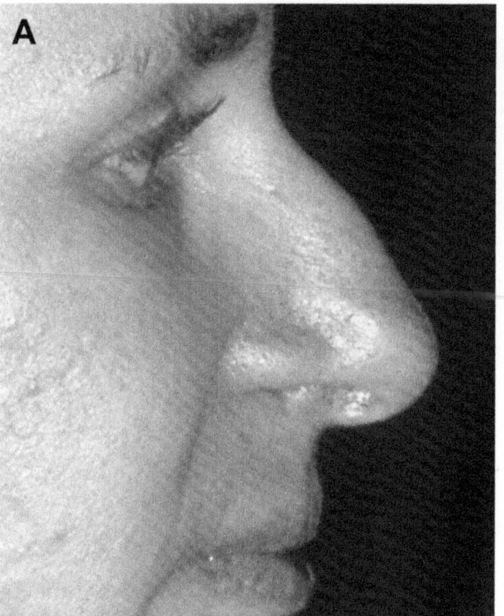

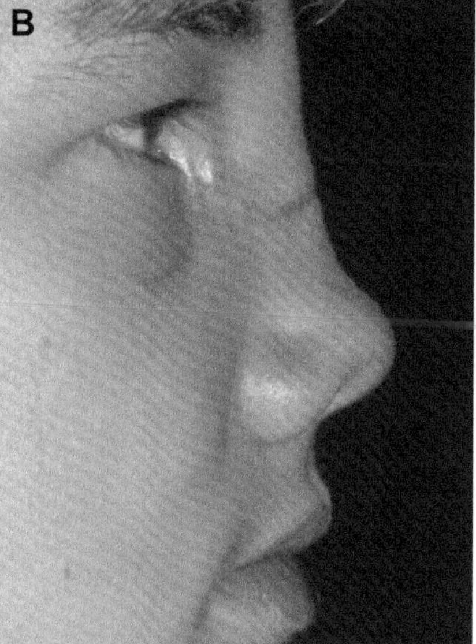

Fig. 4. (*A*) Lateral view of a patient with cephalically malpositioned alar base. (*B*) Lateral view of a patient with caudally displaced alar base.

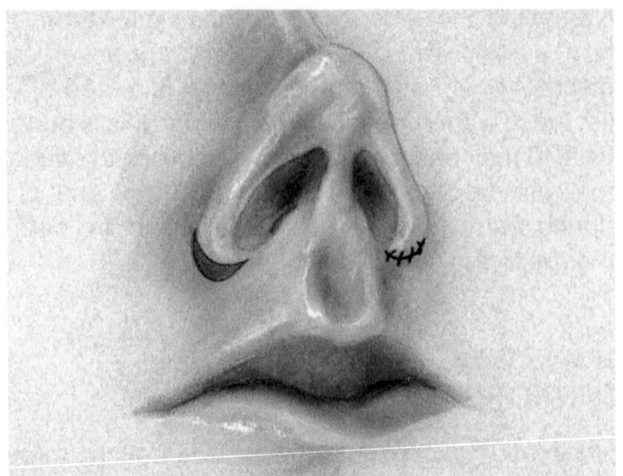

Fig. 5. Design of the lateral extension to correct excess alar flare.

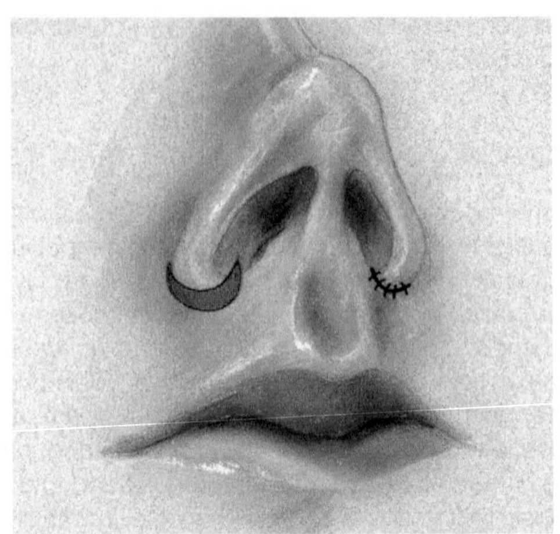

Fig. 7. Excision of excess nostril sill and lateral alar base in combination.

TECHNIQUE

Alar base modification should always be performed as the last stage of rhinoplasty, after all incisions have been closed. Deprojection of the nose and augmentation change the alar flare. Deprojection causes the extra soft tissue to extend in the least resistant direction, which is caudal and lateral. This often exaggerates a preexisting wide alar base. Augmentation of the nasal projection often reduces a wide alar base, nullifying the need for narrowing of a preoperatively wide alar base. Dynamic changes in the nasal base can also arise from surgery on adjacent structures of the nose. Maxillary advancement widens the alar base, and retraction of the maxilla narrows this part of the nose. Lengthening of the maxilla displaces the alar base caudally and reduces the distance between the alar bases. Intrusion of the maxilla results in cephalad displacement and widening of the alar base.[10]

Correction is best done in the same setting as the primary rhinoplasty for balanced nasal aesthetics, provided the patient has been informed before the operation regarding the external surgical scars. Conservatism in excision is advised, as once the tissue is removed, it is difficult to replace it and correction is aesthetically difficult in the alar base area.

The procedure is often performed under general anesthesia in conjunction with a more extensive rhinoplasty or reconstructive procedure. Minor alar base modifications can be performed under local anesthesia in an office setting. The senior author (BG) uses 6-0 plain catgut to negate suture removal from an extremely tender site. In select patients, he also uses a single pass of the CO_2 laser on the suture line at the conclusion of the alar base modification only if visibility of the scar

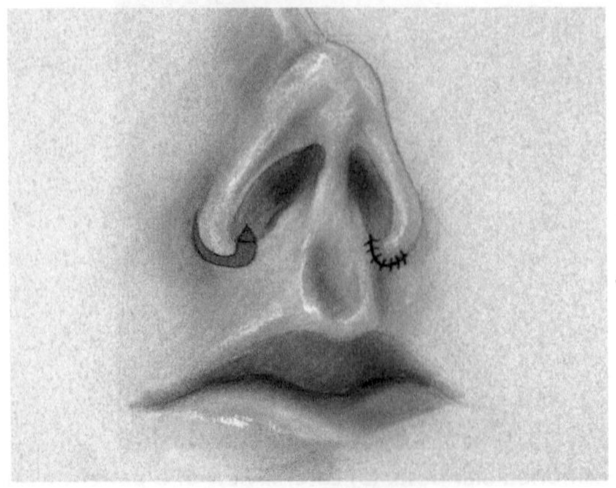

Fig. 6. Excision of excess nostril sill width and repair.

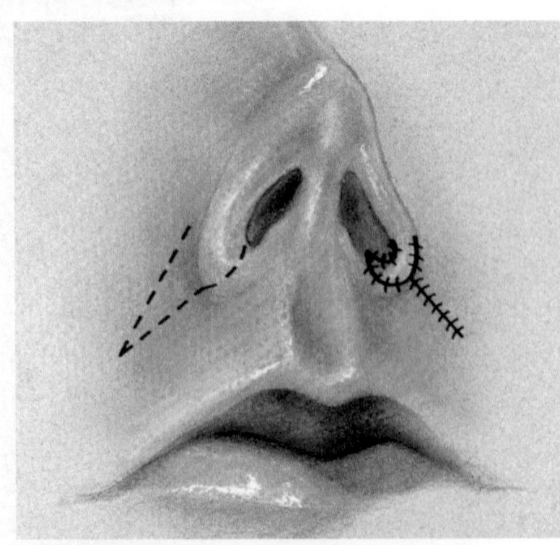

Fig. 8. An L-shaped excision where the anteroposterior limb of the L reduces thickness, and the cephalocaudal excision will narrow the nostril. A mirror image is made on the left nostril, shown completed.

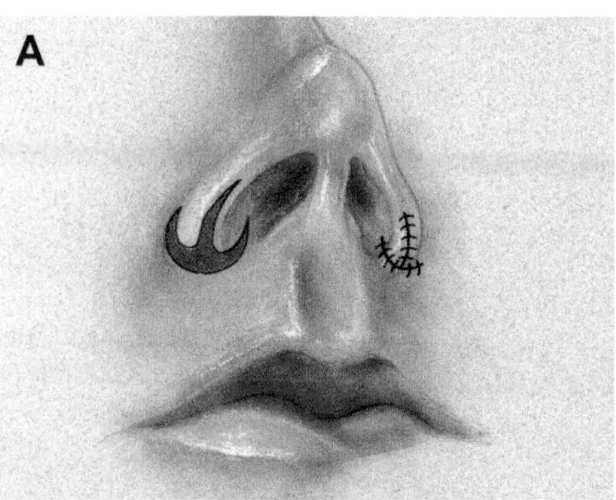

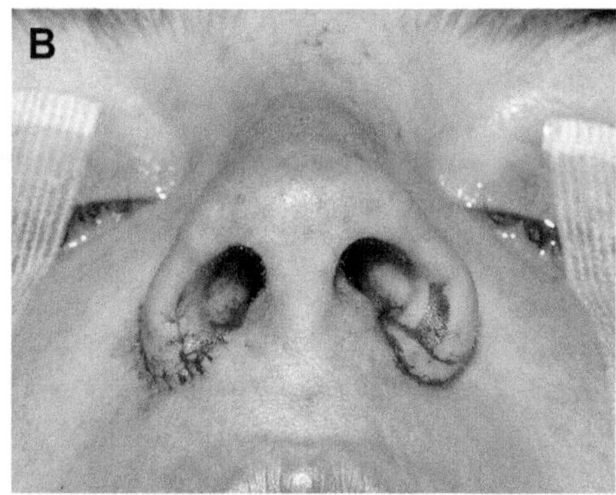

Fig. 9. (*A*) Inverted T excision for combined wide and thick alar base. (*B*) Intraoperative view of a patient undergoing the inverted T excision with comparison to the uncorrected left side.

is considered likely. In some cases, postoperative dermabrasion is used to minimize the visibility of the scar.[13]

Excess Alar Flare (Horizontal Deformity)

An elliptical excision is designed on the lateral nasal base starting at the nostril sill and extending to the cephalic margin of the alar-facial groove. This reduces the amount of alar flare, keeping the nostril sill intact (**Fig. 5**).

Wide Nostril Sill (Horizontal Deformity)

This is the most common abnormality. The excess nostril sill to be excised is marked by 2 lines that are almost parallel to each other and connected by a horizontal line placed at the junction of the nostril sill and the upper lip and extended laterally along the alar-facial crease sufficiently enough to avoid a dog-ear deformity (**Fig. 6**). This should be done in such a way that the final scar ends up being in the alar crease (and not above the crease). An incision is made using a No. 15 blade, and the excess tissue is excised. There should be adequate tissue left laterally to assure a graceful transition from the alar base to the nostril sill and to avoid a pinch deformity. A microneedle monocautery is used to release the soft tissue within the thickness of the ala just enough to facilitate medial transposition of the alar base tripod. The incision is repaired using 6-0 plain catgut.[14] Adjusting the alar base is one of the most delicate components of rhinoplasty. Even a 0.5-mm discrepancy between the 2 sides could be discernable. Some surgeons caution that aggressive removal of more than 2 to 3 mm may effectively reduce the nostril aperture enough that the nasal airway flow is affected.[13] The senior author (BG) concurs that in most cases it would likely require a significant reduction to affect the nasal airway.[15]

Excess Alar Flare and Wide Nostril Sill (Horizontal Deformity)

Correction of a wide nasal base and excessive alar flaring requires excision of an external alar base with extension to the nostril sill in varying proportions by following the principle mentioned in the earlier section (**Fig. 7**).

Thick Alar Base, Thick Rim

The thickness of the alar base can be reduced with an L-shaped excision whereby the anteroposterior limb of the L decreases in thickness, and the cephalocaudal excision will narrow the nostril. A mirror image of the incision is made on the left nostril (**Fig. 8**). The bulkiness of the alar rim can also be reduced by removal of the excess soft tissue

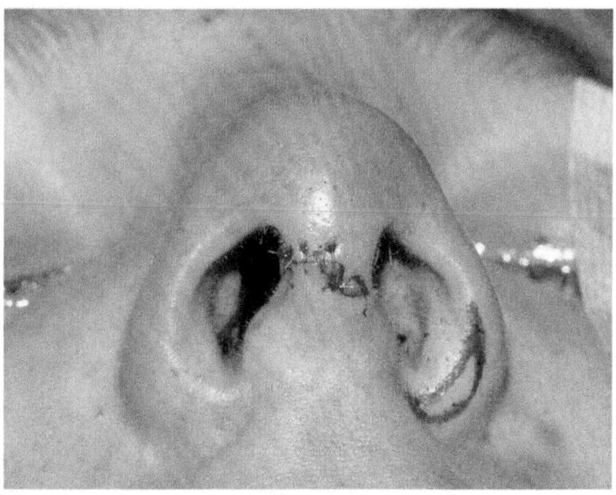

Fig. 10. An intraoperative view of an elliptical skin excision drawn as planned to correct a faceted alar base on the left side of the patient's nose is shown above. The right side is left intact for comparison.

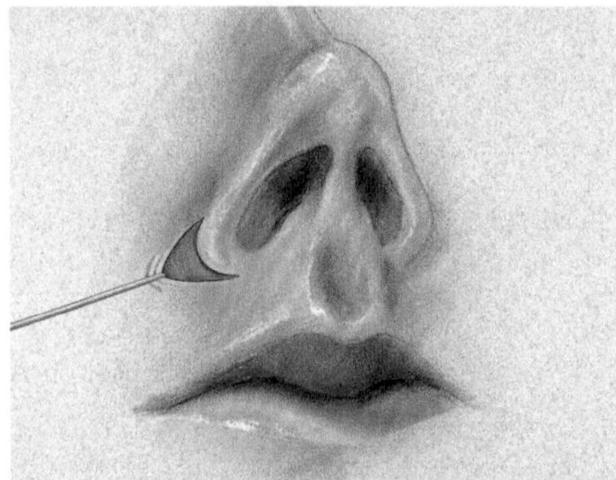
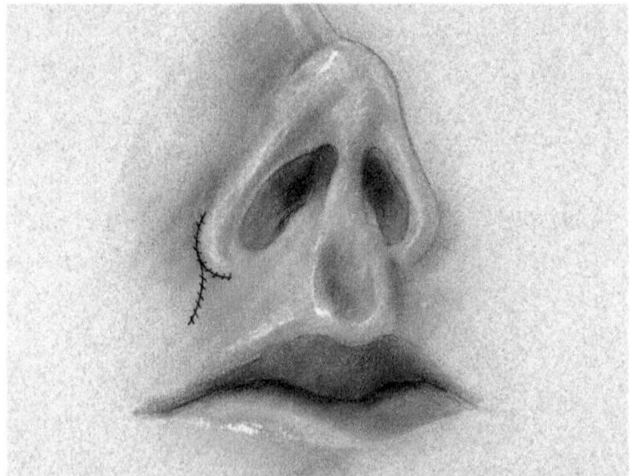

Fig. 11. V-Y advancement where the hook is used to retract the lateral aspect of the wedge incision along the direction of the nasolabial fold. After suturing, the Y of the V-Y is aligned with the nasolabial fold. The left side shows the preoperative view.

between the skin and intranasal lining through an incision along the alar rim.

Combination of Wide Nostril and Thick Alar Base (Horizontal Deformity)

For combination flaws of a wide nostril sill and thick alar rim, the inverted T excision is used. An incision is made at the alar-facial crease and continued around the base of the nostril. A posteriorly based, narrow triangular incision is designed to join the incision that will be used to narrow the alar base (**Fig. 9**). Excess tissue is removed, and the margins are reapproximated using 6-0 fast-absorbing plain catgut. A pass with the CO_2 laser is made along the suture line on patients with sebaceous skin.

Faceted Alar Base

A variation of the thick alar rim is the faceted alar base. An elliptical excision along the vestibular aspect of the alar base can be used to correct this (**Fig. 10**).

Wide Interalar Distance (Horizontal Deformity)

Bernstein described the use of V-Y advancement for a persistently wide interalar distance after wedge and sill excisions.[16] This technique is performed after the nostril rim is reapproximated by

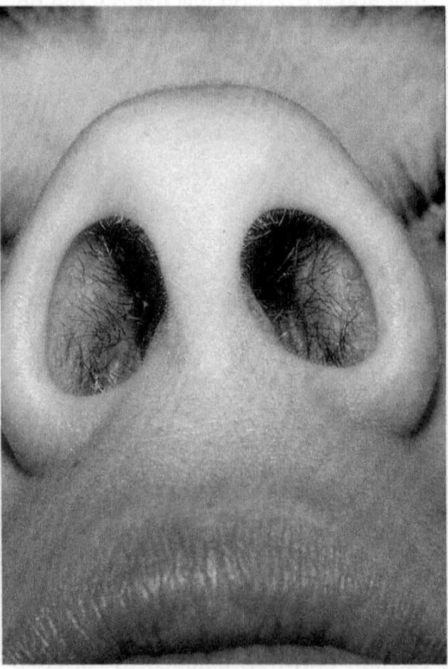
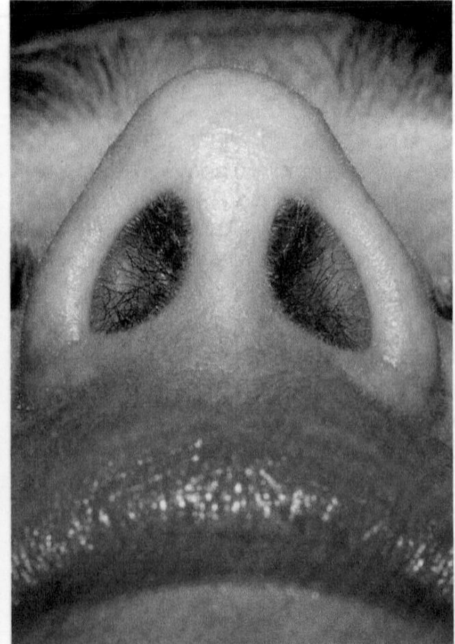

Fig. 12. Patient with flaring of the alar rims and a wide nostril floor, which is a common alar base abnormality. The right side depicts the healed appearance 1 month after surgery.

using a single-prong skin hook to draw the excess skin into the nasolabial fold. A series of sutures is used to create the "Y" limb of the V-Y advancement which is well hidden within the nasolabial fold. This technique narrows the alar rim, medializing it by about 2 mm on each side (**Fig. 11**).

Narrow Nostrils

Constricted or narrow nostrils are a rarely encountered problem. By restricting airflow, narrowed nostrils are a functional and aesthetic disruption. Maxillary retrusion or excess tip projection is often the underlying cause. Correction of the retrusion by Le Forte maxillary advancement can correct this problem. If the issue is nasal base projection, a reduction of the projection will reverse this abnormality.

SUMMARY

As with most aspects of rhinoplasty, there are many different techniques that are available for the correction of the multitude of alar base dysmorphologies. It is up to the advanced rhinoplasty surgeon to decide which technique would best serve the patient. The goal of this article is to assist the rhinoplasty surgeon in recognizing the problem areas better, and the classification system is intended to facilitate choosing the best surgical technique to correct the alar base flaws. The surgical maneuvers designed to correct the alar base disharmonies cannot be used interchangeably. Careful analysis to identify the deformity and proper selection of the technique will ensure a pleasing outcome (**Fig. 12**).

ACKNOWLEDGMENTS

The authors wish to thank Lauren Barney for her illustrations, Michele Mauser for the photography, and Lisa DiNardo for her editorial assistance.

REFERENCES

1. Guyuron B. Precision rhinoplasty. Part I: the role of life-size photographs and soft tissue analysis. Plast Reconstr Surg 1988;81:489–99.
2. Guyuron B, Ghavami A, Wishnek SM. Components of the short nostril. Plast Reconstr Surg 2005;116: 1517–24.
3. Farkas LG, Hreczko TA, Deutsch CK. Objective assessment of standard nostril types: a morphometric study. Ann Plast Surg 1983;11:381–9.
4. Porter JP, Olson KL. Analysis of the African American female nose. Plast Reconstr Surg 2003;111: 620–6.
5. Anderson JR. A reasoned approach to nasal base surgery. Arch Otolaryngol 1984;110:349–58.
6. Gunter JP, Rohrich RJ, Friedman RM. Classification and correction of alar-columellar discrepancies in rhinoplasty. Plast Reconstr Surg 1996; 97:643–8.
7. Silver WE, Sajjadian A. Nasal base surgery. Otolaryngol Clin North Am 1999;32(4):653–68.
8. Tellioglu AT, Vargel I, Cavusoglu T, et al. Simultaneous open rhinoplasty and alar base excision for secondary cases. Aesthetic Plast Surg 2005;29: 151–5.
9. Gruber RP, Freeman MB, Hsu C, et al. Nasal base reduction: a treatment algorithm including alar release with medialization. Plast Reconstr Surg 2009;123:716–25.
10. Guyuron B, Behmand RA. Alar base abnormalities. Clin Plast Surg 1996;23:263–70.
11. Rohrich RJ, Muzaffar AR. Rhinoplasty in the African-American patient. Plast Reconstr Surg 2003;111: 1322–39.
12. Adamson PA, Smith O, Tropper GJ, et al. Analysis of alar base narrowing. Am J Cosmet Surg 1990;7: 239–43.
13. Kridel RW, Castellano RD. A simplified approach to alar base reduction: a review of 124 patients over 20 years. Arch Facial Plast Surg 2005;7: 81–93.
14. Guyuron B. Alar base surgery. In: Rohrich RJ, Adams WP, Gunter JP, editors. Dallas rhinoplasty: nasal surgery by the masters. 2nd edition. St. Louis (MO): Quality Medical Publishing; 2007. p. 583–90.
15. Adamson PA. Alar base reduction. Arch Facial Plast Surg 2005;7:98.
16. Bernstein L. Esthetic anatomy of the nose. Laryngoscope 1972;82:1323–30.

Alar Cartilage Grafts

Stephen M. Weber, MD, PhD[a,*], Shan R. Baker, MD[b]

KEYWORDS

- Rhinoplasty • Septorhinoplasty • Cartilage graft
- Tip graft • Alar batten • Lateral crural strut
- Alar replacement graft • Columella strut

The initial approach to rhinoplasty begins with complete nasal and facial analysis to fully characterize aesthetic and structural problems. Only then can a surgical plan be created that may or may not involve alar cartilage grafting.

The face can be divided into equal vertical fifths. There is a single region between the medial canthi and paired regions between the lateral aspect of the pinna and lateral canthus as well as paired regions between the lateral and medial canthi. The width of the nasal base should approximate the intercanthal distance and is approximately one fifth of the facial width. The vertical height of the face can be divided into horizontal thirds spanning the trichion to glabella, glabella to subnasale, and subnasale to menton. Thus, nasal length is ideally one third of facial height. Although these proportions are equal in the aesthetic ideal, the upper third of the face tends to elongate with age because of elevation of the hairline while the lower third contracts due to bony resorption of the mandible.

ANALYSIS OF THE NASAL TIP

The alar cartilages provide the contour and structural support of the nasal tip. Current rhinoplasty concepts support preservation of alar structure with suture techniques[1]; judicious cephalic trim is indicated for tip deformities.

Tip Projection

Multiple methods exist to determine optimal nasal tip projection. These methods often provide different estimations of the aesthetic ideal. Thus, there is no single tool that provides the optimal measure of tip projection. Well-known methods include those of Goode, Simons, and Crumley. In brief, Goode's method predicts an ideal ratio of 0.55 to 0.6 between the length of a line drawn from nasion to nasal tip relative to a perpendicular line from alar–facial sulcus to nasal tip.[2] Crumley suggests that, ideally, the nose represents a 3-4-5 triangle.[3] Lastly, Simons has estimated that the upper lip height (subnasale to vermilion) should approximate tip projection (subnasale to tip).[4] The senior author uses the guideline of 10, 20, and 30 mm when assessing projection of the nasal dorsal line. Ideally, the nasion should project 10 mm anterior to the corneal plane. The rhinion and tip-defining point should project 20 and 30 mm, respectively, from the anterior facial plane, defined by a vertical line tangent to the alar–facial sulcus and nasion.

Tip Rotation

Ideal nasal tip rotation has been described in the literature. A frequently used correlate of tip rotation is the nasolabial angle. As a general rule, tip rotation in the male is a relatively acute, 90° to 105° nasolabial angle, while that in females is more obtuse, 100° to 120°.[5]

PHOTOGRAPHIC DOCUMENTATION

While both film and digital photographic systems are available, most surgeons have transitioned to the digital format. This provides for rapid acquisition, processing, and printing of images. Further, current 35 mm digital systems provide excellent

[a] Division of Facial Plastic and Reconstructive Surgery, Department of Otolaryngology and Head & Neck Surgery, Oregon Health & Science University, 3181 SW Sam Jackson Park Road, Portland, OR 97239, USA
[b] Division of Facial Plastic and Reconstructive Surgery, Department of Otolaryngology–Head and Neck Surgery, University of Michigan Medical Center, 1500 East Medical Center Drive, Ann Arbor, MI 48199, USA
* Corresponding author.
E-mail address: webers@ohsu.edu

Clin Plastic Surg 37 (2010) 253–264
doi:10.1016/j.cps.2009.12.005

image quality. Typical views included in rhinoplasty photography include a frontal projection, base view, and lateral and oblique images. Some surgeons routinely include smiling lateral views to better assess dynamic tip movement with facial animation. It is critical that all lateral and oblique images are acquired in the Frankfort horizontal plane (a line connecting the superior aspect of the tragus to the infraorbital rim should be parallel to the horizontal), which allows precise comparison between pre- and postoperative images.

COMPUTER IMAGING

Although a discussion of computer imaging is beyond the scope of this article, this tool can provide an estimation of ideal postoperative results. Patients must be cautioned, however, that prediction of rhinoplasty results is fraught with difficulty and that modified images represent the ideal outcome rather than a guarantee. Please refer to the following source for discussion of the utility and accuracy of computerized imaging in prerhinoplasty consultation.[6]

SOURCES OF GRAFT MATERIAL

Autogenous cartilage harvested from the nasal septum, conchal bowl or rib is the ideal graft material (**Fig. 1**). These grafts have very low risk of infection or extrusion compared with an alloplast. Cartilage grafts are tolerated well by nasal tissue and can be sculpted precisely to adapt to the recipient site. Scoring, morselization, or crushing of cartilage grafts also may be performed to create a more malleable graft material.

Nasal Septum

Septal cartilage represents the gold standard material for alar cartilage grafting. It can be accessed in the same operative field during rhinoplasty. The entire quadrangular cartilage with the exception of a 1 cm dorsal and caudal strut may be harvested without compromising dorsal or tip support (**Fig. 2**). The available cartilage typically is robust, and beveling the edges of septal cartilage grafts can help soften their appearance and minimize their visibility and palpability. The occurrence of infection or extrusion is uncommon. The unoperated patient typically has a generous supply of septal cartilage. In cases of revision rhinoplasty, however, there is often inadequate cartilage available to the surgeon for required alar cartilage grafts. Preoperative palpation of the septum with a cotton swab may reveal the extent of submucous resection in previously operated patients, alerting the surgeon to the potential need to access non-nasal cartilage donor sites.

Auricular Cartilage

The conchal bowl provides an easily accessible source of cartilage or composite graft material. While requiring a second operative site, it can be easily incorporated within the surgical field prepared during rhinoplasty. Both medial and lateral approaches can be used to harvest the entire concha cymba and cavum without compromising the appearance of the pinna or structure of the cartilaginous ear canal. The medial approach (**Fig. 3**) places a scar on the postauricular portion of the pinna, which is well-hidden from the casual observer. Alternatively, the lateral approach, which places a scar on the antihelical fold, heals well with minimal scarring. The appearance of the pinna is unaltered by either approach as long as the structure of the antihelical fold cartilage is preserved.

When used in rhinoplasty, conchal cartilage has similarly low rates of infection and extrusion compared with septal cartilage. Crushing or morselization of conchal cartilage is more likely to

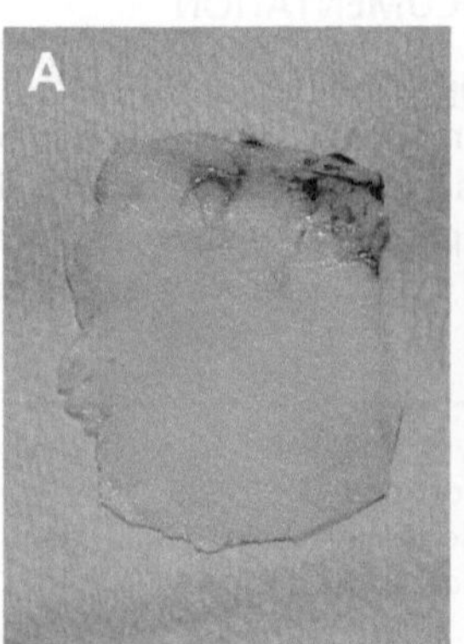

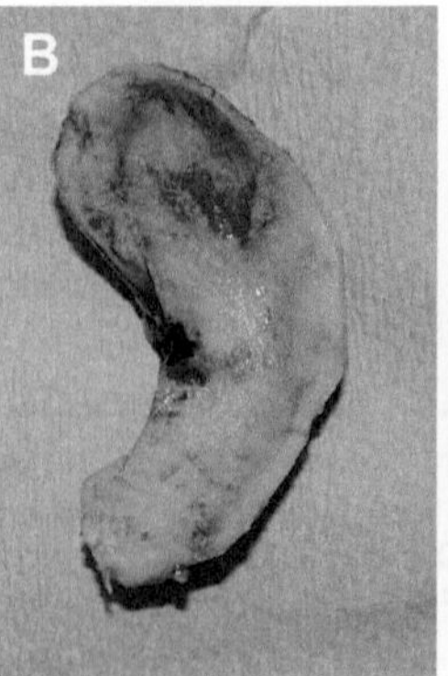

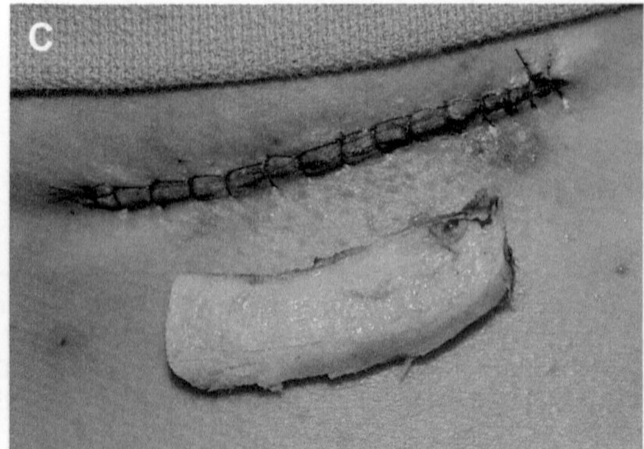

Fig. 1. Common sources for cartilage grafts include septal quadrangular cartilage (*A*), conchal bowl (*B*), and costal cartilage (*C*).

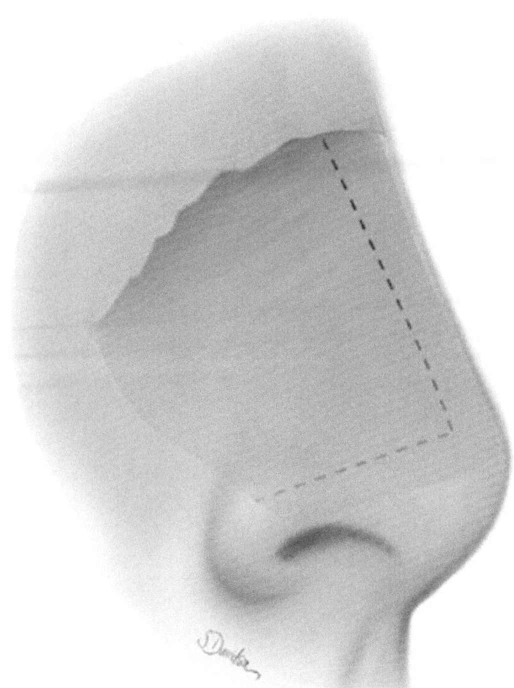

Fig. 2. The entire quadrangular cartilage with the exception of 1 cm dorsal and caudal strut (*broken line*) can be harvested without compromising nasal support.

cause fragmentation as conchal cartilage tends to be weaker than septal cartilage. As a result, the cartilage often must be folded or doubled-over to achieve adequate rigidity. Concha cymba has the disadvantage of being bowl-shaped, which can result in few straight segments of cartilage. The contour of the concha cymba, however, makes this an ideal graft for replacing the lateral crus or the entire alar cartilage. The most common complications of conchal cartilage harvest are auricular hematoma and perichondritis. Hematoma is prevented by quilting with transauricular sutures or using a bolster dressing at the time of wound closure (**Fig. 4**). Perichondritis is evidenced by erythema, edema, and induration of the cartilage-bearing portions of the pinna (not the lobule) and is managed with antipseudomonal antibiotics.

Rib Graft

A generous amount of costal cartilage is available for grafts. The senior author prefers to harvest costal cartilage from the sixth rib, as this allows incision placement within the inframammary crease. If required, cartilage from the seventh rib can be harvested through the same incision.[7] The perichondrium is removed in its entirety, followed by concentric carving[8] of the graft in balanced cross-sections.[9] Despite these maneuvers, the most consistent complication of costal cartilage grafts is the propensity for warping. Many surgeons carve the graft immediately after harvest and allow initial warping of the graft before implantation. Thus, the initial tendency of the graft to warp can be recognized and countered with additional contouring. It has been shown experimentally, however, that grafts continue to warp on a long-term basis.[10] To counteract this risk, some authors place a Kirschner wire along the longitudinal axis of the costal cartilage graft if it is being used as a dorsal onlay graft or columella strut.[11]

Costal cartilage harvest requires general anesthesia, adding to total operative time and expense. In addition, the elderly are poor candidates for rib grafting, as ossification can interfere with graft harvest and carving.[7] Although there is a risk of pleural violation and pneumothorax, these complications are uncommon and can be recognized intraoperatively with the Valsalva maneuver. Through the same exposure for harvesting the rib graft, a red rubber catheter is placed in the chest to evacuate intrathoracic air. As long as the visceral pleura remains intact, a thoracostomy tube is unnecessary. Patients undergo a postoperative chest radiograph if the Valsalva maneuver suggests violation of the pleura and are routinely discharged on the same day of surgery unless a pneumothorax develops.

Irradiated Costal Cartilage

Cadaveric rib cartilage, which has been gamma-irradiated to minimize the risk of infection and tissue rejection, is readily available. A necessary point of discussion with the patient is the implantation of cadaveric tissue. Although rarely a point of major concern, some patients are not agreeable to cadaveric tissue grafts despite the low risk of transmission of infectious disease. Controversy exists as to the long-term survival of this homograft material, but some authors demonstrate predictable, robust long-term results in correction of saddle nose deformity.[12] Further, the severity of warping of fresh and irradiated cadaveric rib appears to be comparable.[10] Although there is justifiable concern of long-term resorption of irradiated costal cartilage grafts, there is evidence that replacement with fibrous tissue can maintain the aesthetic appearance.[13]

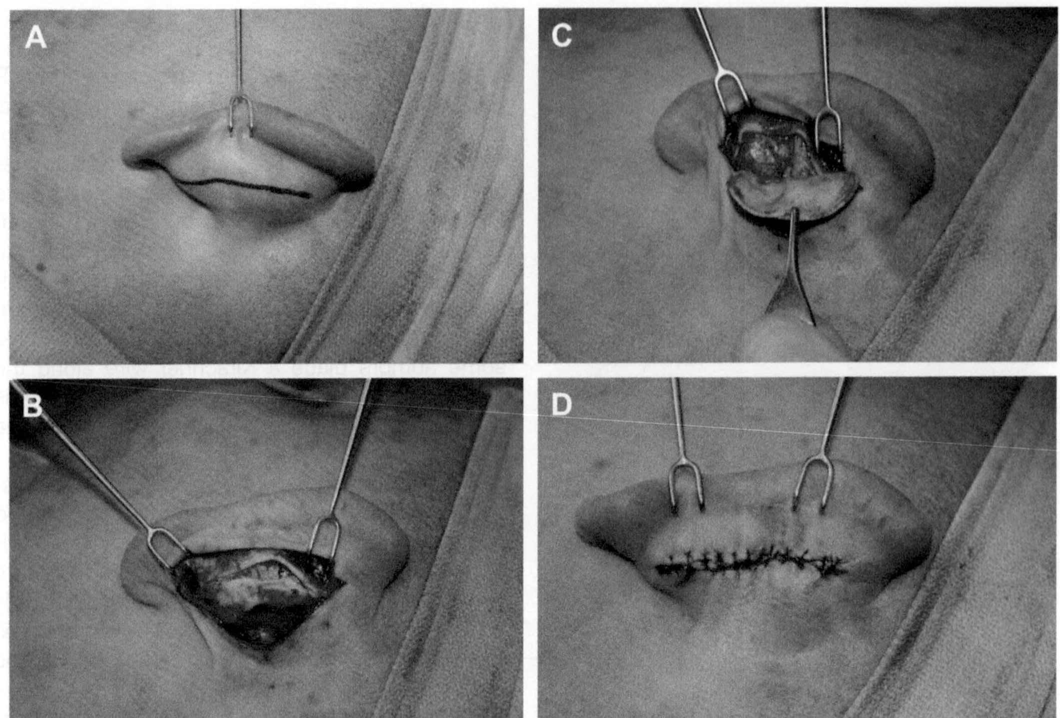

Fig. 3. A medial approach for conchal cartilage harvest requires a postauricular incision placed medial to the antihelical rim (*A*). Following subperichondrial dissection of the medial surface of auricular cartilage, an incision is made through the cartilage, preserving the structure of the antihelical fold (*B*). Dissection on the lateral surface frees the conchal cartilage (*C*), which can be removed in its entirety. The wound is closed with absorbable suture (*D*).

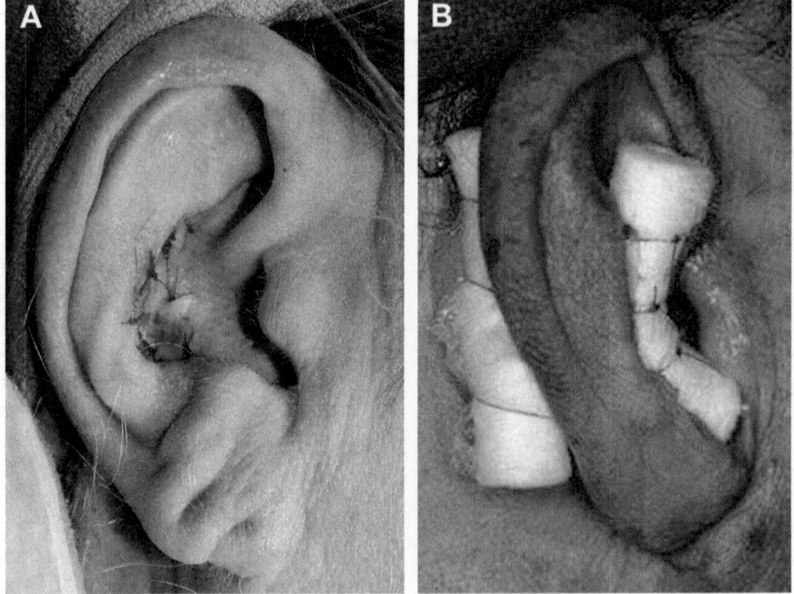

Fig. 4. Auricular hematoma may be prevented with either absorbable quilting sutures (*A*) or a bolster comprised of either dental rolls (*B*) or xeroform gauze secured with transauricular monofilament suture.

Alloplast

Medpor

Medpor is comprised of high-density polyethylene. This biomaterial is highly compatible with human tissue and commercially available preshaped for various nasal graft applications. The pore size of roughly 100 μm allows fibrovascular tissue ingrowth. This helps reduce the risk of implant migration, extrusion, and infection. The porosity of the implant also may allow bacterial colonization and potential graft infection. Thus, many surgeons soak the implant in dilute Betadine or antibiotic solution before implantation. The main drawback of using Medpor is the risk of extrusion caused by infection or implant mobility. Implants may be difficult to excise because of the fibrovascular tissue ingrowth.

APPROACHES TO THE NASAL TIP

The nasal tip can be addressed by either endonasal or external rhinoplasty techniques. Significant tip modification or reconstruction is addressed best by means the external approach given the advantages of direct visualization and modification of the alar cartilages in situ. This is particularly helpful in the revision patient, where the required tip modifications may not be evident based on external examination. The main drawbacks to the external approach are added operative time to elevate the skin, soft tissue envelope, and postoperative edema. Although there is an added transcolumellar scar not required by endonasal techniques, this is rarely a source of postoperative concern for the patient.

Endonasal techniques can be used for more limited tip modification and tip grafting, but this requires the surgeon to be facile with this approach. Both delivery and nondelivery approaches can be used. Although the delivery approach allows direct inspection of the alar cartilages, this level of exposure is more destructive to tip-supporting mechanisms than the nondelivery approach. Further, tip delivery can distort the normal anatomy, potentially compromising alar cartilage grafting techniques. However, many authors referenced herein use exclusively endonasal techniques to place alar cartilage grafts.

COLUMELLA STRUT

The columella strut is likely the most familiar alar cartilage graft known to rhinoplasty surgeons. In most external rhinoplasty approaches, the columella strut is used to maintain tip support and prevent tip ptosis during wound contracture.[14] The main exception is when a long septum is used in a tongue-in-groove technique[15] to position and support the medial crura on the caudal septum. The columella strut is placed in a soft tissue pocket dissected between the medial crura (**Fig. 5**). It is important to dissect the pocket toward but not onto the nasal spine, as placement of the graft on the spine can result in clicking of the graft when the nasal tip is compressed. The columella strut stabilizes the position of the nasal tip. Advancement of the medial crura anteriorly or

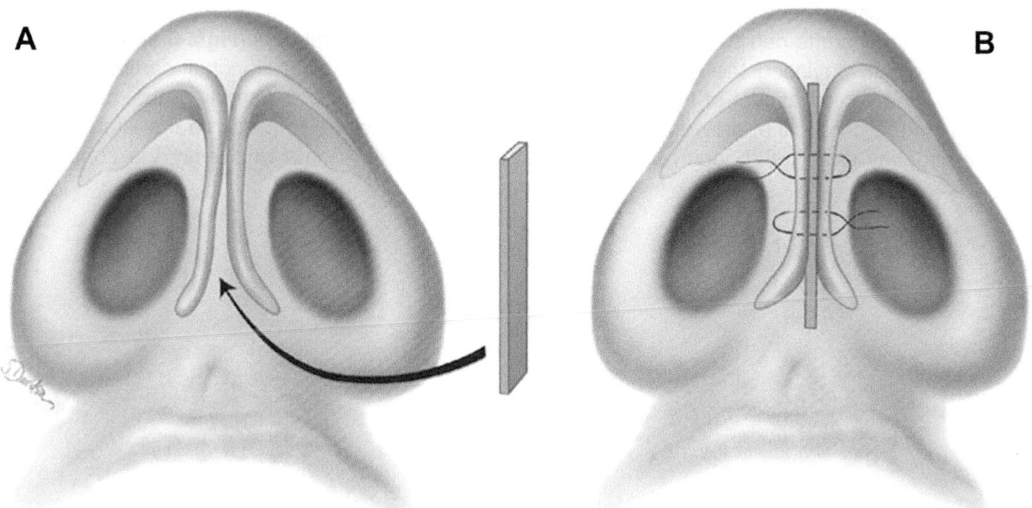

Fig. 5. Columella strut grafts are placed within a soft tissue pocket created between the medial crura (*A*). After determining the proper position of the intermediate crura, the medial crura are fixated with either transcutaneous plain gut sutures (*B*) or buried absorbable monofilament sutures.

posteriorly on the columella strut can enhance or reduce nasal tip projection, rotation, and columella show. The strut most commonly is carved from septal or costal cartilage and secured with either absorbable monofilament sutures placed deep to the vestibular skin or plain gut sutures passed through and through the nasal vestibular skin. Conchal cartilage may be used as a columella strut but often must be doubled on itself to provide adequate rigidity.

LATERAL CRURAL STRUT GRAFT

The lateral crural strut graft is used to reinforce the ala or reduce the concavity of the lateral crura of the lower lateral cartilages.[16] This technique also can be used to overcome the tendency of the lateral crura to become medially displaced (pinched) after placement of dome sutures to narrow the nasal tip. In the vertically oriented lateral crura, lateral crural strut grafts are used in combination with releasing the crura from their vestibular skin attachments and repositioning them in a more lateral and caudal position.

Lateral crural strut grafts are most often carved from septal or costal cartilage. They typically are placed in a soft tissue pocket on the deep aspect of the lateral crura and secured with mattress sutures (**Fig. 6**). They may be extended onto the pyriform aperture for additional stability. Placing the grafts on the deep aspect of the lateral crura may crowd the nasal airway, necessitating graft removal. Gunter and Friedman,[16] however, did not describe any postoperative nasal obstruction in 88 patients treated with lateral crural strut grafts. Gruber, in discussing these results, suggests that lateral crural strut grafts can be placed successfully as an onlay, obviating the need to dissect a pocket on the ventral aspect of the lateral crura and avoiding the potential of crowding the airway with the underlay graft.[17] Although not extending into the airway, these grafts sometimes are visible through the nasal skin, especially in thin-skinned patients. Thus, strut grafts must be used carefully, as an onlay graft and beveled to prevent a visible and palpable step-off at the graft edge.

ALAR BATTEN GRAFT

The alar batten graft is a nonanatomic graft placed either cephalic or caudal to the lateral crus of the lower lateral cartilage to reinforce the internal or external nasal valve, respectively (**Fig. 7**). When placed caudal to the lateral crus, the graft often is referred to as an alar rim graft (discussed separately within this issue). Alar batten grafts extend from the pyriform aperture to a paramedian position and may be sutured in place by means of transcutaneous sutures or placed in a precise soft tissue pocket. Toriumi and colleagues[18] have described the placement of batten grafts to ameliorate both internal and external valve collapse. The authors emphasize the important of preoperative identification of the region of maximal nasal valve collapse to ensure proper graft placement. Batten grafts can be carved from any cartilage source of adequate size or are commercially available as shaped Medpor implants.

ALAR REPLACEMENT (INLAY) GRAFT

Alar inlay grafts represent the last resort for reconstitution of the lateral crura. When suture techniques and alar batten/lateral crural strut grafts are insufficient to meet the surgeon's aesthetic and functional goals, it may be necessary to replace the lateral crus (**Figs. 8** and **9**). This often is performed using conchal cartilage given its natural convexity resembling the native lateral crus. It is helpful to preserve the lateral crus just lateral to the dome to overlay the conchal graft

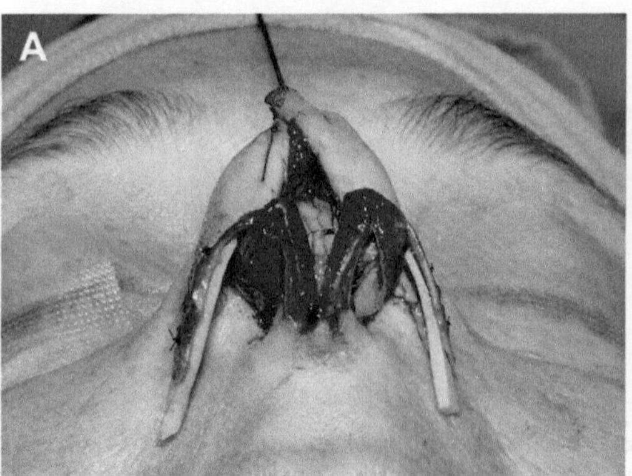

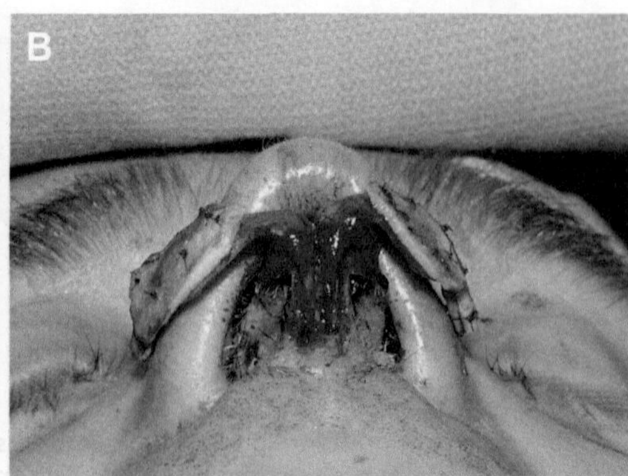

Fig. 6. Lateral crural strut grafts may be placed on either the ventral (*A*) or dorsal surface (*B*) of the lateral crura.

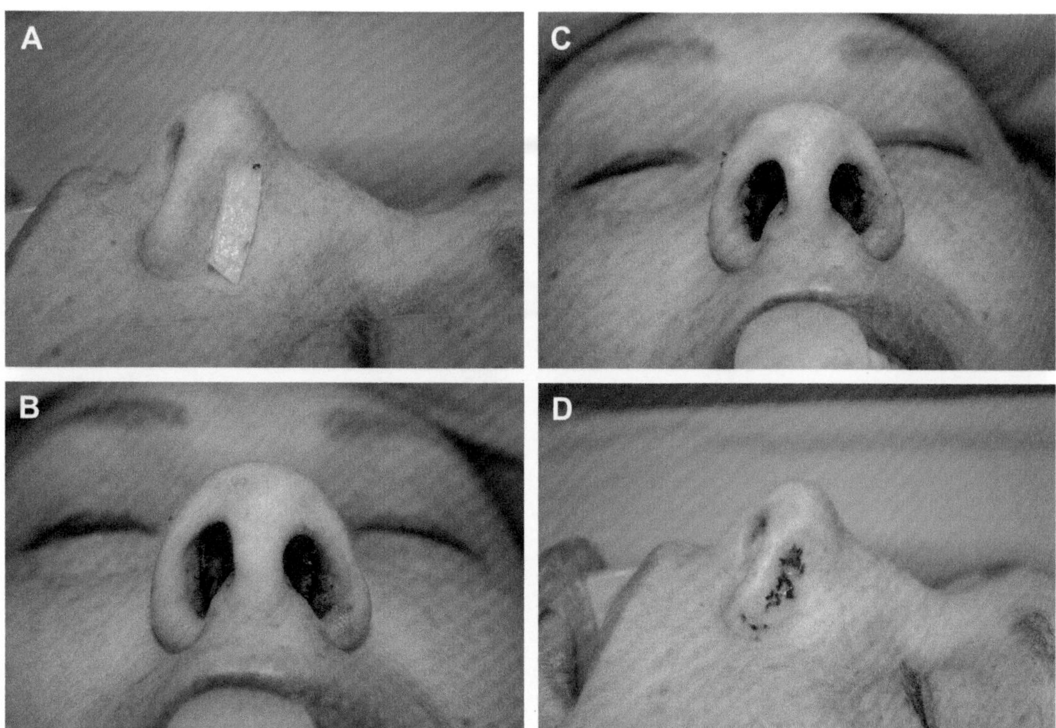

Fig. 7. Alar batten grafts are nonanatomic cartilage grafts (*A*) used to prevent collapse of the nasal valve. Placement of these grafts over the pyriform aperture can prevent medial displacement and collapse of the internal nasal valve (*B, C*). The grafts can be placed in a precise soft tissue pocket or secured with transcutaneous sutures (*D*).

and camouflage its medial border. The lateral extent is placed in a precise soft tissue pocket over the pyriform aperture. Additional horizontal mattress sutures can be placed loosely through the vestibular skin to allow its apposition to the graft.

TIP GRAFTS

Tip grafts are used in cases where increased tip projection is required beyond what can be achieved with medial crural advancement and suture techniques. Alternatively, tip grafts can be used to camouflage persistent tip asymmetry that cannot be repaired with other methods. Grafts also may be used to accentuate the infratip lobule. Papel has described a graduated method of tip graft fixation that correlates the inadequacy of tip projection with the need for progressively more secure graft fixation ranging from placement by endonasal approach in a defined pocket for camouflage/contouring of a normally projected tip to suture fixation via external rhinoplasty approach for severe deprojection.[19]

Sheen Tip Graft

The tip graft initially described by Sheen[20] was created from vomer or septal cartilage. These grafts were designed to achieve optimal tip projection and contour in patients with inadequate native nasal tip structure. Early complications of infection and implant mobility were minimized with increased experience. Further study revealed that tip grafts comprised of bone reabsorbed at an unacceptable rate.[21] The current Sheen type tip graft is shield-shaped to improve nasal tip contour and projection (**Fig. 10**). A variable infratip component allows modification of the infratip lobule and creation of the aesthetic ideal, double break. The borders of the graft are beveled to camouflage the graft, especially in thin-skinned patients. It is often necessary to stack grafts in patients with inadequate projection and a short nose to achieve adequate lengthening and prevent deformation of the graft with wound healing. It is critical that grafts be placed in a precise pocket (endonasal approach) or sutured securely (external rhinoplasty) to prevent migration and unintended contour deformity.[19]

An interesting modification of the tip graft has been suggested by Gruber and colleagues and referred to as an anatomic tip graft. This graft combines a Sheen type graft with an onlay tip graft to simultaneously augment the domes and the infratip region.[22]

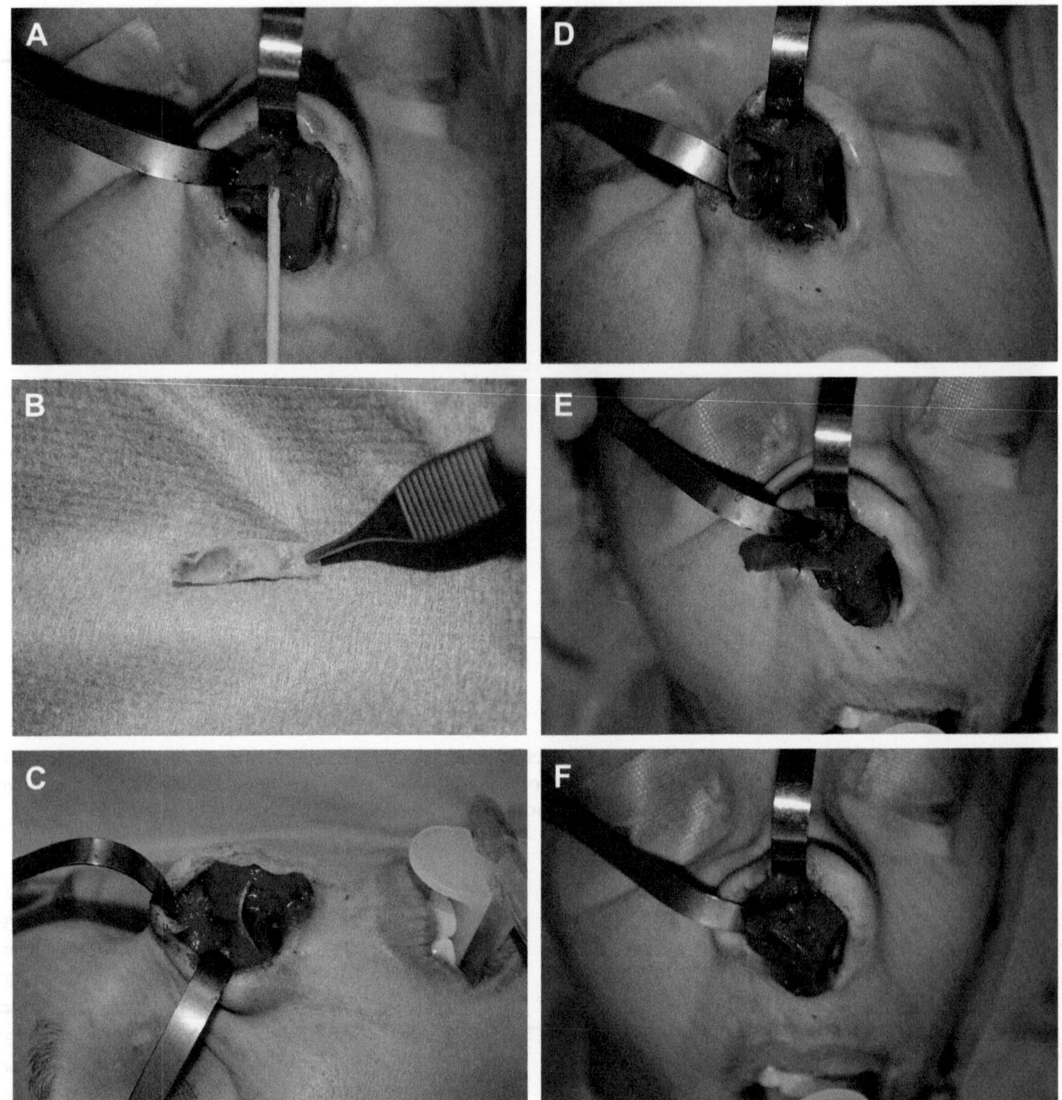

Fig. 8. Lateral crural replacement (inlay) grafts may be used to replace the absent or insufficient lateral crus (*A*). This graft typically is harvested from the conchal bowl (*B*), given its convexity that closely mirrors the native lateral crus (*C*). The grafts are secured just lateral to the intermediate crus (*D, E*) and may be placed in a precise soft tissue pocket laterally (*F*) or secured with suture to the vestibular skin or alar base.

Cap Graft

The cap graft, initially described by Peck,[23] is placed across the domes of the alar cartilages and secured with suture (**Fig. 11**). Given its superficial location, the graft must be beveled so that there is a smooth transition between the borders of the graft and the native alar cartilages. The graft most often is used to increase intrinsic projection of the tip lobule. Cap grafts also can be used to camouflage irregularities or asymmetries of the domes of the alar cartilages. This graft may be created from any sources of cartilage including the alar cartilage removed during cephalic trim of the lateral crura.[24] In this case, because of the thinness of the alar cartilages, there is limited enhancement of projection. Using such grafts, however, lessens the risk of visibility of the graft in thin-skinned patients when compared with cap grafts composed of septal or auricular cartilage.

Infralobular Graft

Infralobular grafts may be used to selectively improve contour of the infratip lobule or to increase columella show. Infralobular grafts typically are created from septal cartilage but may be derived from auricular or costal cartilage. Grafts

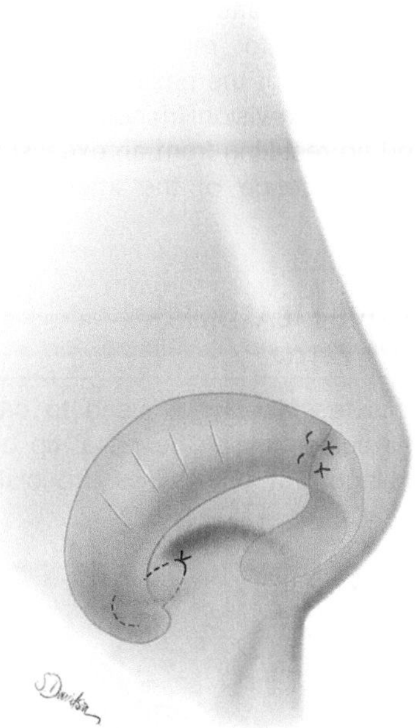

Fig. 9. Schematic representation of lateral crural replacement (inlay) graft.

are placed either in a precise soft tissue pocket (endonasal approach) or are sutured to the medial crura to prevent migration via external rhinoplasty approach.

ANCHOR GRAFT

The anchor graft, recently described by Chang and Davis,[25] resembles an inverted marine anchor. The authors prefer conchal cartilage for this graft given its intrinsic convexity that may restore the natural aesthetic contour of the nasal tip. The shank or shaft of the anchor is sutured to the medial crura/columella strut complex as an onlay graft. The wings or flukes of the anchor are secured to the caudal border of the lateral crura of the alar cartilages with suture. Thus, in addition to refining the nasal tip, anchor grafts may be used to caudally secure or reposition the retracted lateral crura remedying alar retraction often encountered in secondary rhinoplasty. The authors stress that fixation to a stable columella strut complex is critical to prevent graft migration with associated visibility and palpability. This technique represents an effective approach to management of the complex problem of nostril retraction resulting from excessive alar resection and is worthy of long-term study.

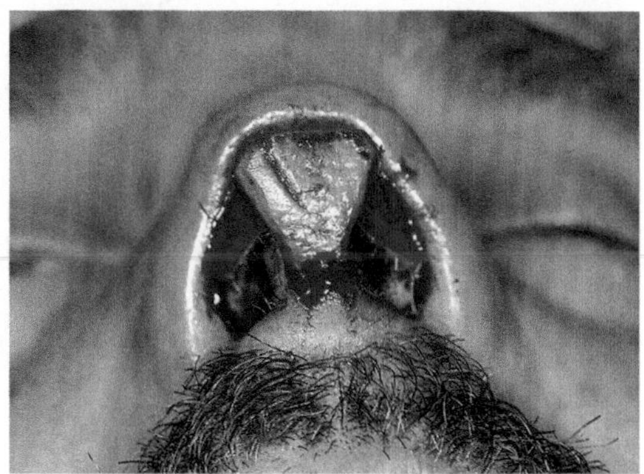

Fig. 10. Sheen-type tip grafts are used when suture techniques are unable to provide adequate tip projection. The grafts are positioned approximately 2 mm anterior to the intermediate crura and secured to the medial crura with absorbable monofilament suture.

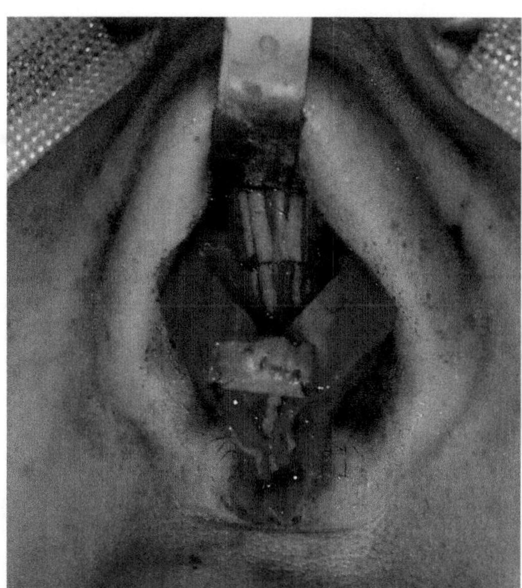

Fig. 11. Peck-type tip grafts are placed over the intermediate crura to increase projection of the tip lobule and may be used to camouflage irregularities of the domes of the alar cartilages.

UMBRELLA GRAFT

The umbrella graft is used to simultaneously provide increased nasal tip projection and support.[26,27] This technique requires a columella strut to ensure tip support, as described previously. The umbrella graft is an onlay nasal tip graft (approximately 4 × 9 mm) that overlies the columella strut and domes of the alar cartilage placed via an endonasal rhinoplasty approach. While Peck described placing the tip graft and columella strut as individual units,[27] other authors have created the entire umbrella graft ex vivo before implantation of the graft construct.[26,28] Thus, the umbrella graft can simultaneously increase nasal tip support and projection in the nose with deficient cartilaginous support and structure. As with other tip grafting methods, the most common complication is visibility of the graft material, which required revision in 5% of patients.[27]

DOME SPREADER GRAFT

The dome spreader graft is a rectangular graft placed between the cartilage of the dome and underlying vestibular skin (**Fig. 12**). The graft is placed deep to the dome in a precisely dissected pocket and secured with monofilament suture. Dome spreader grafts can be used to reliably reshape, reorient, or reinforce the domes and prevent pinching of the nasal tip. They are used most often in revision rhinoplasty to correct a pinched tip resulting from an excessively acute angle of divergence of the intermediate crura (domes).

ADJUNCTIVE MEASURES

Temporalis Fascia

Temporalis fascia may be used to camouflage contour irregularities of the nasal tip or dorsum after cartilage grafting. This is especially helpful

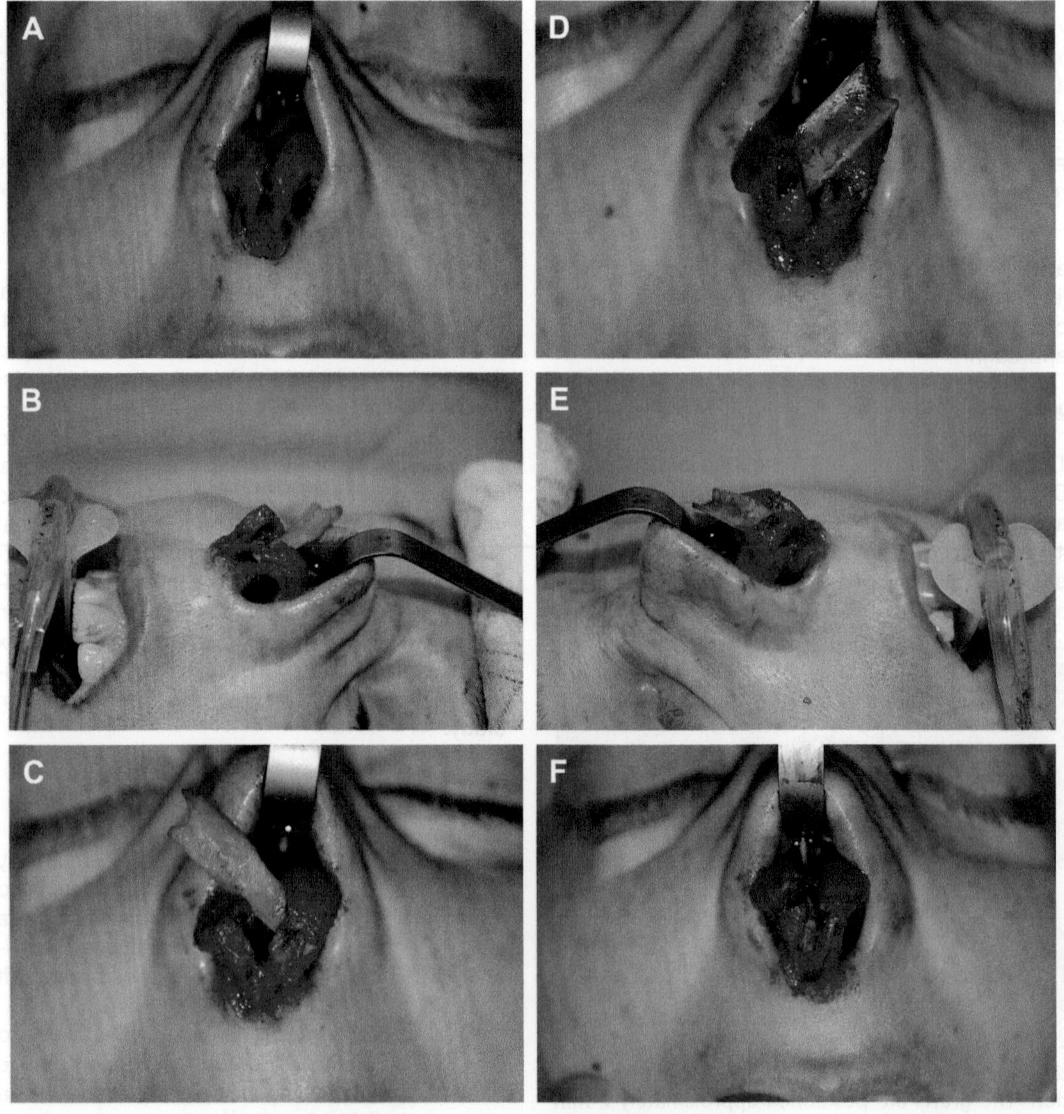

Fig. 12. Dome spreader grafts may be used to remedy pinching or asymmetry of the nasal tip (*A*). After dissecting the vestibular skin from the intermediate crura, dome spreader grafts of appropriate size are secured with horizontal mattress sutures to the intermediate crura (*B–E*) to prevent pinching of the domes of the alar cartilages (*F*).

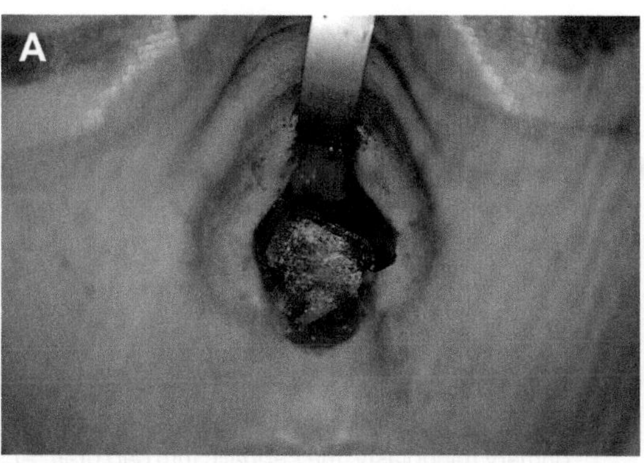

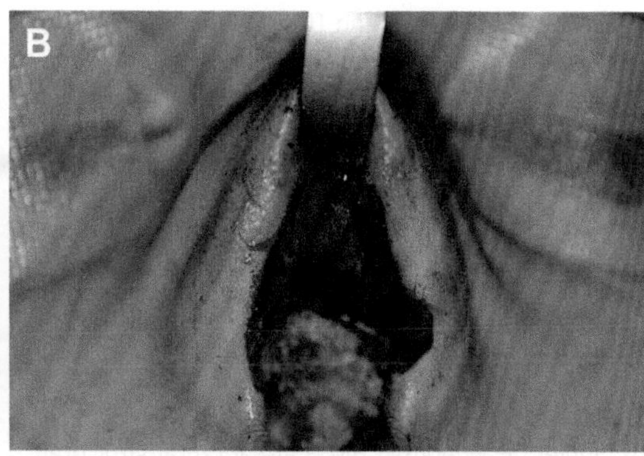

Fig. 13. Compressed and dried temporalis fascia may be trimmed and placed over the nasal tip (*A*) or dorsum (*B*) to camouflage subtle contour deformities in thin-skinned patients.

in the patient with thin skin where there is minimal tolerance for imperfections of the nasal cartilaginous framework. The graft material is harvested via a temporal scalp incision, which easily can be prepared into the rhinoplasty surgical field. Although the temporoparietal fascia also can be harvested, the senior author prefers to harvest the temporalis fascia, as it has greater thickness and tissue strength. After exposing an adequate amount of the fascia, it is incised and bluntly dissected free from the underlying temporalis muscle with an elevator. The graft then is spread into a single sheet, pressed, and dried. Alternatively, if a fascia press is unavailable, the graft may be compressed between two tongue blades. The compressed and dried material then is placed over the nasal tip or dorsum (**Fig. 13**) as a sheet and is rehydrated rapidly by the fluids of the surrounding tissue. It is expected that the temporalis fascia will swell significantly, and these patients can have prolonged edema of the grafted regions.

Crushed Cartilage

As an alternative or addition to temporalis fascia grafts, crushed or bruised cartilage grafts can be used to plump or camouflage areas of soft tissue deficiency or contour irregularity. Drawbacks include contour deformity, migration, and resorption.

SUMMARY

The primary modalities for creation of an aesthetic and structurally sound nasal tip are suture techniques and conservative resection of the cephalic portion of the lateral crura. This luxury is often unavailable in the secondary rhinoplasty patient who has had excessive removal or alteration of the alar cartilages. In these cases, cartilage grafting, often in combination with suture techniques, is required to achieved the desired cosmetic and functional results. This article described the most common cartilage grafts used to restore and contour the alar cartilages. Although not an exhaustive catalog of graft choices, the previously noted methods should provide the beginning and expert rhinoplasty surgeon with various techniques to achieve the desired goals in difficult primary or secondary rhinoplasty.

REFERENCES

1. Baker SR. Suture contouring of the nasal tip. Arch Facial Plast Surg 2000;2:34–42.
2. Goode R. A method of tip projection measurement. New York: Thieme-Stratton; 1984.
3. Crumley RL, Lanser M. Quantitative analysis of nasal tip projection. Laryngoscope 1988;98:202–8.
4. Simons R. Nasal tip projection, ptosis, and supratip thickening. Ear Nose Throat J 1982;61:452–5.
5. Quatela VC, Slupchynskyj OS. Surgery of the nasal tip. Facial Plast Surg 1997;13:253–68.
6. Adelson RT, DeFatta RJ, Bassischis BA. Objective assessment of the accuracy of computer-simulated imaging in rhinoplasty. Am J otolaryngol 2008;29:151–5.
7. Marin VP, Landecker A, Gunter JP. Harvesting rib cartilage grafts for secondary rhinoplasty. Plast Reconstr Surg 2008;121:1442–8.
8. Kim DW, Shah AR, Toriumi DM. Concentric and eccentric carved costal cartilage: a comparison of warping. Arch Facial Plast Surg 2006;8:42–6.
9. Gibson T, Davis WB. The distortion of autogenous cartilage grafts: its cause and prevention. Br J Plast Surg 1957;10:257–74.
10. Adams WP Jr, Rohrich RJ, Gunter JP, et al. The rate of warping in irradiated and nonirradiated homograft rib cartilage: a controlled comparison and clinical implications. Plast Reconstr Surg 1999;103:265–70.
11. Nakamura A. Control of grafted rib cartilage warping. Eur J Plast Surg 1995;18:188–9.

12. Weber S, Cook TA, Wang TD. Irradiated homologous costal cartilage in augmentation rhinoplasty. Operat Tech Otolaryngol Head Neck Surg 2007;18:274–83.
13. Welling DB, Maves MD, Schuller DE, et al. Irradiated homologous cartilage grafts. Long-term results. Arch Otolaryngol Head Neck Surg 1988;114:291–5.
14. Anderson JR. New approach to rhinoplasty. A five-year reappraisal. Arch Otolaryngol 1971;93:284–91.
15. Kridel RW, Scott BA, Foda HM. The tongue-in-groove technique in septorhinoplasty. A 10-year experience. Arch Facial Plast Surg 1999;1:246–56 [discussion: 57–8].
16. Gunter JP, Friedman RM. Lateral crural strut graft: technique and clinical applications in rhinoplasty. Plast Reconstr Surg 1997;99:943–52 [discussion: 53–5].
17. Gruber RP. Discussion—lateral crural strut graft: technique and clinical applications in rhinoplasty. Plast Reconstr Surg 1997;99:953–5.
18. Toriumi DM, Josen J, Weinberger M, et al. Use of alar batten grafts for correction of nasal valve collapse. Arch Otolaryngol Head Neck Surg 1997; 123:802–8.
19. Papel ID. A graduated method of tip graft fixation in rhinoplasty. Arch Otolaryngol Head Neck Surg 1995; 121:623–6.
20. Sheen JH. Achieving more nasal tip projection by the use of a small autogenous vomer or septal cartilage graft. A preliminary report. Plast Reconstr Surg 1975;56:35–40.
21. Sheen JH. Tip graft: a 20-year retrospective. Plast Reconstr Surg 1993;91:48–63.
22. Gruber RP, Grover S. The anatomic tip graft for nasal augmentation. Plast Reconstr Surg 1999;103:1744–53 [discussion: 54–8].
23. Peck GC. The onlay graft for nasal tip projection. Plast Reconstr Surg 1983;71:27–39.
24. Rohrich RJ, Deuber MA. Nasal tip refinement in primary rhinoplasty: the cephalic trim cap graft. Aesthet Surg J 2002;22:39–45.
25. Chang CW, Davis RE. The anchor graft: a novel technique in rhinoplasty. Arch Facial Plast Surg 2008;10:50–5.
26. Mavili ME, Safak T. Use of umbrella graft for nasal tip projection. Aesthet plast surg 1993;17:163–6.
27. Peck GC Jr, Michelson L, Segal J, et al. An 18-year experience with the umbrella graft in rhinoplasty. Plast Reconstr Surg 1998;102:2158–65 [discussion: 66–8].
28. Erdogan B, Ayhan M, Gorgu M, et al. Umbrella graft of columella tip: 20 years' experience. Aesthetic plastic surgery 2002;26:167–71.

Rhinoplasty[5] Pearls: Value of the Endonasal Approach and Vertical Dome Division

Robert L. Simons, MD[a,b,*], Ryan M. Greene, MD, PhD[c]

KEYWORDS

- Rhinoplasty • Endonasal approach • Vertical dome division
- External restructuring technique

What separates rhinoplasty from other facial plastic surgery procedures?

Why do surgeons rank this operation near the top when rating degree of difficulty or desirability?

The answers rest in the combination of factors leading to successful outcomes in nasal surgery. This is an operation that embraces both the art and science of surgery. Technical expertise alone does not guarantee success. The oft-stated adage that "in rhinoplasty we do a little to achieve a lot" places the emphasis on astute diagnosis, not on prescribed techniques.

If the desirability and demands of rhinoplasty reside in long-term enhancement of facial features without surgical stigmata, then the understanding of the patient's needs takes precedence in achieving these goals. The surgical approach is secondary to the experienced surgeon's primary diagnosis.

There is no better time than the initial consultation to obtain valued information regarding the individual nature of the patient. At the top of the chart, in his or her own words are the patient's stated desires; unwritten but spoken at this time are the surgeon's goals to satisfy the patient with a natural look. The recommendation that every rhinoplasty patient deserves at least 5 operations has been made on many occasions (**Fig. 1**).[1,2] The importance of the initial diagnosis at this earliest encounter is reiterated.

At this first step, the crucial decision is not how but whether the operation should proceed. Are the patient's requests reasonable? Are expectations and demands too high? Through conversation, a comfort zone is either established or not. Open-ended questions about the individual, rather than directed remarks about the nose, begin the dialog. The sensitive listener can distill troublesome comments or remarks.

The prospective patient's body language, along with office staff's observations outside the consultation room, add to the information. Too many red flags and the comfort zone is never entered. Without shared comfort, the operative contract has less chance of a successful outcome and probably should never be signed.

Unthreatening, but vitally important, are the photographs taken at the initial visit. It is the second opportunity to plan the operation. Each of the 6 basic views has a meaningful input in the decision process. There should be standardization of positioning, distance, lighting, background, and camera. Two light sources are preferred to a uni-flash arrangement.

[a] Division of Facial Plastic and Reconstructive Surgery, Department of Otolaryngology—Head and Neck Surgery, University of Miami School of Medicine, 1666 NW 12th Avenue, Suite 314, Miami, FL 33131, USA
[b] The Miami Institute for Age Management and Intervention, 1441 Brickell Avenue, 3rd Floor Sky Lobby, Miami, FL 33131, USA
[c] Advanced Facial Plastic Surgery & Laser Center, Fort Lauderdale, FL, USA
* Corresponding author.
E-mail address: drsimons@miami-institute.com (R.L. Simons).

Clin Plastic Surg 37 (2010) 265–283
doi:10.1016/j.cps.2009.11.005
0094-1298/10/$ – see front matter

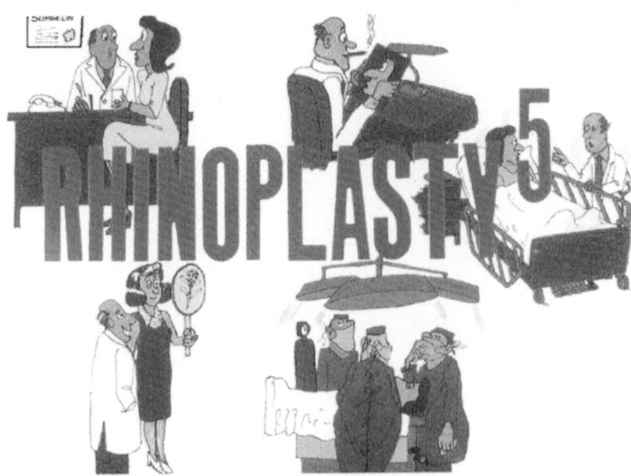

Fig. 1. The rhinoplasty journey allowing for a minimum of 5 steps to assess procedure.

If well taken, the frontal view reinforces impressions about the width, deviation, asymmetries, and length of the nose. The 2 light sources illuminate the presence or lack of meaningful highlights (**Fig. 2**).

The 2 lateral views taken with the Frankfort horizontal plane (tragus to infraorbital rim) parallel to the floor, provide evidence regarding tip projection and overall dorsal height and length. Relationships between the alar rim and columella, favorable or unfavorable angles at the nasofrontal and nasolabial areas, and the appropriate position of the chin are all considered.

Additional information is afforded by the lateral smiling view. The dynamic movement on smiling may enhance the dependency of the nasal tip and length of the nose (**Fig. 3**). The heightened prominence of the septal angle and the acuteness of the nasolabial angle together with the downward displacement of the lower alar cartilage complex defines the ptotic nasal tip. It argues for measures to disrupt the activity of the depressor septi muscle and to reposition the alar complex. The smile may also change the static position of the chin. A protruding mentalis muscle may negate the consideration of chin augmentation.[3]

The three-quarter or oblique view helps to establish the nasal relationship to the surrounding bony and soft tissue features, such as the frontal, zygomatic, maxillary, and mandibular contours. The brow-tip aesthetic line addresses the need for a strong, smooth, dorsal line with appropriate tip position.

However, probably the most important preoperative photograph is the base view (**Fig. 4**). This photograph needs to be taken at right angles and within 45 cm of the patient. Because rhinoplasty is basically an operation of skin redrapage, the best information relating to support and thickness of coverage is afforded by the base view.

Medial support is paramount to good tip projection. The base view evidence of the desired 2:1 relationship of columella to lobule helps the surgeon's understanding of the need to maintain or change tip projection (**Fig. 5**).

Two light sources readily document the distance and symmetry of the 2 lobular apices (**Fig. 6**). Divergent medial crura and the base asymmetries created by functional septal displacement must be appreciated preoperatively.[4] The photographic views are shared with the patient in different ways by various surgeons. In the past, a lateral view was placed against a radiographic view box

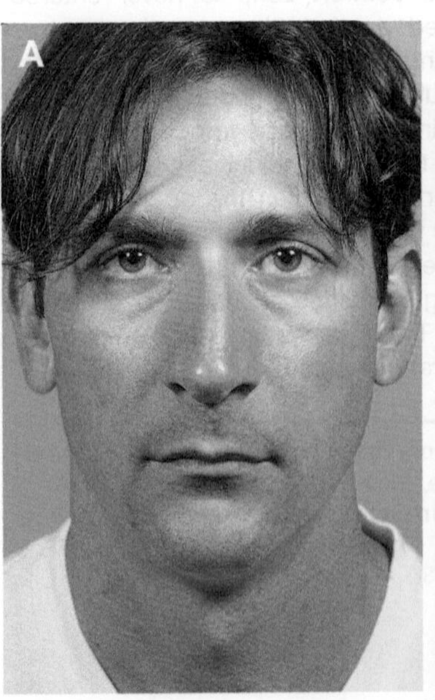

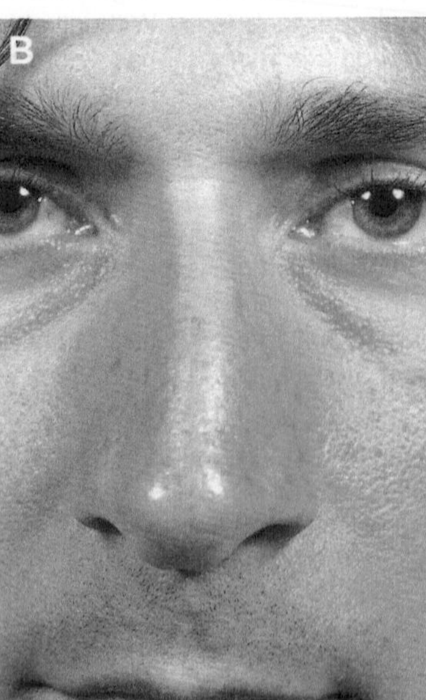

Fig. 2. Preoperative frontal views taken with 2 light sources provide good evidence with shadows and highlights of dorsal height, width, and asymmetries. (*A*) Standard distance. (*B*) Close-up clearly delineating comma-shaped bend in nasal dorsum and dorsal asymmetry.

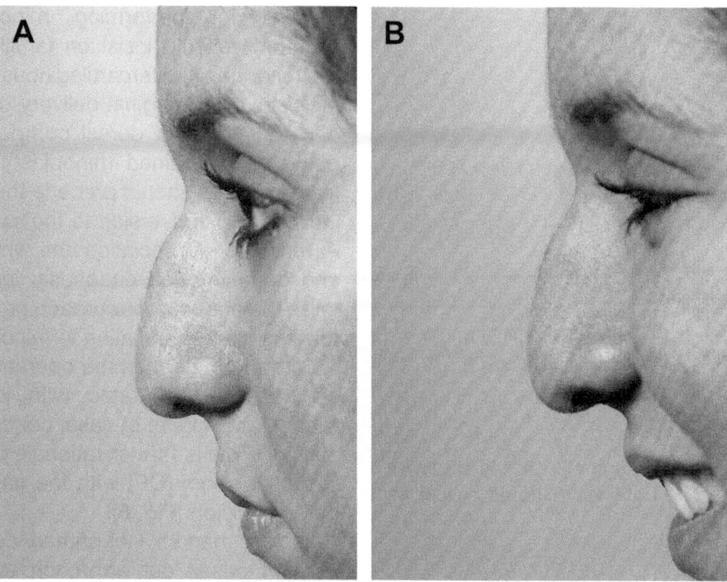

Fig. 3. (*A, B*) Lateral views emphasizing the importance of the smiling view. (*B*) Smiling accentuates the acuteness of the nasolabial angle, height of the anterior septal angle, and nasal length.

and the desired profile changes sketched in with a black marker. Computers are now used to create the anticipated changes.

In an era of virtual reality, the immediate sense of personal change and gain afforded by computer imaging is a powerful tool. It has educational benefits for both patient and surgeon. However, the line drawings must be reasonable and are not guaranteed. The healing in rhinoplasty is too variable to give the patient a sense of the final result, similar to the promises of a plan presented by an architectural draftsman.

Our use of the computer is limited to sharing with patients the results for other patients with similar problems (**Fig. 7**). Establishing a problem-specific database takes time and effort, but is

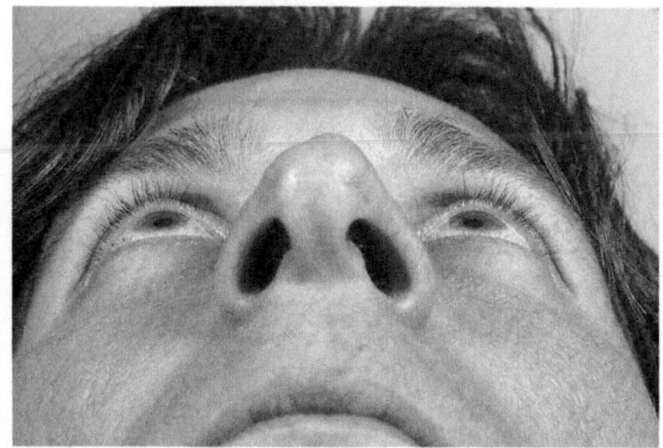

Fig. 4. Close-up base view shows separation of medial crura, deviation of caudal septum, asymmetric domal highlights, and thin skin.

most rewarding. Whether the issue is one of size, width, deviation, trauma, aging, ethnicity, revision, or adjunctive procedures, cases can be provided to show patients what is possible in their specific situation. This is also another opportunity to reassess the game plan and gauge the level of comfort.

Rhinoplasty is routinely performed as an outpatient procedure. Using your own surgical facility or an ambulatory center comfortable for your needs is beneficial to the patient and the surgeon. A relaxed situation is provided by familiarity and appropriate preparation.

Anesthesia protocol depends on the repeated provision of safety and comfort. During the first 35 years in practice, we successfully used local anesthesia injections with assisted intravenous sedation. For the last 6 years, we have routinely used general endotracheal anesthesia. The operation works well in either situation. The change to general anesthesia was due primarily to the experience and background of the anesthesia providers.

Sometime before the operation, possibly in the preoperative holding area or at the scrub sink, there is again the opportunity to readdress the game plan. The preoperative analysis based on photographic review and physical examination should provide an almost x-ray assurance of what will be found and what must be done. Surprises are not the norm, and waiting until the nose is opened to decide what to do is rarely acceptable. The approach to rhinoplasty depends largely on the background and skills of the

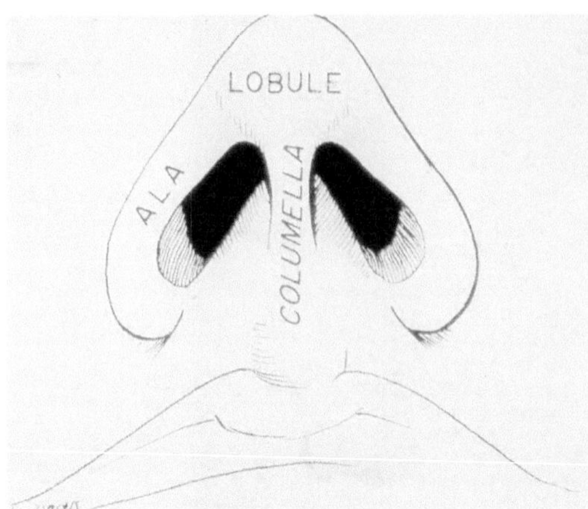

Fig. 5. The length of the columella should be twice that of the lobule. The base view should reveal an equilateral triangle.

surgeon. Neither the endonasal nor the external approach is inherently superior or inferior. Both approaches have their advantages and the choice in most cases depends on the training and experience of the surgeon.

In the early 1960s and 1970s everybody approached the nose through endonasal and transfixion incisions.[5–10] The senior author's continued preference for the endonasal, marginal delivery and incisional tip techniques was strongly influenced by Irving Goldman MD during residency years at Mount Sinai Hospital in New York City.

The swing of the pendulum to the external approach occurred in the late 1970s when many surgeons became enchanted with newfound exposure, especially in the intradomal area.[11–15] Visualization, mobilization, suturing, and restructuring seemed easier and training programs suffered the loss of teachers with endonasal skills. Rather than lose or have to rediscover a beautiful method for performing rhinoplasty, training programs should insist on familiarity and use of the endonasal intercartilaginous and transfixion incisions, the marginal delivery of alar cartilages, and visualizion of dorsal components. In developing a well-trained rhinoplasty surgeon, these learning steps should precede the transcolumellar incision and conversion to the external approach. A renewed appreciation for what can be seen and done through endonasal incisions will revitalize the endonasal approach or at least eliminate the illogical differentiating terminology of "closed."

With the patient on the operating table, supine, sedated, and infiltrated with local anesthesia, preoperative areas of nasal concern become less distinct. This is further rationale for arriving in the operating room (OR) with the game plan in hand before incision (**Fig. 8**).

In more than 95% of primary cases and 90% of revision cases our approach to the surgery is endonasal. With complete transfixion and marginal incisions, the endonasal approach affords excellent visualization of all areas except the lateral osteotomy site, allows variation of technique, permits delicate touch evaluation, limits pocket size for grafts, and avoids any external scar. Final profile adjustments and the appropriate relationship of tip to dorsum are made easier with the skin envelope intact.

The external approach is used in unique situations of extreme scarring, tissue deficiency, or marked curvature of the dorsum. Usually the placement of spreader grafts or the need for high septal repositioning is more easily approached and controlled from above.

In most instances the operation begins with the transfixion of the nose. Separation of caudal septum from columella, combined with elevation of dorsal skin through intracartilaginous incisions, is as old as the text of Jacques Joseph,[16] but it

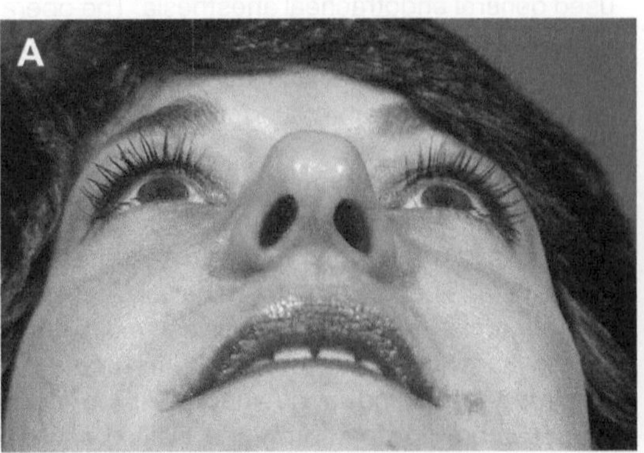

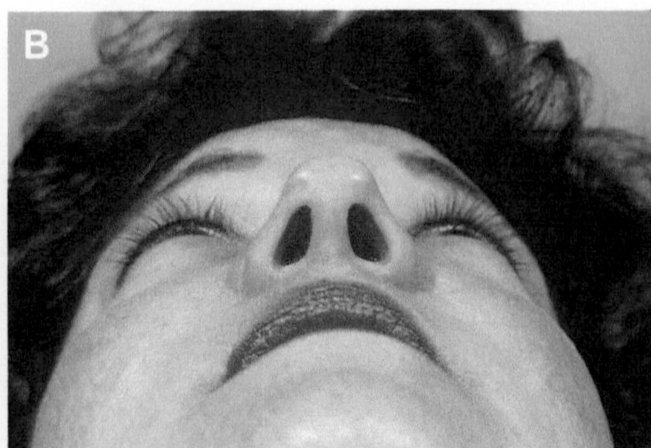

Fig. 6. Base view documentation of bossae formation. (*A*) Preoperative photograph shows 4-mm separation of domal highlights, firm cartilage, and thin skin. (*B*) Six years postoperatively with lateralization of domes following tip procedure consisting solely of cephalic excision of lower lateral alar crura.

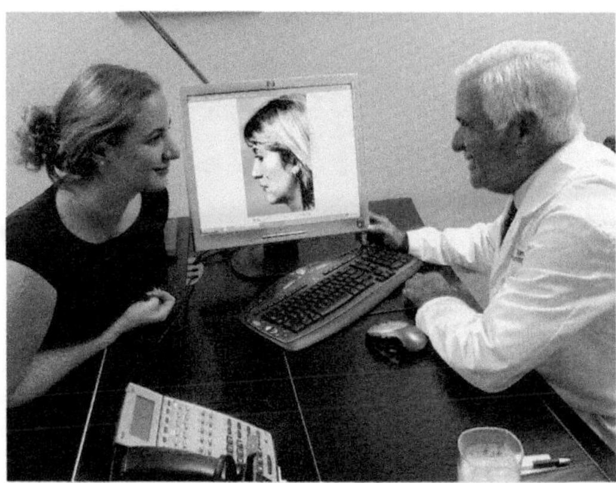

Fig. 7. Dr Simons sharing with a prospective patient preoperative and postoperative views of another patient with similar concerns, using the computer with a problem-specific database.

remains effective and utilitarian. Planes of elevation hugging the perichondrium or periosteum lessen bleeding and aid healing.

The extent of the transfixion incisions at the base of the columella may vary from partial to full with the latter preferred in cases where the caudal septum must be shortened or straightened, where the depressor septi muscle attachment to premaxilla is transected, or where over projection of the tip may benefit from medial crural feet retrodisplacement.[17,18] A retrograde dissection into the columella to remove soft tissue from between the medial crura to help narrow a widened columella, is most easily performed at this time.

Beyond initial transfixion or uncovering of the dorsum there is no universal sequence of steps in rhinoplasty. In cases where dorsal height and central length is excessive it makes sense to start with an initial paring down of these elements. Shortening the caudal septum along with overhanging mucoperichondrium must be judicious and limited to situations presenting with columellar hang, nasal crowding of the upper lip, or the desirability of more tip rotation.

Similarly, the lowering of the dorsal profile must be conservative.[19] One of the major mistakes of earlier days was the excessive lowering of the cartilaginous and bony dorsum to achieve the illusion of projection for a dependent or inadequately projected nasal tip.

In most cases, dorsal reduction is accomplished by removal of more cartilage than bone (**Fig. 9**). If the nose is generally wide, dividing the upper laterals just lateral to their septal attachment makes the careful lowering of the septal angle a bit easier. This maneuver will also help later in narrowing the wide middle third when lateral osteotomies are performed.

The excess bony pyramid is discerned by palpation and visualization. From the slight depression at the rhinion to the desired height of the nasofrontal angle or nasion, a line of over projection is now demarcated. This distinction is easily made when the skin envelope is intact. The cephalic extent of the bony excision depends on the preoperatively determined, desired position of the nasofrontal angle.

Deepening a shallow nasofrontal angle is one of the more difficult maneuvers in rhinoplasty. To be effective, it is necessary to be aggressive and remove a portion of the solid root leading to the frontal bone. Our preferred method is to first use Mayo scissors to free the procerus muscle from its frontal attachment. Then, with decreasingly wide Rubin osteotomes (from 15 to 10 mm), we shave-excise en bloc the excess bone with muscle attached (**Fig. 10**). Rasps are helpful in smoothing

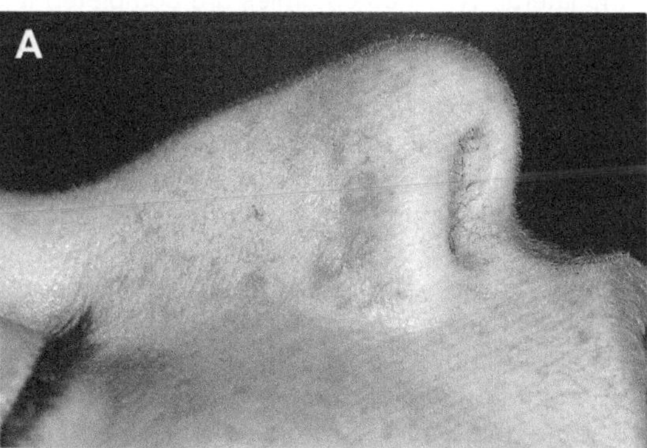

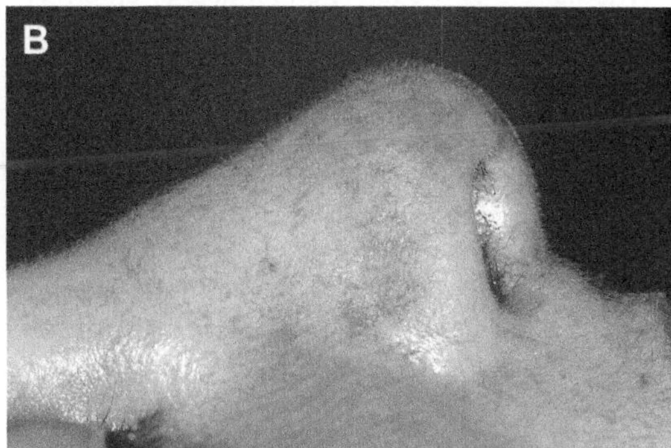

Fig. 8. Changes following local anesthesia infiltration. (*A*) Preoperative profile in supine position. (*B*) One minute later following injection of 10 mL of local anesthetic. Further evidence of the need for preoperative game planning.

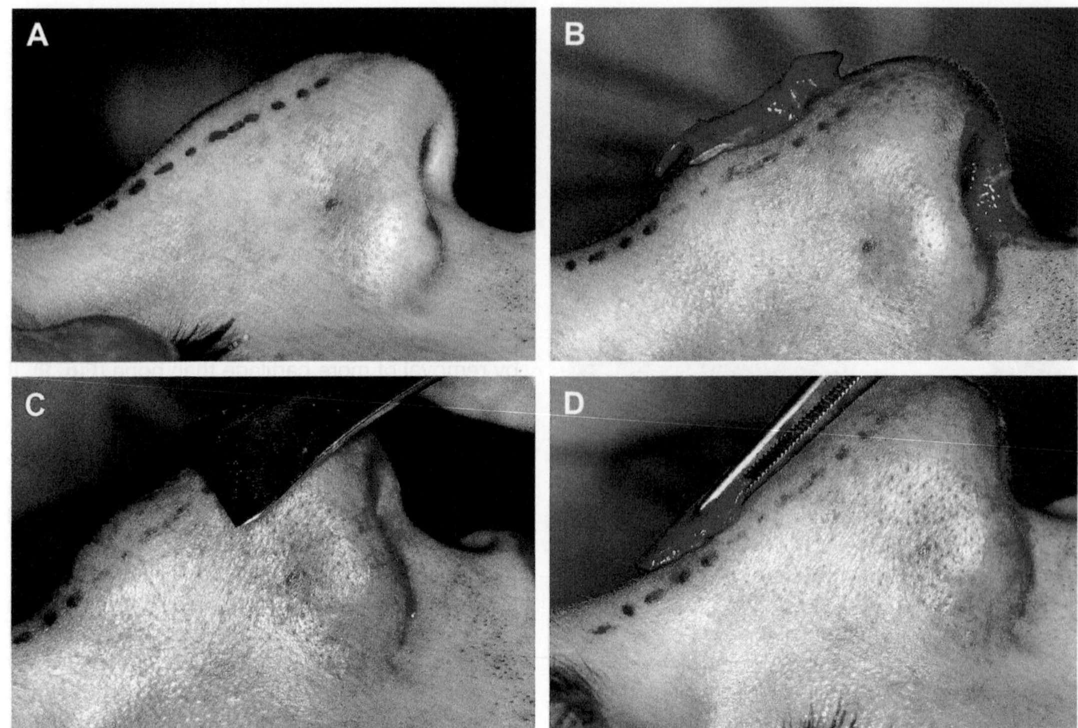

Fig. 9. Intraoperative photos showing the planned dorsal resection with osteotome. Staged dorsal reduction with cartilage and then bone removed.

but are more traumatic and less satisfactory in providing a measurable change in the bony pyramid.

In cases where the middle third is narrow or of normal height there is no reason to separate the upper laterals from the septum. Proceeding with septal work with preliminary lowering of the dorsum allows a better gauge for maintenance of adequate septal support. A relatively straight septum for both functional and aesthetic purposes is achieved before the lateral osteotomies.

Whether the approach is endonasal or external, the lateral osteotomies are beyond the surgeon's view, and therefore, often a struggle for the less experienced surgeon. From our perspective, lateral osteotomies are a necessary part of rhinoplasty any time the bony pyramid is lowered. We prefer using the laterally guarded, v-shaped (Parkes) chisel. Although the instrument is straight, the osteotomy line should be curved from high to low to high. To stay on course and low in the nasofacial groove, the caudal portion of the frontal process of the maxilla should be engaged at right angles. With a downward and outward direction (approximately 45°), the chisel should engage the bone just above a palpable notch at the base of the pyriform aperture (**Fig. 11**).

Staying as low as possible in the nasofacial groove and hugging the maxilla, the chisel should follow the curvature of the bone and turn inward at the medial canthus. This is the time for the surgeon to lower the hand and let the chisel cut through the nasal bone to the nasion. A high to low to high osteotomy should be complete and not "greenstick" in nature.

Intermediate and medial osteotomies used to help straighten or narrow excessively wide or asymmetric nasal bones are performed before the lateral. When osteotomies are completed it is natural for the dorsal profile line to change. Attached to the undersurface of the nasal bones are the upper lateral cartilages, and inward movement of the bones brings the upper lateral cartilages medial and upward, at times, creating a previously unnoted bump in the cartilaginous dorsum.

The cartilage resting above the septal line and below the intercartilaginous incision may be judiciously removed. This type of conservative tailoring done after the osteotomies does not lead to mid-vault constriction or upper lateral collapse. Is appreciation for a smooth dorsal line to tip more easily assessed with the skin envelope intact? For the authors, the answer is yes.

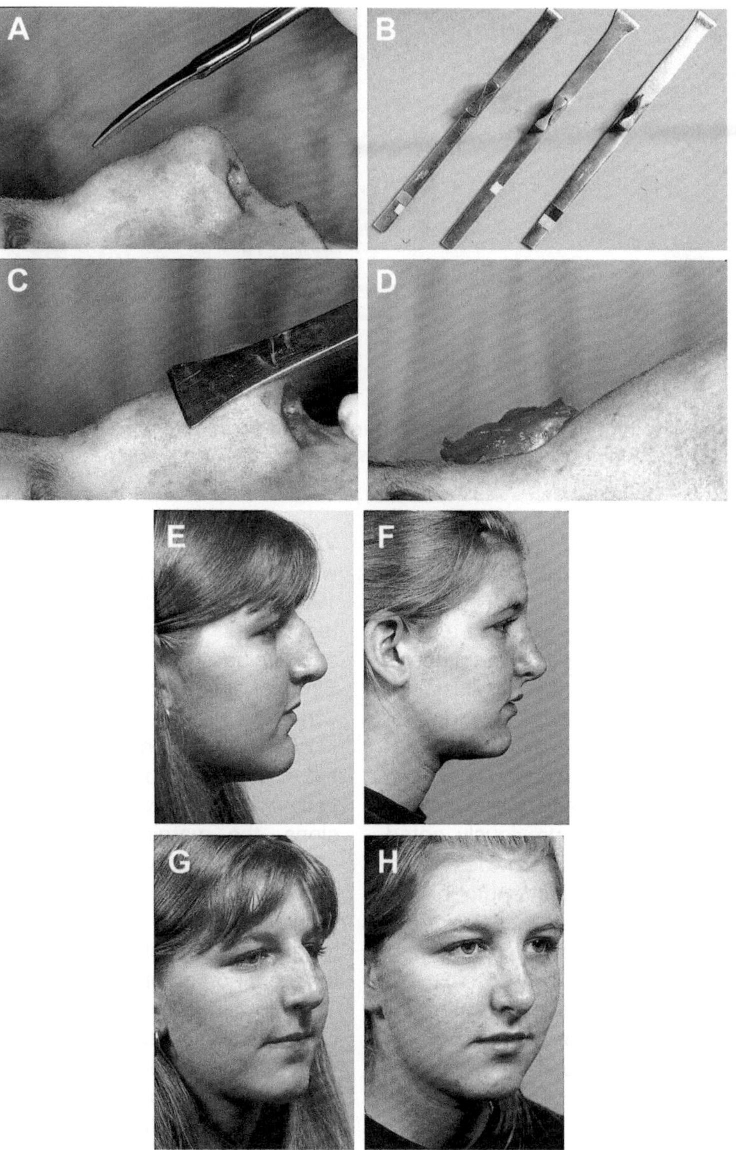

Fig. 10. (*A–D*) Intraoperative photos of deepening of a shallow nasofrontal angle. (*E, G*) Preoperative view of patient. (*F, H*) 1-year follow-up of patient, (*H*) improved brow-tip aesthetic line in oblique view.

For many surgeons, the essence of rhinoplasty resides in nasal tip surgery. Original teachers, including Sam Fomon and Irving Goldman, have observed that "he who masters the tip masters rhinoplasty." In many respects, the changes in tip surgery mirror the general transformation in rhinoplasty teaching and practice.[20–28]

From the days when the excision of lateral crura in varying amounts was limited only by the sanctity of the intact alar strip, there has been a jump to the era of prophylactic surgery in which primary grafting of potentially weak alar cartilages is routinely recommended. During this philosophic pendulum swing, the majority of rhinoplasty procedures have shifted from an endonasal to an external approach. For many young surgeons the need for significant tip surgery is the raison d'être for the external approach.

Somewhat lost between the philosophies of excisional and grafting techniques is the methodology of incisions and repositioning of tissue. Known generically as vertical dome division (VDD), these procedures can be readily accomplished through either the endonasal or external approach. The philosophic tenets of this incisional school, as initially taught by Irving Goldman, MD, at Mount Sinai Hospital, New York, in the 1950s and 1960s, include good visualization of the alar

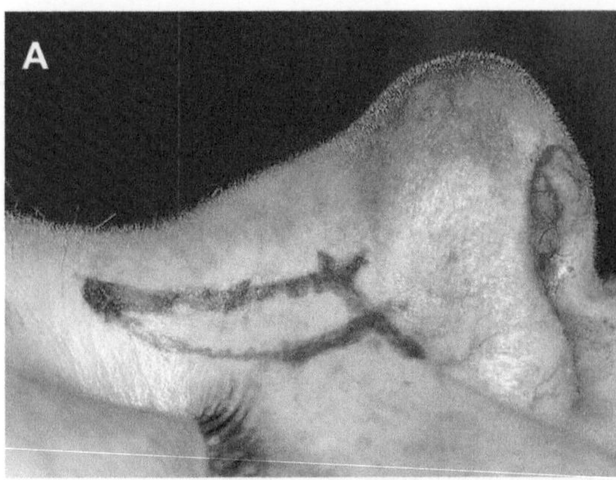

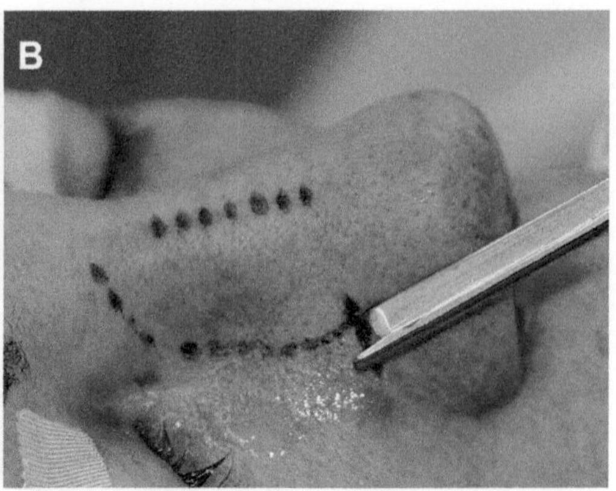

Fig. 11. (*A*) High to low to high lateral osteotomy outlined, with occasional preceding intermediate osteotomy line drawn above. (*B*) Positioning of chisel for lateral osteotomy.

cartilages, minimal excision, and medial stabilization, a prescription for almost every modern-day tip procedure.

Before tip technique however, we need a diagnosis. How do you determine whether a tip needs an actual change in projection or a mere illusion of such through upward or downward rotation? Of the many suggestions for determining tip projection,[29–31] we prefer the 1:1 relationship between the length of the nasal base and the upper lip (**Fig. 12**). This, along with the previously noted examination of the base view, provides good evidence as to the length and strength of the medial crura that naturally form the basis for the desired double break and good tip support (**Fig. 13**).

If the preoperative diagnosis shows a need for actual change in tip projection or if there is divergence of the medial crura, we use some form of

TIP PROJECTION

> 1:1 <

Fig. 12. Adequate tip projection will have a 1:1 ratio between the length of the base of the nose and the upper lip, as demonstrated in the center figure.

VDD in more than 80% of cases. The term VDD was introduced by the senior author in the late 1970s,[32,33] as a generic reference to various tip techniques. The prototype is the Goldman, but also included and used more frequently are the Simons modification and the hockey-stick variations.

With any of these tip alignments done through the endonasal approach wide exposure is critical. Following the previously outlined transfixion incisions, the marginal delivery technique readily allows for good visualization of the medial and lateral crura. For easier delivery of the entire lobular complex, it is important to extend the medial portion of the marginal incision along a decent portion of the anterior columella (**Fig. 14**).

No incisions are made in the dome until both chondrocutaneous arches have been delivered. With thick skin the undermining is more superficial so that subcutaneous fat can be removed from the cartilage en bloc. In all cases, but especially those presenting with medical crural divergence, it is beneficial to remove the fat from the intradomal space. Here, postoperative scarring helps with medial stabilization.

In the Goldman tip technique, the importance of the medial crura leading the lateral is critical.[34] The division of medial from lateral is made through the cartilage and the underlying vestibular mucosa and skin (**Fig. 15**). The right angle hook helps to deliver the lobular dome and mark its apex. Two to three millimeters along the caudal border is the borrowing boundary and it represents the extension of tip projection (**Fig. 16**). The medial components delivered into the right nostril are sutured together with 4-0 chromic catgut, providing an excellent, natural chondrocutaneous strut.

If there is question of need for additional support, a cartilaginous strut is placed sagittally between the

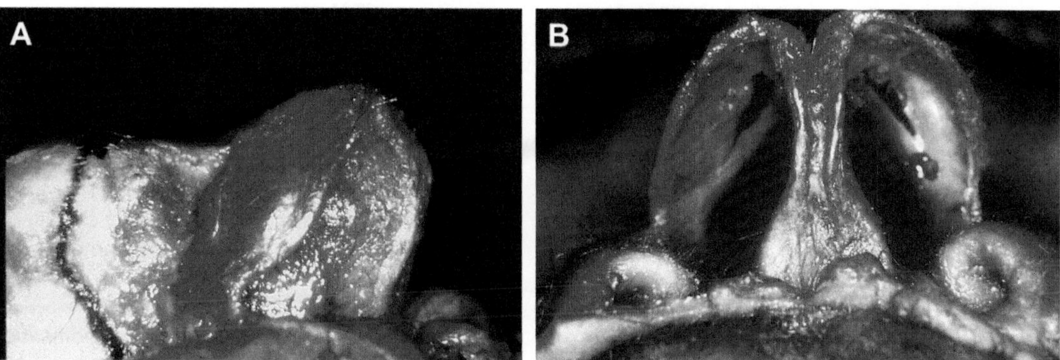

Fig. 13. Anatomic evidence of desired medial and lateral support provided by lower alar cartilage.

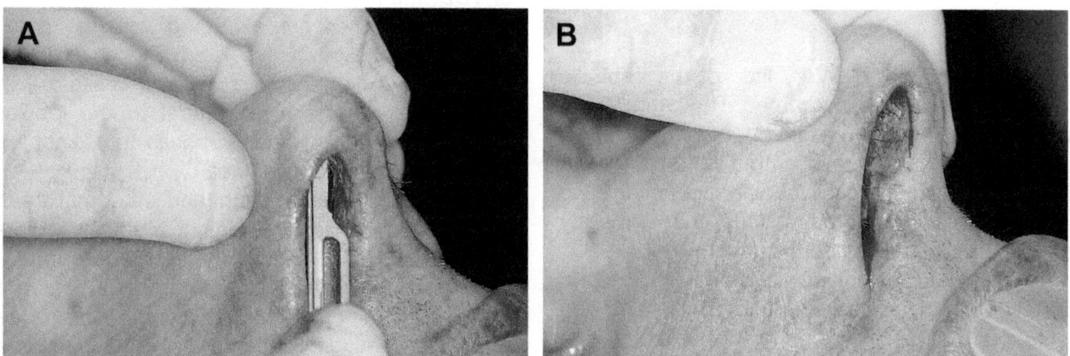

Fig. 14. The marginal incision is begun behind the facet and extended 50% along the anterior columella.

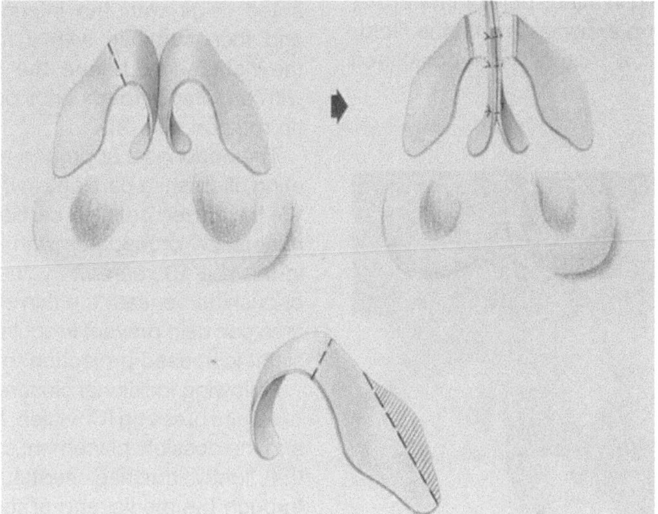

Fig. 15. Schematic representation of Goldman tip technique, with suturing together of augmented medial crura, including vestibular skin. Note small amount of excised lower lateral cartilage.

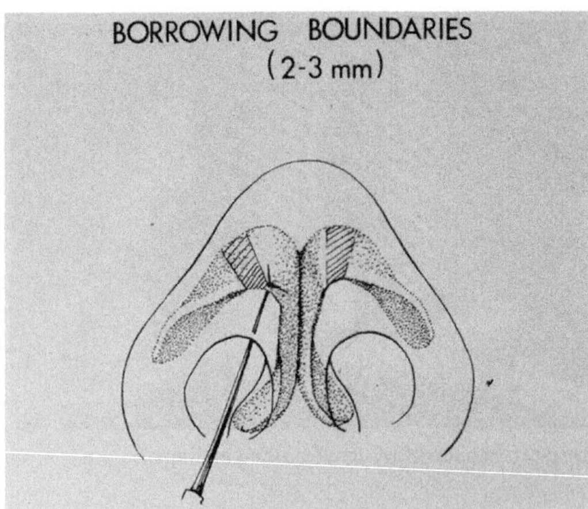

Fig. 16. Drawing of right-angled hook at dome. Notice the figuratively planned vertical dome division (as shown by diagonal lines) borrowing no more than 2 to 3 mm along the caudal border.

medial crura (**Fig. 17**). Very little of the cephalic border of lateral crus is trimmed. The lateral crura are repositioned by closure of the marginal incisions with 4-0 chromic catgut sutures placed obliquely to encourage medial movement. No attempt is made to reconstitute the dome by suturing the medial to lateral cut ends.

The Goldman technique,[35] used in approximately 13% of our cases, is superb for achieving increased projection or changing the direction of a plunging, ptotic nasal tip. Its use in the older patient with a perceived dorsal hump caused by increasingly poor tip support, allows for a more youthful appearance without any significant modification in the dorsal line (**Figs. 18** and **19**).

Rather than resulting in a tent-pole or lateral alar collapse, our long-term experience with the Goldman tip attests to a natural well-positioned appearance.[36,37] These results are accomplished by adhering to the incisional, repositioning tenets of avoiding significant excisions, that is, the minimal removal of lateral crus or cephalic or caudal septum.

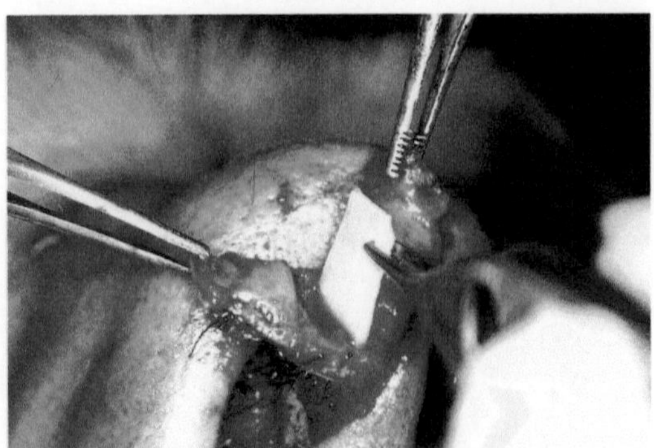

Fig. 17. Intraoperative photo of cartilaginous strut placed between medial crura.

Obviously, no one tip technique is appropriate in all cases. We use some form of VDD in more than 80% of primary noses. For the majority of patients for whom tip rotation, narrowing, symmetry, and modest changes in projection are indicated, our modification of VDD is most effective.[38]

Similarities between the Simons modification and the Goldman technique include cartilage incision and mobilization with little tissue excision. Differences involve preserving the intact underlying bridge of skin and mucosa and the use of a permanent nylon suture to approximate and influence the rotation of the medial crura (**Fig. 20**).

In the Simons modification, as with other forms of VDD, the lobular apices are identified individually when domes are extracted with the right-angled hook. Soft tissue is invariably removed from the intradomal space. In most cases a V of cartilage is removed just lateral to the lobular apex, along with a small cephalic trim, keeping the underlying mucosa intact.

It is important that the right and left domal areas be incised at similar positions. It is equally important that the placement of the suture to approximate the domal area, is made so that it does not create asymmetry. By delivering the medial edge of the left domal incision into the right nostril, fine visualization and control of both medial cuts is achieved.

Generally using a 5-0 clear nylon suture placed in a buried horizontal mattress fashion, it is important to place the superior bite closer to the transected edge with the inferior exit more medial, and then continue with a mirrored passage on the right edge, before the suture is tied down with an inferior to superior pull to enhance better tip rotation (**Fig. 21**).

The endonasal approach also allows the pocketing of crushed cartilage in the infralobular space. We have used crushed cartilage as a final touch in rhinoplasty procedures with increasing frequency in the last 15 years. Its value as a softening filler or cushion beneath the thin skin of the infralobular area can help prevent irregularities or even provide slight increased projection to the tip.

Following incisional closure, internal positioning of a Telfa dressing (Covidien, Mansfield, MA, USA), and the possible placement of a columellar batten, the lightly crushed septal cartilage is placed through the medial end of the right marginal incision and manually molded into place. It is this use of pockets and crushed cartilage fillers that

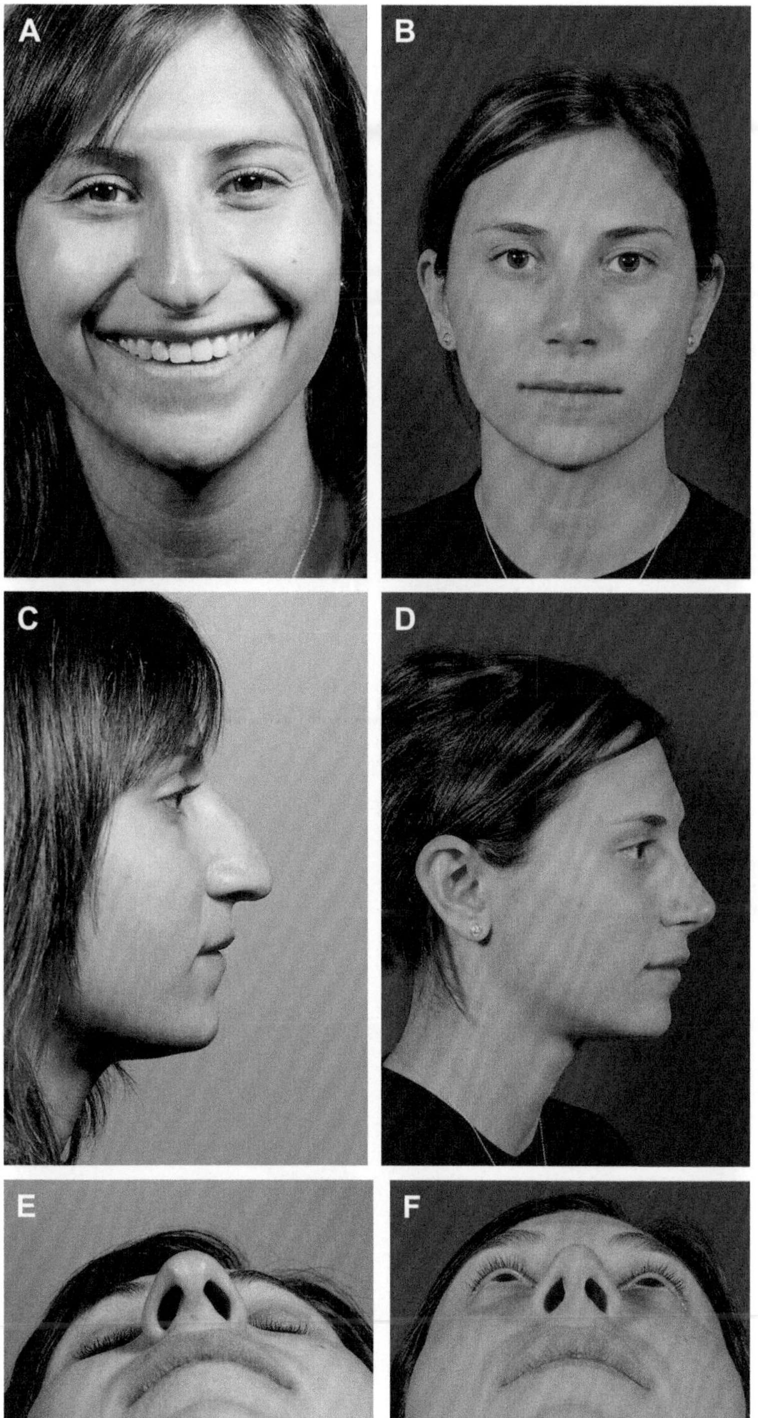

Fig. 18. (*A, C, E*) Preoperative views of young woman with dorsal hump and underprojected tip. (*B, D, F*) 2-year postoperative views of same woman after rhinoplasty with the Goldman technique.

benefits greatly from the endonasal approach in both primary and secondary cases (**Fig. 22**).

Our third variation of VDD, the hockey-stick technique, is used in patients with an over-projected tip. The domal excess is excised symmetrically, using 2-mm boundaries laterally and medially from the lobular apex.[39,40] The underlying mucosa is kept intact and the medial

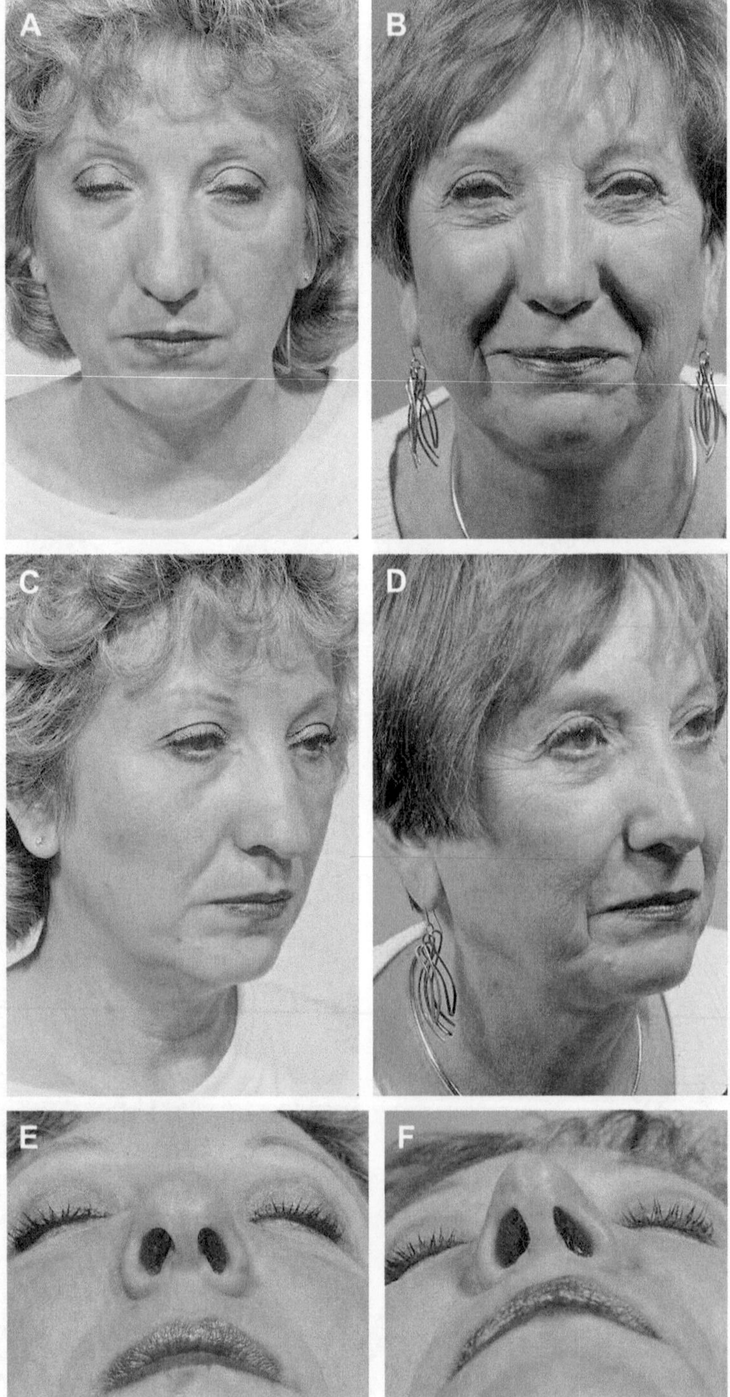

Fig. 19. (*A, C, E*) Preoperative views of older woman with under-rotated tip. (*B, D, F*) 17-year postoperative views of the same woman after rhinoplasty with the Goldman technique. The change in tip direction and dorsal strength are maintained long-term.

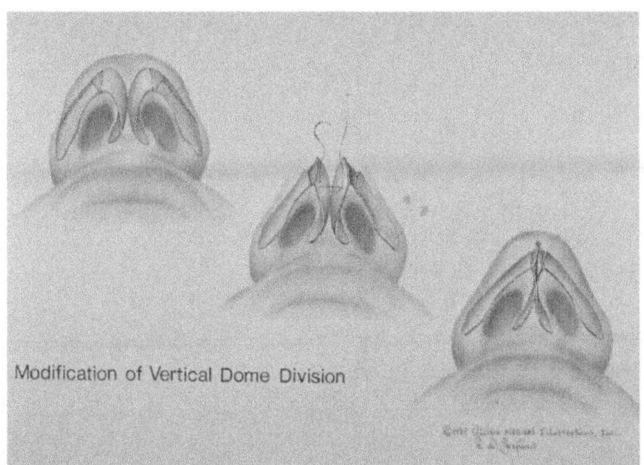

Fig. 20. Simons modification of vertical dome division. V-excision with conservative removal of cartilages is shown on the left. In the center diagram, note that the suture is placed in a horizontal mattress fashion with the needle closer to the superior edge than the more medial inferior exit. The diagram on the right demonstrates the results of Simons modification after suture placement. The alar cartilages are returned to the natural position. The pyramidal appearance of the base is achieved.

cartilages are coapted with suture. By shortening the medial crura de-rotation and de-projection of the tip are created (**Figs. 23** and **24**).

With the hockey-stick technique, more alar cartilage may be debulked or removed than with other procedures.[41] It is extremely important, however, to abide by the old adage "leave behind more than you take." When treating the over-projected tip, the concepts of conservative surgery and facial harmony may well prompt the use of dorsal and chin augmentation with grafts or implants. Frequently in the heavy ethnic base, the tip may also benefit from defattening. Superficial delivery of the lobular complex through endonasal marginal incisions allows ready removal of the fatty soft tissue overlying the alar cartilages.

At the end of the operation, a lobular cinch dressing of clear tape is used to medialize the lobule, with Telfa pads as internal dressing for 2 to 3 days. The tape and plaster cast external dressing is removed approximately 4 to 6 days postoperatively. A flesh-colored tape dressing is reapplied for a few more days for comfort, to further encourage reduction of swelling, and provide a cautionary sign to avoid trauma.

Before surgery, every patient is counseled about the postoperative period. Although most patients return to work and normal activities within 1 to 2 weeks following surgery, all patients must be reassured that full recovery generally takes months, not days or weeks, to occur. With the expected natural resolution of swelling and its concomitant subtle changes, it is generally best to resist desires for revision for at least 1 year.[42] The exceptions for

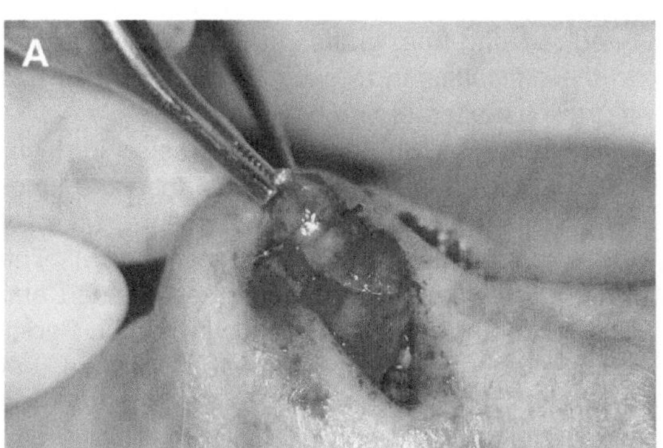

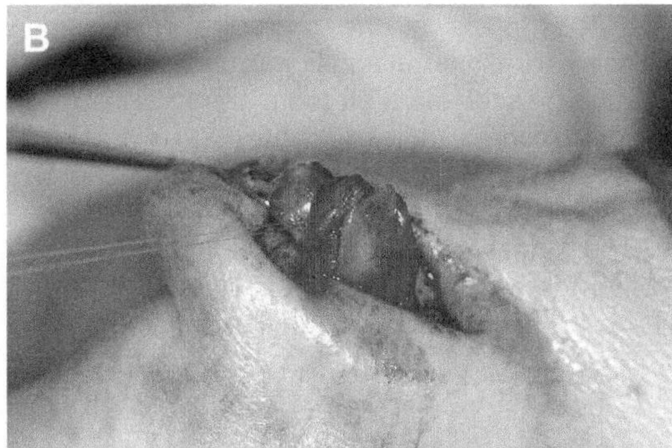

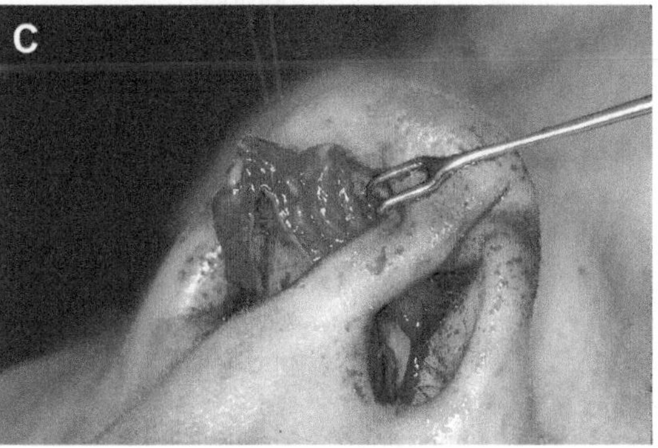

Fig. 21. Intraoperative photos of Simons modification as shown in **Fig. 20**.

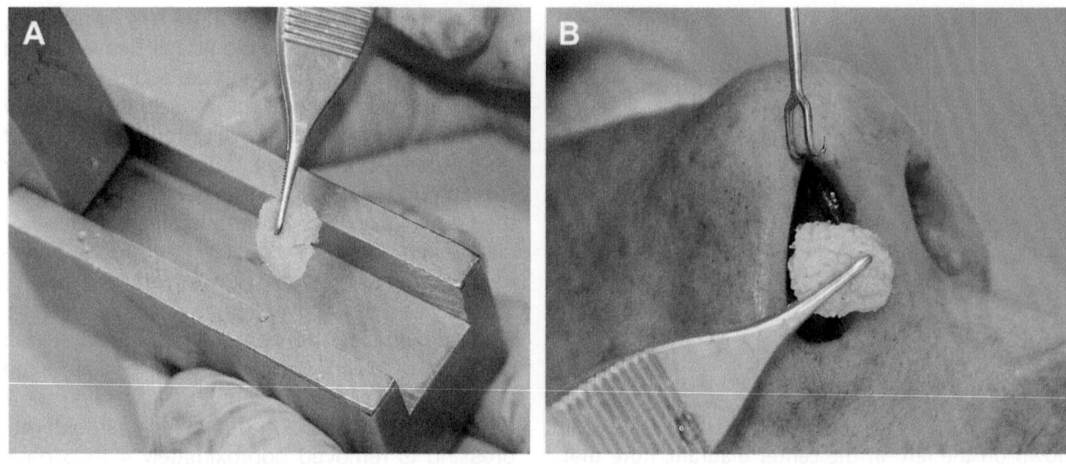

Fig. 22. (*A*) Septal cartilage morselized in Cottle crusher and (*B*) placed into infralobular area.

the 1-year revisional wait rule are infrequent, but may include graft or cartilage displacement, bony asymmetry because of a poor osteotomy, prolapsed lower laterals, or intranasal septal synechiae.

Revision of one's own work is measurably different from the revision of another surgeon's efforts. Emotions, cost, prior approach may all be involved in heightening the concerns when assuming the care of a patient dissatisfied with the work of a previous surgeon. The ongoing relationship with the patient and family, knowledge of what took place at the original surgery, and a desire to minimize additional charges makes the revision scenario a bit more comfortable. The authors' records indicate about 5% revision of primary cases, which doubles when operating on the twisted nose.

As in primary cases, the principal author also prefers the endonasal approach in revisions.[43] It allows for adjustments of addition or subtraction through direct, smaller pockets without completely dismantling the previous surgery. It is only in the case of patients presenting with extreme scarring, loss of tissue, and need for major reconstruction that the authors favor the external approach.

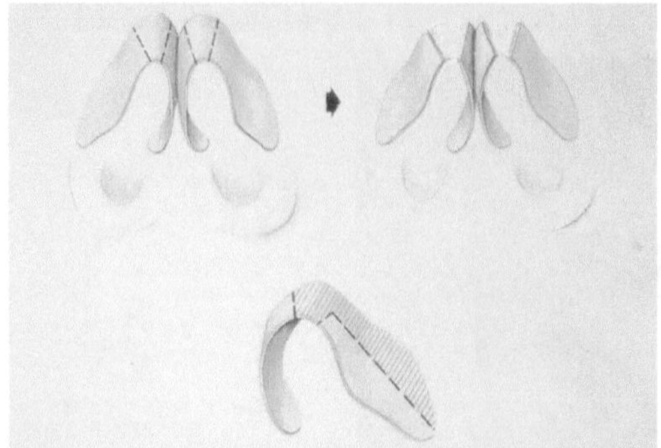

Fig. 23. The hockey-stick technique shows de-bulking of cartilage, with preservation of underlying mucosa.

One would imagine that tissue loss would not be a problem in noses originally operated on by the open-structured approach. However, it is disturbing to find the precious septal cartilage reserve can be generally depleted by the previous external procedure. Lack of grafting material and heightened scarring from grafts in the tip area may add to the difficulties in revising a nose that has had a previous external procedure.

For surgeons who are truly interested in rhinoplasty, there is no better teacher than the long-term follow-up of one's own patients. Most of these encounters are pleasant (**Fig. 25**). The majority of rhinoplasty patients are pleased and grateful for the surgery 10 to 20 years later. Rarely is the surgeon-student completely satisfied, but a fifth or sixth opportunity to reassess work is wonderfully instructional, albeit at times, humbling.

The less frequent examples of unfavorable sequelae generally bespeak a missed diagnosis, unexpected healing, or too aggressive surgery. The long-term problems of excessive scarring or shrink-wrappage continue to challenge and frustrate the experienced surgeon. The authors expect a greater use of fillers or cushioning agents to offset extreme redrapage problems in the future.

Where else are surgeons heading with rhinoplasty? It is an operation that will remain the number one personal preference for most facial plastic surgeons. Scientifically, technological advances will most likely involve more computer

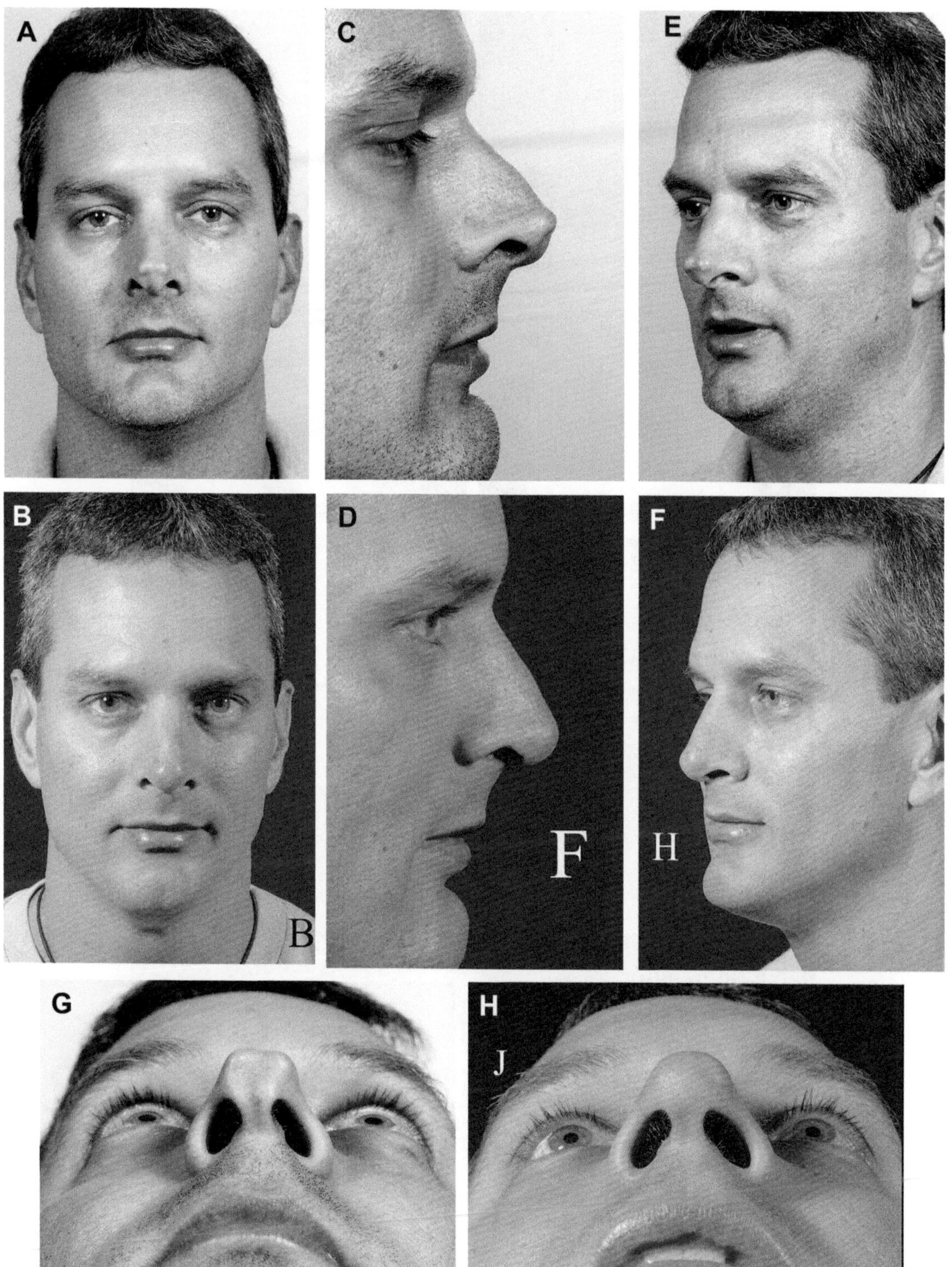

Fig. 24. (*A, C, E, G*) Preoperative view of patient with pre-existing natural bossae and over-rotated and over-projected tip. (*B, D, F, H*) 1-year postoperative view of same patient. Tip is de-projected and bossae are effaced with hockey-stick excision, lateral alar battens, and crushed cartilage in the infradomal area.

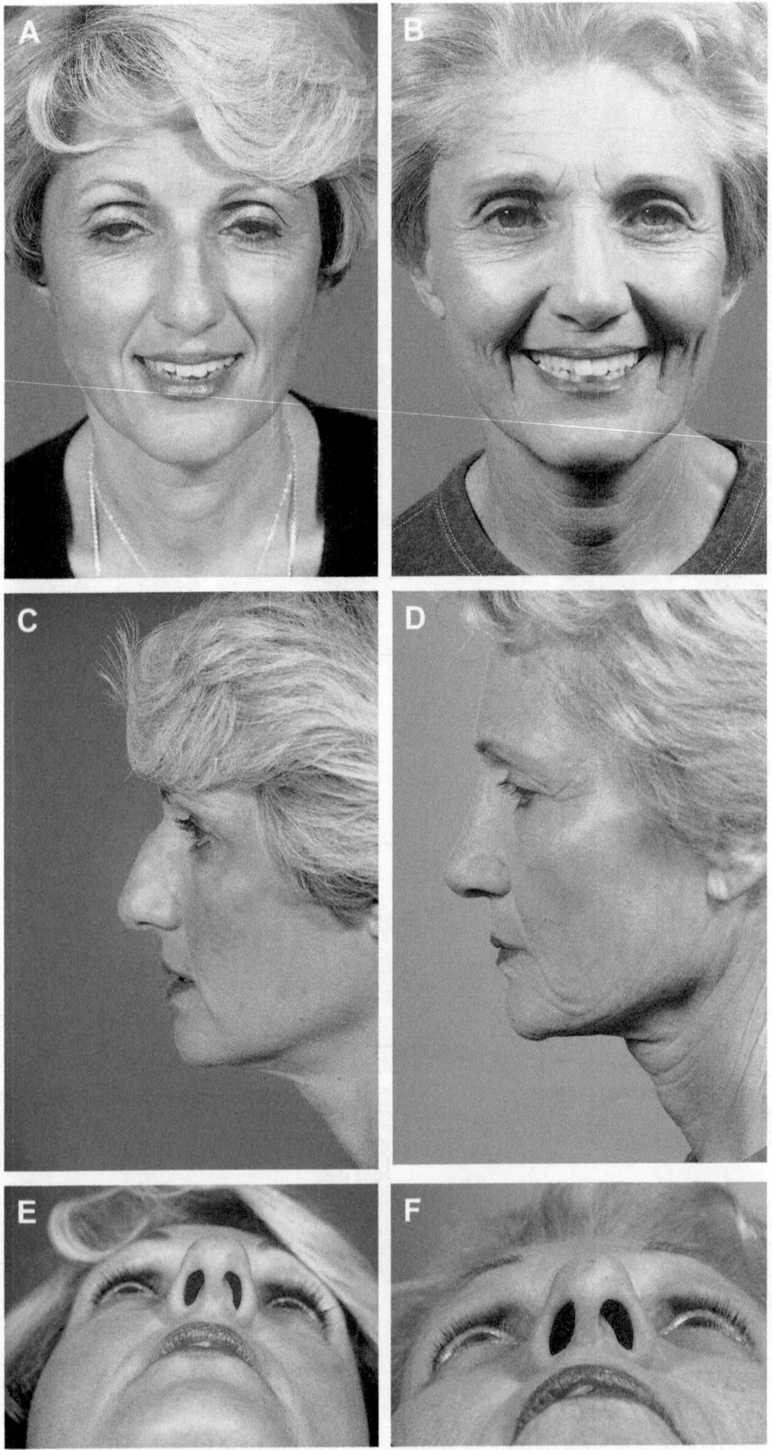

Fig. 25. Three happy patients with greater than 20-year follow-ups using different tip techniques. (*A–F*) Complete strip. (*G–L*) Simons modification, (*M–R*) Hockey-stick.

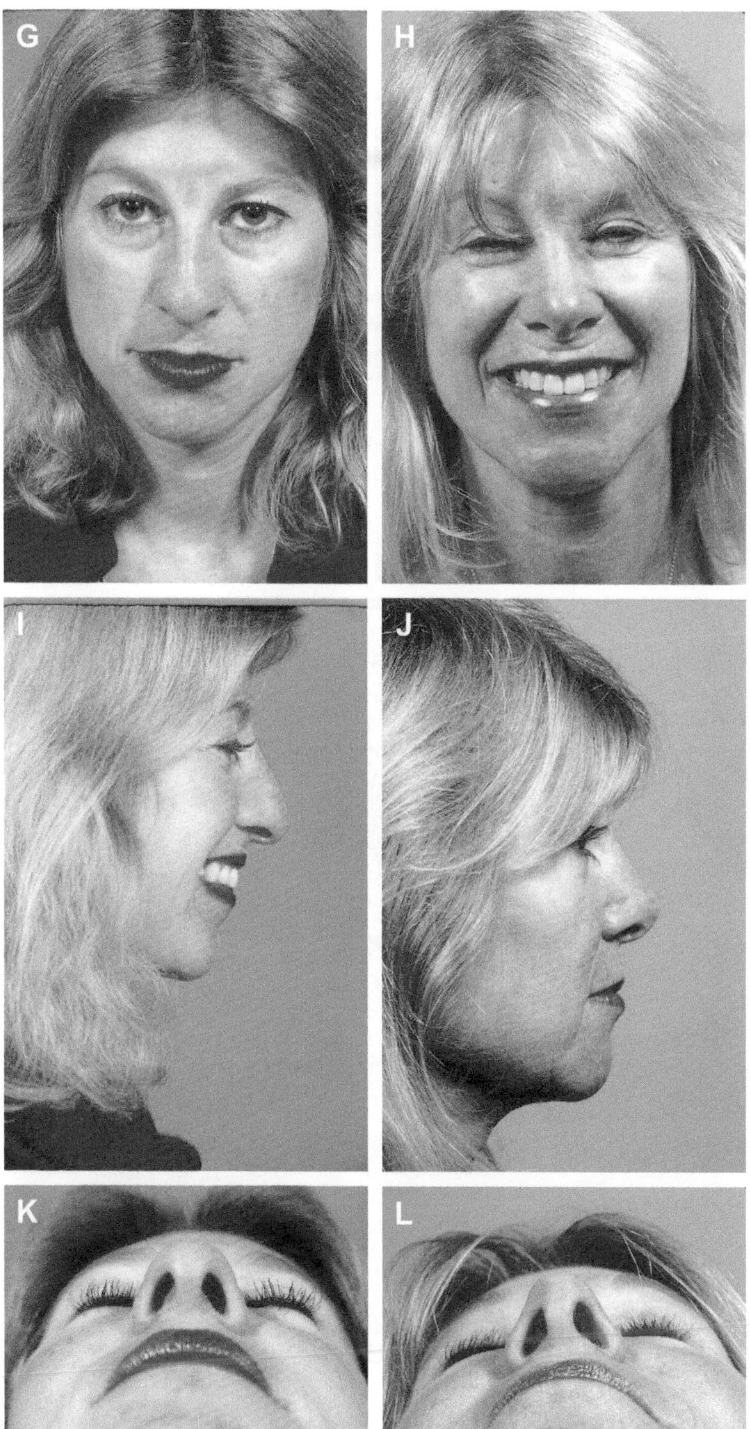

Fig. 25. (*continued*)

assistance and improved choices for implant materials. Artistically, the rational appeal of various approaches and techniques will continue to engage the student of rhinoplasty.

The institutional pendulum, having swung widely toward the external approach and structural grafts, will ultimately rebalance. In the future there will be a rediscovery and renewed enthusiasm for the

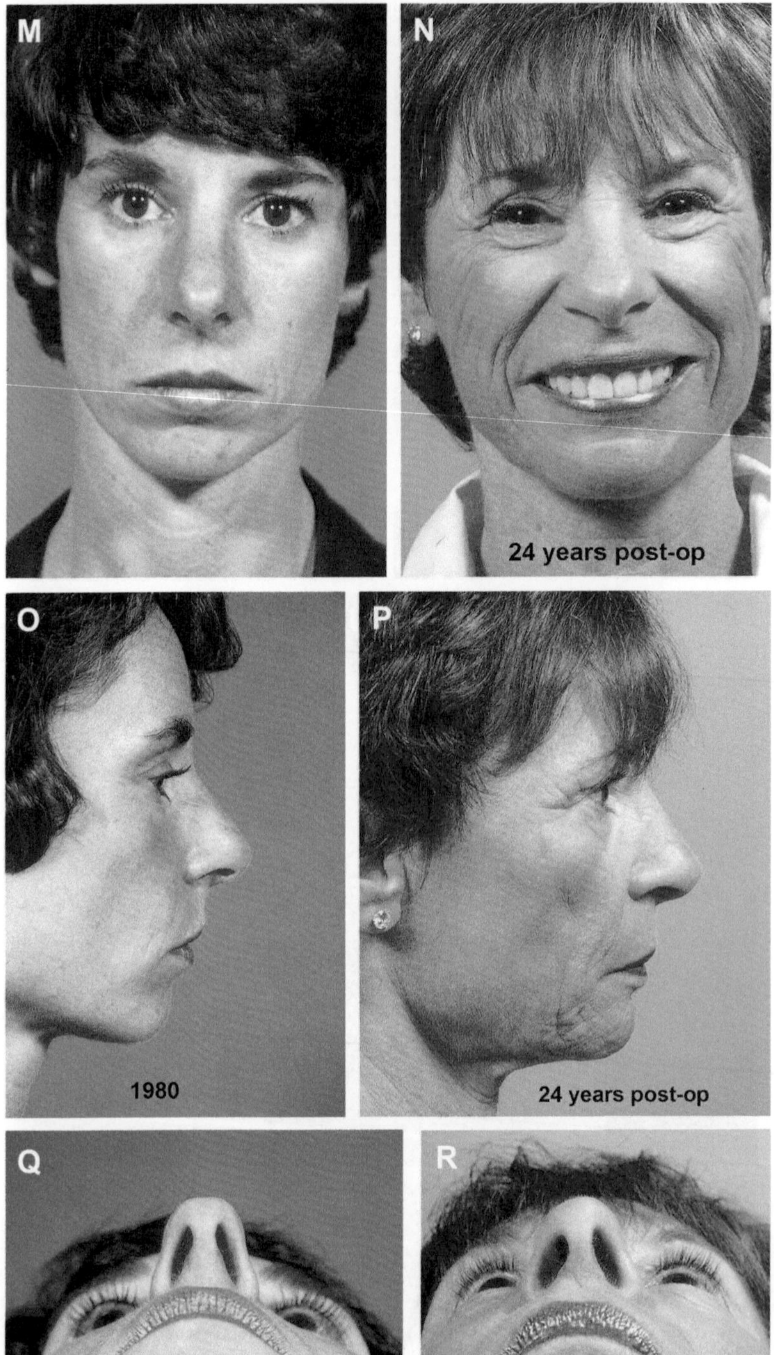

Fig. 25. (*continued*)

beauty, artistry, delicacy, and versatility of rhinoplasty performed through the endonasal approach.

REFERENCES

1. Simons RL. A personal report: emphasizing the endonasal approach. Facial Plast Surg Clin North Am 2004;12(1):15–34.
2. Simons RL, Rhee JS. Surgery of the nasal tip: vertical dome division. In: Papel ID, Frodel JL, Holt GR, Larrabee WF, et al, editors. Facial plastic and reconstructive surgery. New York: Thieme; 2009. p. 577–88.
3. Simons RL. Adjunctive measures in rhinoplasty. Otolaryngol Clin North Am 1975;8(3):717–42.
4. Gillman GS, Simons RL, Lee DJ. Nasal tip bossae in rhinoplasty: etiology, predisposing factors, and

management techniques. Arch Facial Plast Surg 1999;1(2):83–9.
5. Fomon S. The surgery of injury and plastic repair. Baltimore (MD): The Williams and Wilkins Company; 1939. p. 1409.
6. Fomon S, Goldman IB, Neivert H, et al. Management of deformities of the lower cartilaginous vault. Arch Otolaryngol 1951;54:467.
7. Cottle MH. Nasal roof repair and hump removal. Arch Otolaryngol 1954;60:408.
8. Safian J. Deceptive concepts of rhinoplasty. Plast Reconstr Surg 1956;18:127.
9. Goldman IB. Surgical tips on the nasal tip. EENT Monthly 1954;33:583–91.
10. Fomon S, Bell J. Rhinoplasty – new concepts: evaluation and application. Springfield (IL): Charles C Thomas; 1970. p. 314.
11. Padovan LF. External approach in rhinoplasty (decortication). Symp ORL 1960;4:354–60.
12. Padovan LF. External approach in rhinoplasty. Proceedings of the 1st International Symposium AAFPRS. New York, Grune and Stratton; 1972. p.143–6.
13. Goodman WS. External approach to rhinoplasty. Can J Otolaryngol 1973;2:207.
14. Anderson JR, Ries WR. Rhinoplasty: emphasizing the external approach. New York: Thieme Inc; 1986.
15. Johnson CM Jr, Toriumi DM. Open structure rhinoplasty. Philadelphia: WB Saunders; 1989.
16. Joseph J. Nasenplastik und sonstige Gesichtsplastik, nebst einem Anhang uber Mammaplastik. Leipzig (Germany): Curt Kabitzsch Publishers; 1931.
17. Sedwick JD, Lopez AB, Gajewski BJ, et al. Caudal septoplasty for treatment of septal deviation: aesthetic and functional correction of the nasal base. Arch Facial Plast Surg 2005;7(3):158–62.
18. Simons RL, Gillman GS. Rhinoplasty in the older patient. Aesthetic Plast Surg 2002;1(Suppl 26):S1.
19. Simons RL, Adelson RT. Rhinoplasty in male patients. Facial Plast Surg 2005;21(4):240–9.
20. Anderson JR. A reasoned approach to nasal base surgery. Arch Otolaryngol 1984;110:349–58.
21. Sheen JH. Aesthetic rhinoplasty. St. Louis (MO): CV Mosby; 1978.
22. Webster RC. Advances in surgery of the tip. Otolaryngol Clin North Am 1975;10:615–44.
23. Tardy ME. Rhinoplasty: the art and the science. Philadelphia: WB Saunders; 1996. p. 858.
24. McCullough EG. Surgery of the nasal tip. Otolaryngol Clin North Am 1987;20(4):769–84.
25. Kridel RW, Konior RJ. The underprojected tip. In: Krause C, Mangat D, Pastorek N, editors. Aesthetic facial surgery. Philadelphia: Lippincott-Williams and Wilkins; 1991. p. 191–228.
26. Gunter JP, Friedman RM. Lateral crural strut graft: technique and clinical applications in rhinoplasty. Plast Reconstr Surg 1997;99:943–55.
27. Toriumi DM. New concepts in nasal tip contouring. Arch Facial Plast Surg 2006;8(3):156–85.
28. Adamson PA, Litner JA, Dahiya R. The M-Arch model: a new concept of nasal tip dynamics. Arch Facial Plast Surg 2006;8(1):16–25.
29. Crumley RL, Lanser M. Quantitative analysis of nasal tip projection. Laryngoscope 1988;98(2):202–8.
30. Powell HP, Humphries B. Proportions of the aesthetic face. New York: Thieme-Stratton Inc; 1984. p. 72.
31. Simons RL. Nasal tip projection, ptosis and supratip thickening. Ear Nose Throat J 1982;61(8):452–5.
32. Simons RL. Nasal tip projection through vertical dome division. Proceedings of the Third International Symposium; 1979.
33. Simons RL. The difficult nasal tip. In: Gates G, editor. Current therapy in otolaryngology – head and neck surgery. Philadelphia: BC Decker; 1983. p. 122–5.
34. Goldman IB. The importance of the medial crura in nasal tip reconstruction. Arch Otolaryngol 1957;65: 143–7.
35. Simons RL, Beeson WH. Rhinoplasty. In: Beeson WH, McCullough EG, editors. Aesthetic surgery of the aging face. St. Louis (MO): Mosby; 1986. p. 296–350.
36. Simons RL, Fine IB. Evaluation of the Goldman tip in rhinoplasty. In: Sisson G, Tardy ME, editors. Plastic and reconstructive surgery of the face and neck, vol. I. Proceedings of the 2nd International Symposium; 1977. p. 38–46.
37. Davis AM, Simons RL, Rhee JS. Evaluation of the Goldman tip procedure in modern-day rhinoplasty. Arch Facial Plast Surg 2004;6(5):301–7.
38. Simons RL. Vertical dome division in rhinoplasty. Otolaryngol Clin North Am 1987;20(4):785–96.
39. Brown JB, McDonnell F. Plastic surgery of the nose. St. Louis (MO): CV Mosby; 1951.
40. Smith T. Reliable methods of tip reduction. Arch Otolaryngol 1978;104:6.
41. Chang CW, Simons RL. Hockey-stick vertical dome division technique for overprojected and broad nasal tips. Arch Facial Plast Surg 2008;10(2):88–92.
42. Simons RL, Gallo JF. Rhinoplasty complications. Facial Plast Surg Clin North Am 1994;2(4):521–9.
43. Simons RL, Grunebaum LD. The endonasal approach to rhinoplasty. In: Stucker FJ, De Souza C, Kenyon GS, et al, editors. Rhinology and facial plastic surgery. New York: Springer; 2009. p. 713–21.

Humpectomy and Spreader Flaps

Ronald P. Gruber, MD[a,b,*], Stephen W. Perkins, MD[c,d,e]

KEYWORDS

- Upper lateral cartilage • Rhinoplasty
- Humpectomy • Spreader grafts

Sheen,[1] Constantian and Clardy,[2] and others[3–9] established the importance of preserving the internal nasal valve area and reconstructing the middle one-third of the nose by spreader grafts. That concept was extended some years ago by trying to preserve the upper lateral cartilage (ULC) in a primary rhinoplasty and using it to act as a spreader graft, thereby minimizing the need to harvest additional cartilage. One of the first techniques to use the ULC as spreader grafts was described by Berkowitz[10] and Oneal and Berkowitz,[11] who gave it the name of "spreader flap." Seyhan[12] and Lerma[13] described the operation in an almost identical fashion. Rohrich and colleagues[14,15] described a variation of this operation, which they referred to as the "autospreader" or "turnover flap." Similarly, Fayman and Potgeister[16] (and also Sciuto and Bernardeschi[17]) recommended releasing the ULC from the dorsum, reducing the dorsal septum as needed, and then folding the ULC over the dorsum in a pants-over-vest fashion. Recently Byrd and colleagues[18] reviewed the entire spreader flap concept.

For many years, the concept of spreader flap was not popular. This was because of the fact that the original procedures involved complete scoring of the folded-over ULC. Doing so caused the flap to become very thin. It provided some width to the middle one-third of the nose, but it was often not enough. Only in recent years did it become apparent that scoring should be limited to the caudal end of the flap, where it normally narrows as the tip cartilages are approached.[19]

INDICATIONS

Any patient who has a hump that is to be resected is a candidate for the spreader flap/humpectomy approach. Most patients will be of the primary type, and the operations are easier to perform with an open approach. If, for some reason, the hump is too small to provide a substantial spreader flap, the surgeon can always replace the released ULC up against the dorsal septum to recreate the proper width and structural integrity of the middle one-third of the nose. Nothing is lost by attempting the spreader flap. Release of the ULC from the dorsal septum allows for a much easier humpectomy.

METHOD

Open Approach

1. After hyperinfiltration of the underside of the ULC and dorsal septum several minutes before actual dissection, the dorsal skin is elevated off the dorsum exposing the keystone area.
   - The periosteum is cleaned off the ULC/bone junction with a scalpel or periosteal elevator.
2. Beginning at the anterior septal angle, a tunnel is created with a Cottle elevator deep to the ULC at its junction with the dorsal septum. This tunnel continues all the way up to and just under the nasal bone (**Fig. 1**). The ULC is released from the dorsal septum with a scalpel

[a] Division of Plastic & Reconstructive Surgery, University of California (SF), San Francisco, CA, USA
[b] Division of Plastic & Reconstructive Surgery, Stanford University, Stanford, CA, USA
[c] Meridian Plastic Surgeons, 170 West 106th Street, Indianapolis, IN 46290, USA
[d] Meridian Plastic Surgery Center, 170 West 106th Street, Indianapolis, IN 46290, USA
[e] Department of Otolaryngology–Head and Neck Surgery, Indiana University School of Medicine, Indianapolis, IN, USA
* Corresponding author. 3318 Elm Street, Oakland, CA 94609.
E-mail address: rgrubermd@hotmail.com (R.P. Gruber).

Clin Plastic Surg 37 (2010) 285–291
doi:10.1016/j.cps.2009.12.004

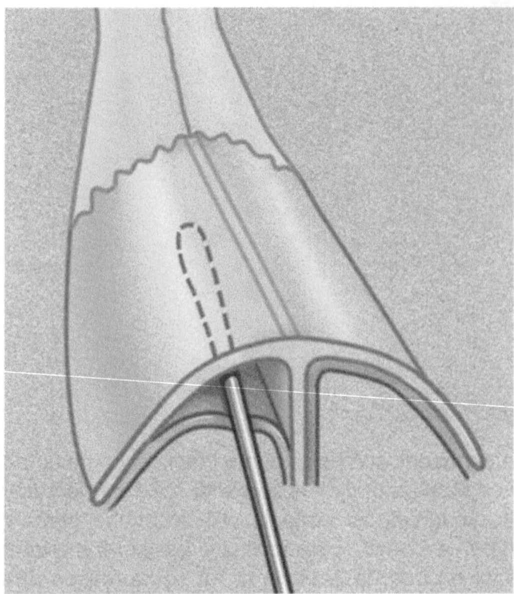

Fig. 1. Beginning at the anterior septal angle, a tunnel is created with a Cottle elevator deep to the ULC at its junction with the dorsal septum. This tunnel continues all the way up to and just under the nasal bone.

(**Fig. 2**). The mucoperichondrium of the septum is elevated off the septum for a distance of at least 2 cm. Doing so allows for better mobilization of the released ULCs. If a septoplasty is planned, the entire mucoperichondrium is released off both sides of the septum.

3. The medial aspect of the ULC is freed (disarticulated) from its attachment to the nasal

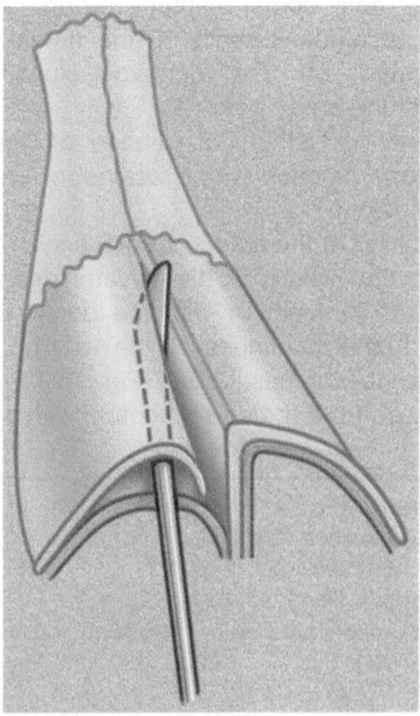

Fig. 2. The upper lateral cartilage is released from the dorsal septum with a scalpel.

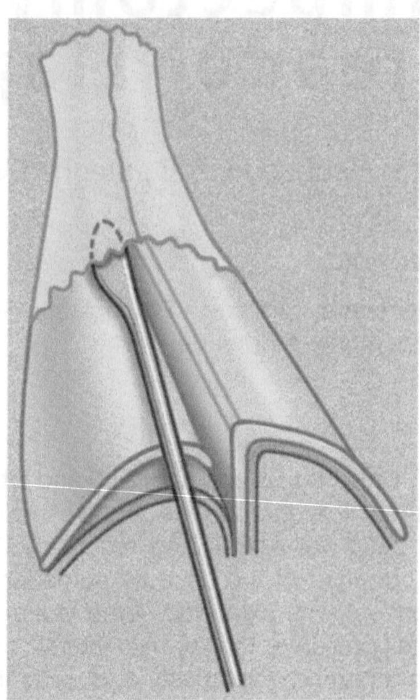

Fig. 3. The upper lateral cartilage is disarticulated from its attachment to the nasal bone with a Joseph periosteal elevator or scalpel.

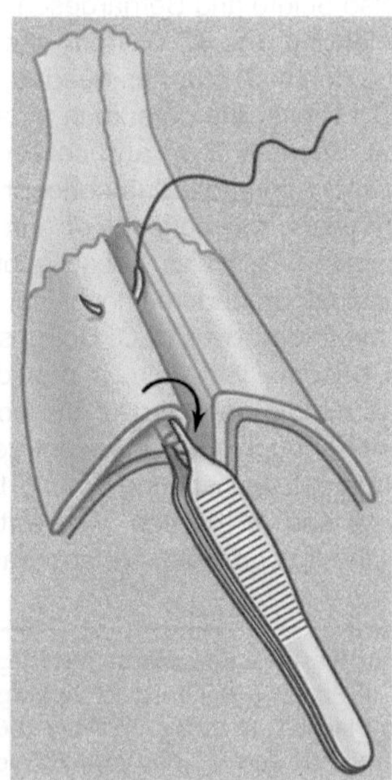

Fig. 4. The caudal end of the upper lateral cartilage is grasped with a clamp or Brown-Adson forceps and folded over. To maintain the folded over ULC, 5-0 polydioxone horizontal mattress sutures are placed in the ULC.

bone with a Joseph periosteal elevator or scalpel (**Fig. 3**). The caudal end of the ULC is grasped with a mosquito clamp (**Fig. 4**) and folded over. Mobility of the flaps is enhanced if there is an intercartilaginous incision. Even a very limited intercartilaginous incision is helpful so that a clamp can be applied to the caudal aspect of ULC where it is to be folded.

- Two 5-0 polydioxone (PDS) narrowly spaced sutures are used to maintain the fold of the ULC. The knot should not be so tight that the newly folded over spreader flap is narrowed more than desired.
- The more the ULC is folded over the lower it drops.
- If the ULC cannot be folded easily for any reason, the dorsal edge of the ULC is scored. This is seldom the case.
- Scoring is more appropriate (and may be essential) at the caudal end where the ULC normally tapers as it reaches the lateral crus.

4. The hump of the dorsal septum is incised (not removed yet) with a scalpel by placing it at the keystone area and removing the dorsal septum in retrograde fashion. The amount to remove is dictated by preoperative measurements with imaging.
5. An osteotomy is placed between the dorsal septum and cartilaginous hump. It is driven into the bone in a cephalic direction. The result is a humpectomy of a single unit consisting of cartilaginous septal hump and bony hump. Additional rasping is often necessary but should be done with a push rasp so that the cartilaginous septum is not disarticulated from the bone at the keystone junction.
6. The skin of the nose is redraped to assess adequacy of hump reduction.
7. Despite the fact that the ULC is usually no more than 1 mm thick, the width after being folded over can be substantial (**Figs. 5** and **6**) and

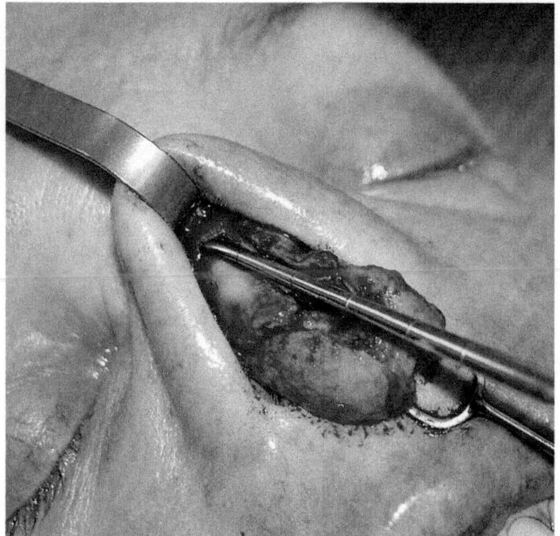

Fig. 5. Intraoperative view demonstrating folding over of the upper lateral cartilage to make a spreader flap.

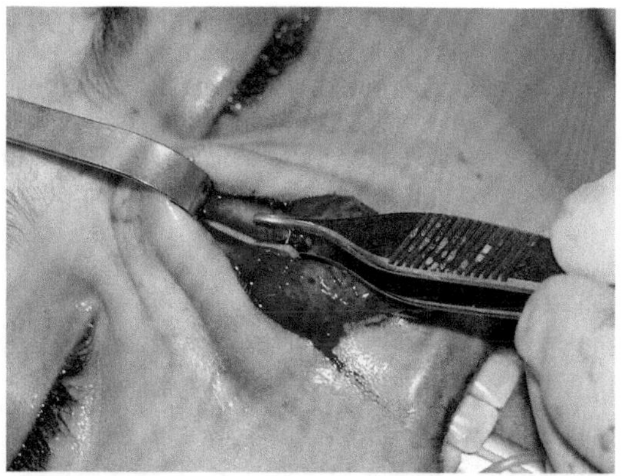

Fig. 6. Intraoperative view demonstrating the disarticulation of the upper lateral cartilage from the nasal bone so that it can be folded over to make a spreader flap.

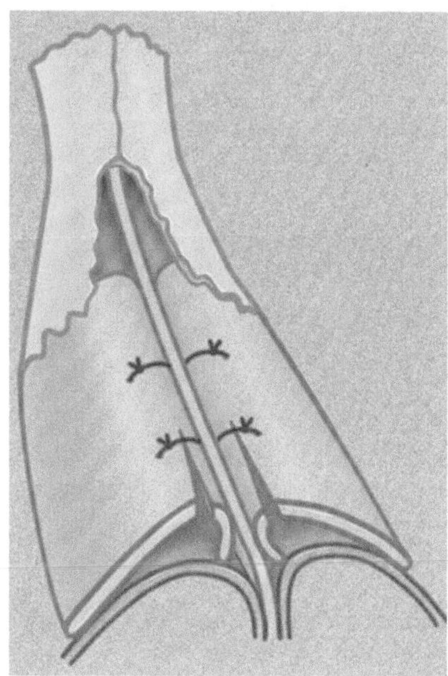

Fig. 7. The dorsal cartilaginous hump is shaved with a scalpel. The bone is removed with an osteotome. If a rasp is used, it should be a push rasp so as to not pull the cartilages off the bone. The newly made spreader flaps are secured to the dorsal septum with 5-0 PDS sutures. The caudal end may need to be narrowed as it approaches the lower lateral cartilages. This is done by scoring the caudal end of the spreader flaps.

can easily be up to 3 mm. Therefore, scoring is often necessary to narrow the flap, particularly at the caudal end where the ULC normally tapers. On average, the width of the completed spreader flap (in the middle portion) is 2 mm. In the event that the dorsal hump is small, there may not be enough ULC cartilage to make a flap. In that case the ULC is simply returned to the dorsal septum and secured with sutures.

8. Any septal straightening that needs to be done should be done at this time. Immediately afterward, the spreader flaps can be used to help

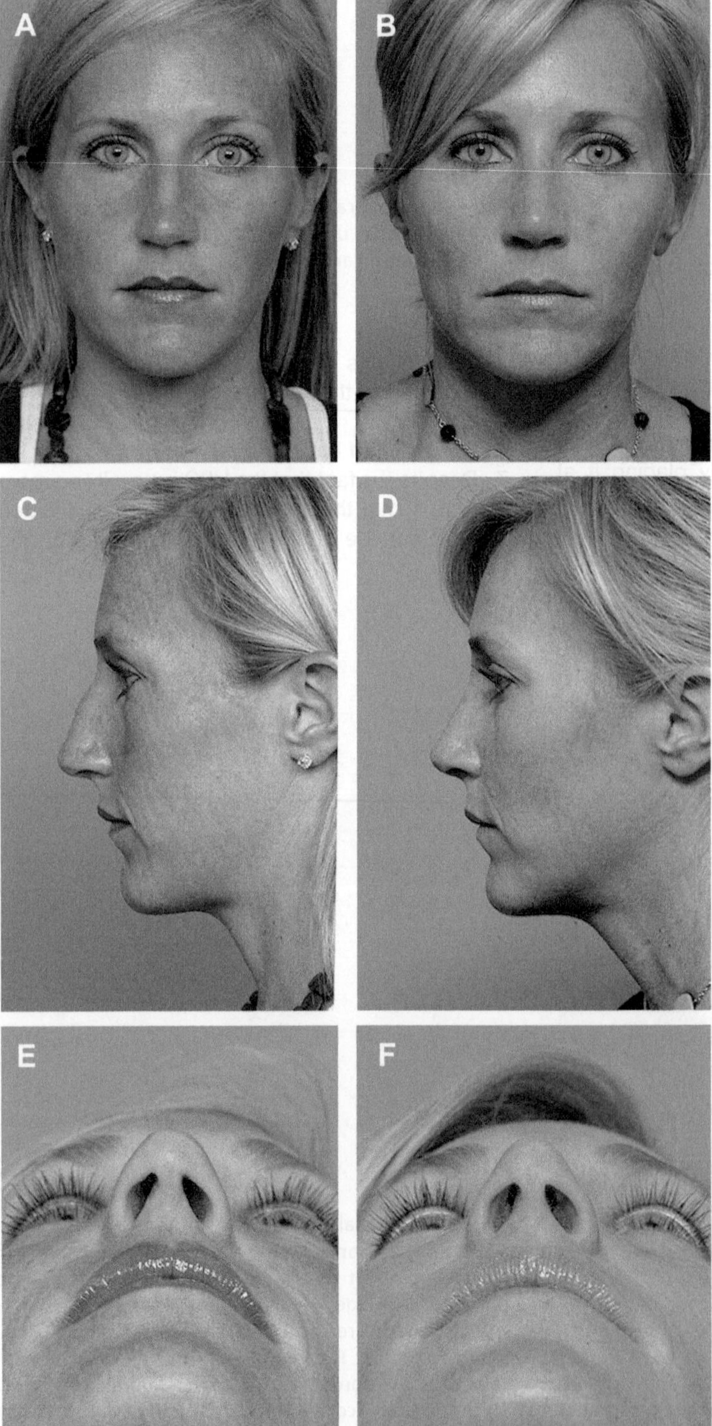

Fig. 8. Frontal (*A*), lateral (*C*), and basal (*E*) preoperative views of a patient who required a primary rhinoplasty, including humpectomy. Frontal (*B*), lateral (*D*), and basal (*F*) views of the patient 1 year postoperation, exhibiting proper width of the dorsum of the middle one-third of the nose without airway obstruction.

maintain septal straightness. The mosquito clamps act as the reins of a horse. By pulling them in one direction or another one can use them to line up a slightly crooked septum. A long No. 27 needle is used to skewer both spreader flaps and septum after all 3 are lined up in a straight fashion. Then 5-0 PDS sutures are used to secure the caudal ends of the

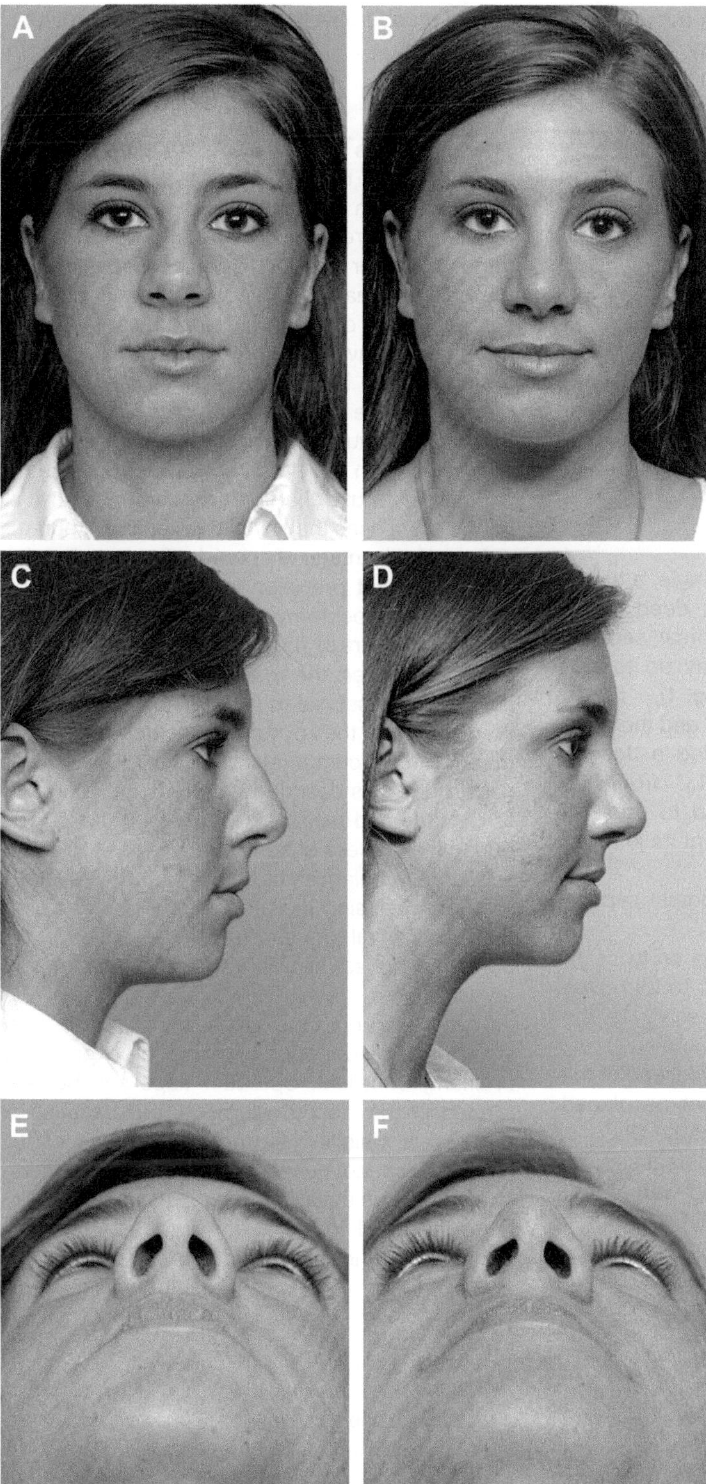

Fig. 9. Frontal (*A*), lateral (*C*), and basal (*E*) preoperative views of a patient who required a primary rhinoplasty, including humpectomy. The patient received spreader flaps as described. Frontal (*B*), lateral (*D*), and basal (*F*) views of patient 1 year postoperation, showing proper width of the dorsum of the middle one-third of the nose without airway obstruction.

spreader flaps to the dorsal septal cartilage (**Fig. 7**).[20]

9. If, for any reason, the spreader flaps are too small to permit the construction of a proper width flap, they can be returned to the dorsal septum and simply sutured in place. If there is still inadequate width to the middle one-third of the nose, one simply resorts to spreader grafts as is conventionally done.
10. The intraoperative views in **Figs. 5** and **6** show the process of disarticulation of the ULC from the nasal bone and folding over the ULC to make a spreader flap.

Closed Approach

The spreader flap is difficult in the closed approach and should not be attempted until after one is comfortable with doing it in the open approach. It is usually too difficult to apply a mattress suture to the dorsum of the spreader flap except at its caudal end. It is also usually difficult to visualize and free the ULC from its attachment to the nasal bone. Therefore, the following maneuvers are performed:

1. Beginning at the anterior septal angle, a tunnel is created with a Cottle elevator deep to the ULC at its junction with the dorsal septum. This tunnel continues all the way up to and just under the nasal bone (see **Fig. 1**).
2. The attachment between the ULC and the nasal bone is blindly released by using a Joseph elevator to disarticulate the ULC from the bone. A Joseph elevator is used to press in a posterior direction on the ULC at its junction with the bone.
3. The ULC is released from the dorsal septum with a knife (see **Fig. 2**).
4. The dorsal edge is scored once or twice to allow the dorsal edge of the ULC to fold over. Scoring is almost always necessary in the closed approach.
5. A suture is applied only at the caudal end of the folded-over ULC. A suture cannot be placed easily in the more cephalic part of the ULC.
6. After removing the hump of the dorsal septum with a scalpel and the bony hump with an osteotome, the caudal end of the ULC is sutured to the dorsal septum (with 5-0 PDS sutures).
7. A spreader graft is used if the spreader flap method fails to provide adequate width to the middle one-third of the nose.

EXAMPLES

Fig. 8 is an example of a patient who underwent a primary rhinoplasty, including humpectomy and spreader flaps, using an open approach. At approximately 1 year postoperation, the patient exhibited an appropriate width to the middle one-third of the nose. The patient exhibited no subjective evidence of airway obstruction. **Fig. 9** is a similar example of a patient with thinner skin, shown preoperatively and 1 year postoperation.

DISCUSSION

Spreader grafts[1,2] are the gold standard for reconstructing the middle one-third of the nose. However, when a hump exists, spreader flaps can invariably be created and can act as a substitute for the spreader graft. The spreader flap minimizes the need for harvesting additional material. The spreader flap can prevent functional problems (such as an inverted V deformity) by increasing the size of the internal nasal valve angle and by maintaining the width of the middle one-third of the nose. Because scoring has been minimized or eliminated from the old spreader flap technique, it is possible to use the spreader flap in almost all rhinoplasty cases that involve a significant hump.

A great advantage of spreader flap construction is the resultant precision in humpectomy. Traditionally, humpectomy has been considered a mundane part of rhinoplasty in contrast to tipplasty. However, the reality is that humpectomy is frequently associated with postoperative dorsal irregularities at the keystone area. Before a procedure for the accurate release of the ULC from the nasal bone was described, there was a tendency to damage and tear the cephalic end of the ULC during the process of bony hump removal. This resulted in irregularities of cartilage at the keystone area. By releasing the medial aspect of the ULC from the nasal bone, the caudal edge of the bone is exposed, allowing accurate placement of an osteotome.

The open approach lends itself well to constructing spreader flaps because the exposure is ordinarily excellent. Spreader flaps can be performed in the closed approach, but because of the poorer visibility, all the components of the technique cannot necessarily be executed. Therefore, scoring is usually needed. One should anticipate the need for spreader grafts if attempting spreader flaps in the closed approach.

REFERENCES

1. Sheen JH. Spreader graft: a method of reconstructing the roof of the middle nasal vault following rhinoplasty. Plast Reconstr Surg 1984; 73:230–9.

2. Constantian MB, Clardy RB. The relative importance of septal and nasal valvular surgery in correcting airway obstruction in primary and secondary rhinoplasty. Plast Reconstr Surg 1996; 98:38–54.
3. Perkins SW. The evolution of the combined use of endonasal and external columellar approaches to rhinoplasty. Facial Plast Surg Coin North Am 2004; 12:35–50.
4. Constantinedes MS, Adamson PA, Cole P. The long-term effects of open cosmetic septorhinoplasty on nasal air flow. Arch Otolaryngol Head Neck Surg 1996;122:1–45.
5. Gunter JP, Rohrich RJ. Correction of the pinched nasal tip with alar spreader grafts. Plast Reconstr Surg 1992;90:821–9.
6. Guyuron B, Varghai A. Lengthening the nose with a tongue-and-groove technique. Plast Reconstr Surg 2003;112:1533–9.
7. Rohrich RJ, Hollier LH. Use of spreader grafts in the external approach to rhinoplasty. Clin Plast Surg 1996;23:255–62.
8. Schlosser RJ, Park SS. Functional nasal surgery. Otolaryngol Clin North Am 1999;32:37–51.
9. Stal S, Hollier L. The use or resorbable spacers for nasal grafts. Plast Reconstr Surg 2000;106: 922–8.
10. Berkowitz, RL. Barrel vault technique for rhinoplasty. Presented at the poster session of the 28th Annual Meeting of the American Society for aesthetic plastic surgery. San Francisco, March 1995.
11. Oneal RM, Berkowitz RL. Upper lateral cartilage spreader flaps in rhinoplasty. Aesthet Surg J 1998; 18:370–1.
12. Seyhan A. Method for middle vault reconstruction in primary rhinoplasty: upper lateral cartilage bending. Plast Reconstr Surg 1997;100:1941.
13. Lerma J. Reconstruction of the middle vault: the "lapel" technique. Cir Plast Iberio-Latinoam 1995; 21:207.
14. Rohrich RJ. Treatment of the nasal hump with preservation of the cartilaginous framework. Plast Reconstr Surg 1999;103:1729–33 [discussion: 1734–5].
15. Rohrich RJ, Muzaffar AR, Janis JE. Component dorsal hump reduction: the importance of maintaining dorsal aesthetic lines in rhinoplasty. Plast Reconstr Surg 2004;114:1298–308.
16. Fayman MS, Potgieter E. Nasal middle vault support-a new technique. Aesthetic Plast Surg 2004;28:375–80.
17. Sciuto S, Bernardeschi D. Upper lateral cartilage suspension over dorsal grafts: a treatment for internal nasal valve dynamic incompetence. Facial Plast Surg 1999;15:309–16.
18. Byrd HS, Meade RA, Gonyon DL Jr. Using the autospreader flap in primary rhinoplasty. Plast Reconstr Surg 2007;119:1897–902.
19. Gruber RP, Park E, Newman J, et al. The spreader flap in primary rhinoplasty. Plast Reconstr Surg 2007;119:1903–10.
20. Guyuron B, Uzzo CD, Scull H. A practical classification of septonasal deviation and an effective guide to septal surgery. Plast Reconstr Surg 1999;104:2202–9.

Rhinoplasty: Dorsal Grafts and the Designer Dorsum

Rollin K. Daniel, MD*

KEYWORDS

• Dorsal graft • Diced cartilage • Fascia • Dermis

Over the last 2 decades, many of the difficulties in shaping primary tips and rebuilding destroyed secondary tips have been solved through the use of tip sutures and grafts. Dorsal grafts have become the single greatest challenge in rhinoplasty for many reasons. Dorsal grafts are a highly visible determinant of the nasal profile and contour, as well as being technically demanding with a high complication rate. Due to these challenges, most surgeons try to avoid using a dorsal graft whenever possible, sometimes to the detriment of the final result. Over the last 7 years, the author's approach to dorsal grafts has dramatically altered because of surgical advances using fascia and diced cartilage, either separately or combined.[1,2] Thus, a new era in rhinoplasty has emerged with the advent of "The Designer Dorsum."

OVERVIEW

Ever since rhinoplasty began, a wide variety of dorsal grafts have been used with respect to composition and indications.[3] Early grafts were composed of virtually any material available, including ivory, gold, paraffin, duck bone, and glass. More recently, modern chemistry has brought in silicone, Gore-Tex (W.L. Gore & Associates Inc, Flagstaff, AZ, USA), Medpor (Porex Surgical Inc, Newnan, GA, USA), and a plethora of new fillers. The problem lies in the selection of the best material for an individual patient. In deciding which material to use, the critical factors are as follows: recipient site requirements, technical difficulty, resistance to infection, and both short- and long-term complication rates. When these factors are taken into consideration, autogenous grafts are clearly superior to alloplastic ones. Even so, the most common autogenous grafts used for dorsal grafts had technical problems rather than viability or compatibility difficulties, which forced surgeons to develop newer techniques.

Septal Cartilage

Septal cartilage is the gold standard of autogenous grafts in rhinoplasty, but its use as a dorsal graft has declined for 2 reasons. In many primary cases among Asians and also most secondary cases, septal material for a full-length dorsal graft (35 × 8 mm) is not available. Other challenges are the requisite height of the dorsal graft, and whether one stacks or bends the septal cartilage. Visibility is a major factor, at least short-term in thin skin patients, and long-term in patients with even an average skin envelope.

Conchal Cartilage

As championed by Sheen and Sheen,[4] auricular cartilage has been used extensively in nasal surgery. When it is used as a dorsal graft, surgeons have adopted the method of either suturing or layering to overcome its intrinsic curvature. Despite excellent results early on, the limitations of the conchal cartilage have become disappointingly apparent to patient and surgeon with time. The layered conchal graft requires

Aesthetic and Plastic Surgery Institute, University of California Irvine, CA, USA
* 1441 Avocado Avenue, SE 308, Newport Beach, CA 92666.
E-mail address: Rkdaniel@aol.com

Clin Plastic Surg 37 (2010) 293–300
doi:10.1016/j.cps.2009.12.009
0094-1298/10/$ – see front matter

dove-tail techniques to achieve length, and stacking to obtain height. Conchal grafts can be sutured transversely to increase their height, but their lateral junction with the underlying dorsum is always visible. Also, as the skin envelope tightens the intrinsic irregularity and asymmetry of the concha become more visible.

Rib Cartilage

Costal cartilage has been the material of choice for nasal reconstruction and repair of complex secondary rhinoplasty deformities.[5] The primary challenge is the prevention of warping of solid costal cartilage grafts.[6] The basic principle is to do "balanced cuts" to offset contracting forces once the peripheral cartilage has been excised during the shaping process. Although conceptually simple, warping will occur. Gunter and colleagues[7] inserted a K-wire into the center of the graft to prevent warping. Although probably effective, the reality is that the K-wire has a 10% morbidity ranging from extrusion to infection. Additional challenges of solid dorsal grafts include technical factors (misalignment, radix fullness, abnormal shape) and long-term issues (warping, visibility through thinned-out skin). Due to its inevitable absorption, cadaver costal cartilage is not recommended except in extenuating situations (older patient, ethnicity).

DESIGNER DORSAL GRAFTS

If all the classic autogenous techniques have major limitations, what is the solution? The answer is to have a highly flexible technique that can be designed to fit a specific defect, rather than inserting the same type of dorsal graft into a wide range of deformities. In the last 7 years, the author has used a combination of fascia and cartilage to fabricate a wide range of dorsal grafts.[5,8] These grafts can be classified in several ways. Based on composition, there are 4 types: (1) fascia, (2) diced cartilage (DC), (3) diced cartilage beneath fascia (DC + F), and (4) diced cartilage encased in fascia (DC – F). The shape of the grafts can vary widely to fit the defect with respect to length (partial or full-length) and thickness (1–8 mm, uniform thickness or tapered). Dermis grafts are used when the overlying skin envelope is damaged. Each of the specific grafts is discussed in detail.

Fascia (F)

Fascia is the ultimate material for concealment under thin skin and subtle augmentations in the 1- to 2-mm range.[9,10] The donor material of choice is deep temporal fascia for 4 reasons: (1) the fascia is ideal in thickness and pliability; (2) the donor site is hidden in the hair; (3) survival and resistance to infection is a virtual certainty; and (4) surgical morbidity is minimal. All alternative sources have limitations. Superficial temporal fascia is too thin, whereas tensor fascia lata leaves a visible scar. Rectus fascia, removed during a rib harvest, is too thick and noncompliant. Cadaver fascia (Tutoplast [IOP Inc, Costa Mesa, CA, USA]) is acceptable, but introduces the problems of cost, and the uncertainty of nonviable material.

Perichondrium, removed during a rib harvest, is considered by some to be an equivalent to fascia but is different as regards thickness, pliability, and perhaps, postoperative thickening.

Applications

The most common application of fascia is reducing dorsal visibility under thin skin in primary and secondary cases, providing concealment and preventing "shrink wrappage" of thin skin. However, it is not a substitute to a smooth underlying osseocartilaginous dorsum. Actual augmentation depends on the number of layers used: 1 layer (0.5 mm), 2 layers (1.0 mm), or 3 layers (1.5 mm). The fascia is pinned to a silicone block and folded as necessary. The free edge is sutured with a running 4-0 plain catgut suture. Two 4-0 plain catgut sutures on small straight needles (ST-1) are placed at the cephalic end, and then used to guide the graft into the dorsal pocket. The graft is then smoothed, and the caudal end is sutured at the anterior septal angle.

Problems

Fascia grafts have had surprisingly few problems. Displacement, visibility, and overgrafting are not issues. However, additional swelling is an important expectation associated with fascia. Also, the patient should "compress" the graft and not massage it, because shearing leads to more fluid accumulation, not less. Rather, the concern should be directed more toward insufficiency Donor site problems are minimal, and include the occasional scar revision (2 in 428 cases) or hematoma (1 in 428 cases).

Diced Cartilage (DC)

Since the 1930s, the viability and effectiveness of DC grafts have been validated in facial and cranial reconstruction. The fundamental concept is that cartilage can be cleanly cut into small pieces and placed into the recipient site, where fibrous tissue creates a semi rigid larger graft. Because the grafts are cleanly cut, the pieces survive. The cartilage is not morselized, bruised, or crushed because this would lead to unpredictable survival. Dicing is usually done using #11 blades to cut it into tiny pieces less than 0.5 mm in length. The pieces should be a fine "paste" and small enough to spurt out of a tuberculin syringe. The grafts are placed into the recipient bed using either an elevator for small areas or a tuberculin syringe for larger areas. It is important that the recipient area is not overgrafted—what you see at the end of the operation is what you get postoperatively.

Applications

It is important to distinguish how one uses DC. Intrinsically, it is used as a filler material rather than a "structured graft." The author uses DC either as a volume or site filler. As a volume filler, DC is placed on the sides of dorsal rib grafts or in peripyriform depressions to alleviate the pyriform contracture that occurs in the cocaine nose. As a site filler, DC can be placed in the infralobule to create a round tip or hide bifidity, but it does not create tip definition. It can be extremely useful for filling dorsal depressions as a closed approach, especially in revision cases.

Problems

If one avoids overgrafting, there are few problems with DC. Absorption is not an issue, but visibility can occur in a thin-skin nose. As regards dorsal corrections, the biggest challenge is decision making. One should never confuse a limited "filler concealment" with secondary rhinoplasty. Many surgeons and dermatologists show results of fillers placed in secondary cases emphasizing what can be done, but do not acknowledge the associated problems or limited benefits. Because DC does not have the risks of absorption or infection, it can be conceptualized as a "permanent autogenous filler" that has its advantages and disadvantages. However, the results would be limited improvement, rather than a major functional and aesthetic change that a complete secondary rhinoplasty can provide. The typical patient would probably be the facial rejuvenation recipient, who would accept an incidental, incomplete improvement in his or her nasal appearance.

Diced Cartilage and Fascia (DC + F)

DC + F grafts have the same standard harvest and preparation as fascia and DC grafts. Once the graft materials are ready, a 2-stage insertion is done. The fascia is inserted first, then the DC is placed underneath until the desired contour is achieved. Essentially, the fascia keeps the DC from being visible.

Applications

DC + F grafts provide a true major volume graft in the radix, and a fine type of dorsal augmentation. The author uses DC + F grafts to correct deep hypoplastic radix area deficiencies. Because the purpose of the fascia is to conceal rather than augment, the amount used is less than that of the standard radix fascia graft. The fascia is inserted and then elevated with an Aufricht retractor; this is followed by placement of the DC against the bare bone that has been stripped of its periosteum to promote fusion with the cartilage. The area is not overcorrected, and is filled precisely. DC + F grafts for the dorsum are done for subtle contour improvements, and not for major augmentations. A single- or double-layer fascia graft is inserted and elevated, and small amounts of DC are placed as "contour fill." Because the cartilage can be easily displaced, this maneuver is often the last step before closure.

Problems

The most common problems are either technical or judgmental errors. In the radix area, one can misjudge the amount of cartilage in either direction or dissect the pocket too laterally, either of which can result in a bulge. The primary risk is displacement and visibility of cartilage pieces over the dorsum. In selected cases, these pieces can be fragmented using a #16 needle in the examination room.

Diced Cartilage in Fascia (DC – F)

When major augmentations are required, the DC is placed in a fascial sleeve. This sleeve acts as a container but also promotes vascularity, and minimizes visibility under thin skin.

The "construct" graft is made to measure on the back table and then placed carefully into the recipient bed, where its volume can be adjusted in situ.

Applications

The range of applications is dramatic. When a combined radix/upper dorsum graft is required, the fascia is pinned to a silastic block, the DC is placed on top, and the fascial edges are sutured together to create a "bean bag" graft. In the recipient site, placing additional DC(s) deep to the fascia against bare bone can increase the volume of the graft. The graft can be reduced in size by "milking out" cartilage from the graft through a small separation of the suture line using the suction cannula. The dramatic flexibility of these grafts is shown in the range of dimensions for dorsal grafts, with thickness being tapered to uniform thickness, height from 2 to 8 mm, and any desired length. Custom-made dorsal grafts are easily created using the DC – F technique. The steps are as follows:

1. A large sheet of deep temporal fascia (4 × 2 cm) is folded transversely and pinned to a silastic block to create a "tube." The free longitudinal edge is sutured with a running 4-0 chromic suture.
2. The cephalic end is closed with 4-0 plain sutures on small straight needles, which are left in place to facilitate percutaneous placement.
3. The DC is then placed from the caudal end. When a uniform graft is required, the author uses a tuberculin syringe filled with compressed DC. The syringe is placed against the closed cephalic end, and the DC is injected as the syringe is removed. The nondominant hand is used to mold the graft to create the desired contour. When a tapered graft is required, the volume of DC is carefully controlled to fit the recipient site defect.
4. The graft is guided into the recipient site using the percutaneous sutures and elevation of the skin envelope with the Aufricht retractor. The graft is carefully placed over the dorsum, and carefully inspected for edges and volume. Any excess volume is milked out of the caudal end.
5. Once the surgeon is satisfied, the graft is sutured, closed, and fixed to the dorsum near the anterior septal angle.

Problems

As long as one avoids using DC – F grafts for structural support, graft problems are minor, and their frequency diminishes as one advances on the learning curve. A common error is to place the graft too high and blunt the radix. Kelly avoided this by using a distinct fascial radix graft above the DC – F graft.[11]

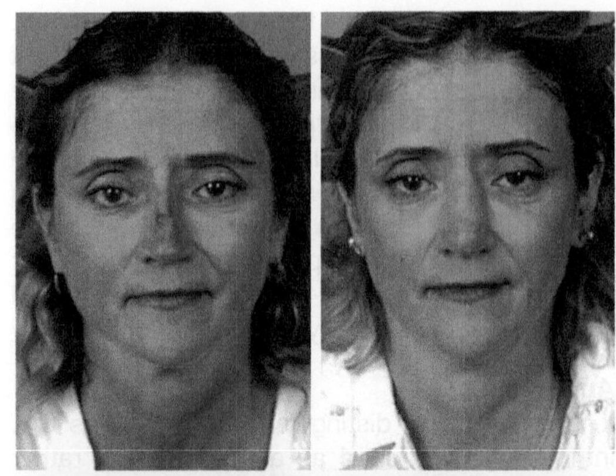

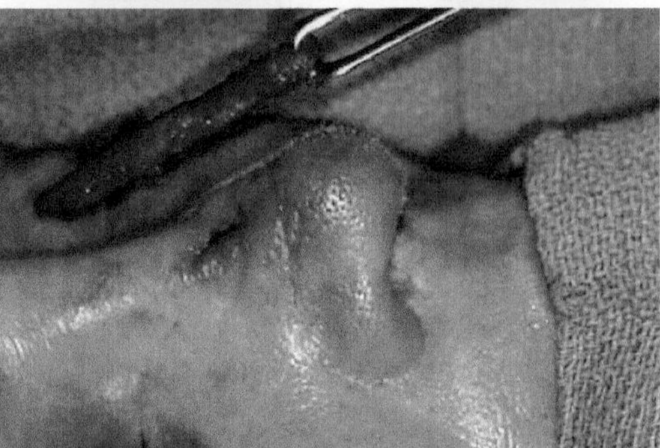

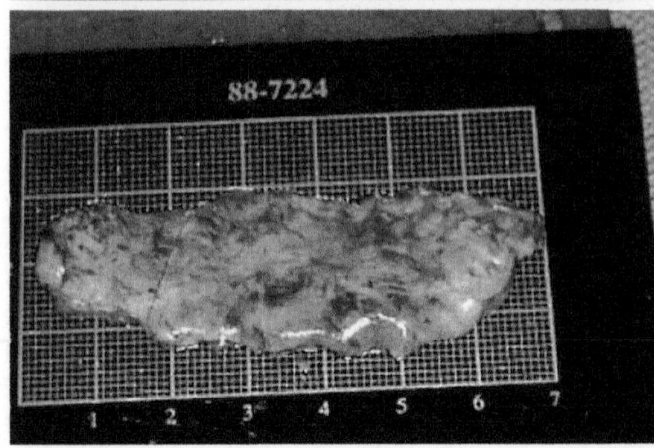

Fig. 1. A 54-year-old woman had an infected Porex dorsal implant with exudate through 2 skin ulcerations. The implant was removed and replaced with a 2-layer full-length dermis graft. The wound healed without difficulty. The patient is shown at 9 months post surgery.

Dermis

When the skin envelope is severely thinned out or attenuated, then a dermal graft is the solution. The objective is not to achieve major augmentation, but to thicken and normalize the skin envelope.[12] These cases are divided into 2 groups: the infected nasal implant, and the multiply operated nose with a crucified skin envelope. For the latter, the first stage is to insert dermis to allow safe elevation of the skin envelope at the second stage of reconstruction (**Fig. 1**). In contrast to Sheen and Sheen,[4] who worried about dermis grafts surviving a possible infection, the author routinely uses dermis when low-grade infection is present because of an extruding alloplastic implant. The implant is removed, the capsule excised, and the wound profusely irrigated with antibiotic solution. The dermis graft is excised from the suprapubic area, often using a Cesarean section scar. The area (as big as 14 × 4 cm) is de-epithelialized first, and then removed at the subdermal plane leaving the fat behind. The graft is turned over, and any hair follicles present are carefully removed. The dermis is guided into the wound with percutaneous sutures. In most cases, the dermis is placed in multiple layers and even "stuffed" into the partially closed incision. The nose is overgrafted because the amount of survival is unpredictable. Thus, until now, dermis grafts have been part of the solution, and not of the problem.

CASE STUDIES

Case Study 1: Fascia

A 39-year-old patient complained that she had a "nose job" look some 24 years after her primary rhinoplasty (**Fig. 2**). Because the skin was paper thin with visible pointed tip cartilages, it was planned to place fascia grafts over the dorsum and tip. At surgery, a prior domal division was found and repaired with sutures. Lateral wall support was achieved with lateral crural strut grafts. A small concealer graft was added to the infralobule to smooth the tip area. A full-length fascia graft was guided into the nose using percutaneous sutures and then incorporated into the suture closure of all the incisions. The purpose of the fascia blanket graftwas to prevent a shrink wrap contracture of the extremely thin skin envelope.

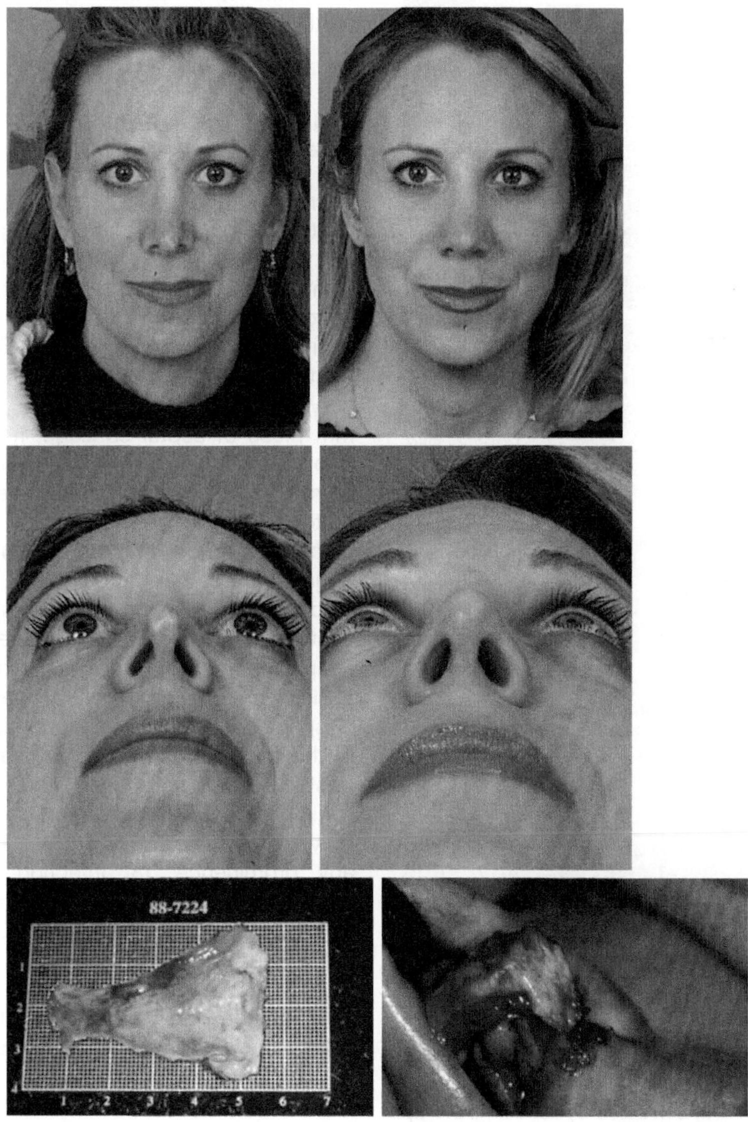

Fig. 2. A patient after a secondary rhinoplasty with a collapsed tip and visible bossa through thin skin. After tip repair, a full-length "fascial blanket" was inserted over the dorsum, and underneath all areas of skin elevation.

Case Study 2: Diced Cartilage Beneath Fascia

A 26-year-old woman of Mexican descent requested a major aesthetic improvement in her nose (**Fig. 3**). She felt that her tip was heavy and droopy. However, the author considered the preexisting inverted-V deformity and hypoplastic upper dorsum a more serious issue. Creating a new unified dorsum would require reducing the cartilaginous dorsum (2 mm) while augmenting the upper bony dorsum. A combined radix and dorsal graft of fascia was used followed by insertion of 0.2 cc of DC in the upper dorsum. The patient is shown at 1 year post surgery.

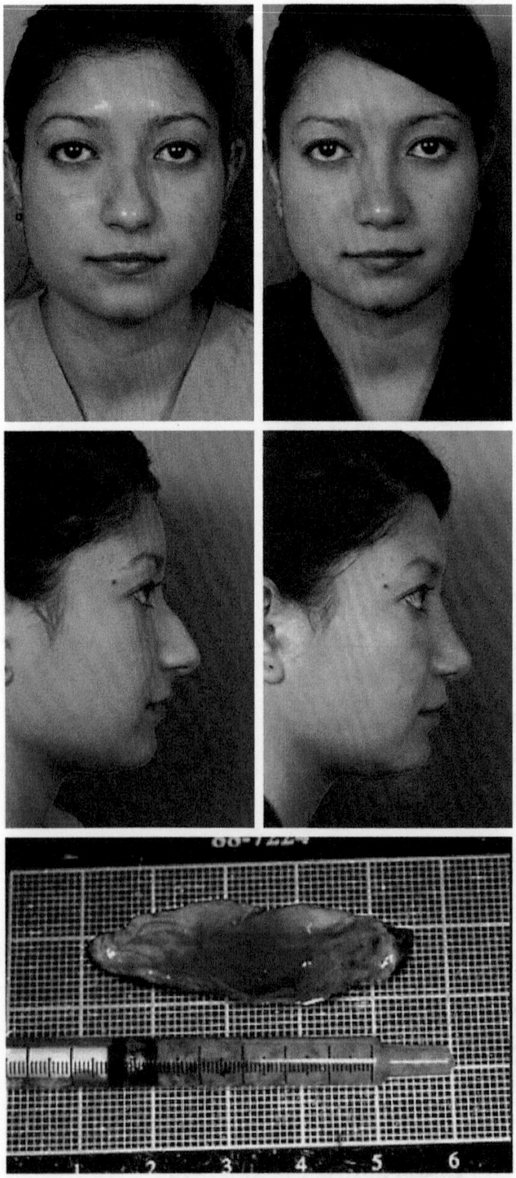

Fig. 3. A young Hispanic girl with marked dorsal base disproportion that was corrected by reducing the tip and then augmenting the dorsum with a DC + F graft, the diced cartilage being placed beneath the fascia.

Case Study 3: Diced Cartilage in Fascia

An 18-year-old girl of Middle Eastern descent sought rhinoplasty. She disliked the profile and the heaviness of her nose (**Fig. 4**). A balanced approach for her nasal deformity required dorsal reduction (bony 1.5 mm, cartilage 5 mm) combined with a radix/upper dorsal augmentation using a DC – F graft. 0.2 cc of diced cartilage was wrapped in fascia and inserted just before closure. Tip definition was increased by tip sutures and a double level add-on graft of excised alar cartilage.

WHY FASCIA AND DICED CARTILAGE GRAFTS?

There are numerous advantages and few disadvantages for these grafts. The advantages are as follows. (1) These grafts are autogenous, using viable fascia and cartilage with no risk of rejection. (2) One can use any combination of excised, septal, conchal, or rib cartilage. In contrast to solid grafts, one does not have to harvest the perfect, and rarely found, 35 × 8 mm piece of septal cartilage, nor fuse together 2 pieces of curvy conchal cartilage. (3) There is no risk of warping, or a need for foreign material (K-wire). (4) The grafts are easily and quickly prepared, with the circulating nurse or a junior assistant dicing the cartilage and loading the syringe. (5) The shape is easily customized as regards thickness (1–8 mm), shape (tapered or uniform), and length. The ability to mold a graft with a specific shape for a specific defect is extraordinary. (6) Molding of the graft is possible intraoperatively and early postoperatively. (7) The graft can be easily revised using a percutaneous #16 needle to remove a sharp edge, or a #15 blade to shave off any prominence. (8) Infection has not been a problem. (9) Absorption has not been observed in more than 300 cases with a maximum follow-up of 7 years. Over a period of months, the DC solidifies. The interspace between the DC bits is filled with fibrous tissue within the fascial sleeve. When removed, the graft is solid and semirigid. The pieces shaved off for shaping purposes are sufficiently solid and can be used even for tip grafts. Histologic studies confirm that the individual pieces of

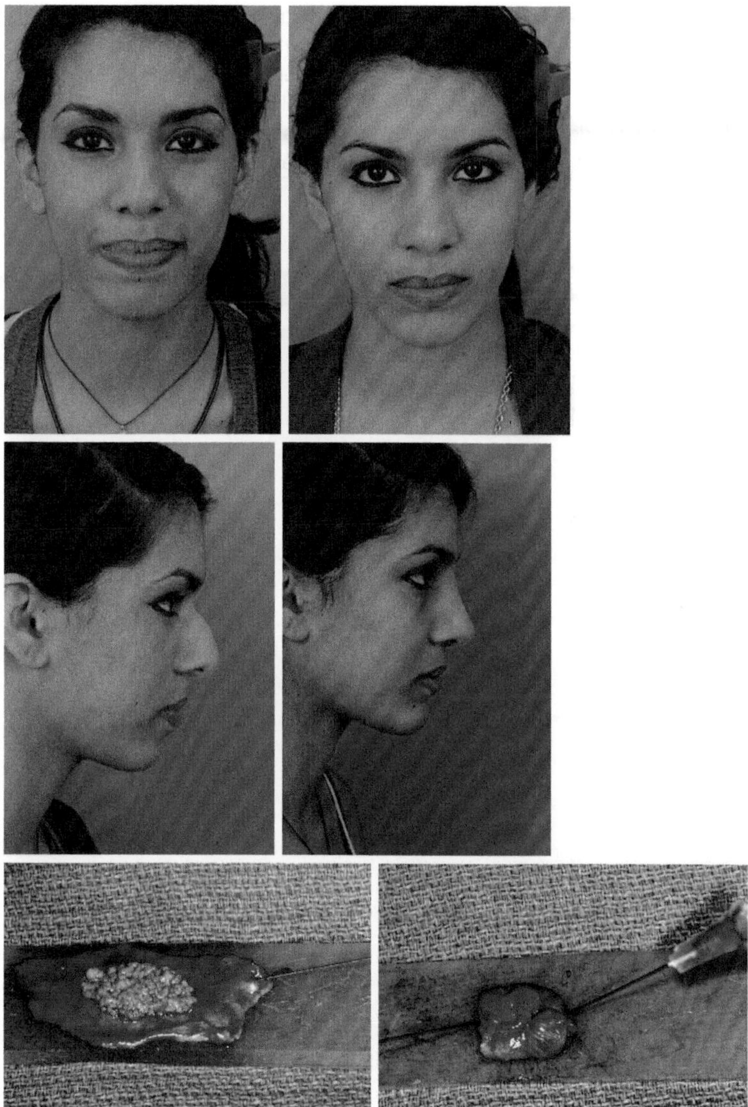

Fig. 4. A Middle Eastern girl with true hypoplasia of the radix and upper dorsum. The cartilaginous dorsum was reduced. The radix/upper dorsum was augmented with a "bean bag" DC – F graft.

cartilage have survived, and suggest that the fascia has become a neoperichondrium.[13]

REFERENCES

1. Daniel RK. Rhinoplasty: an atlas of surgical techniques. New York: Springer; 2002.
2. Daniel RK, Calvert JW. Diced cartilage grafts in rhinoplasty surgery. Plast Reconstr Surg 2004;113:2156.
3. Daniel RK, Brenner KA. Saddle nose deformity: a new classification and treatment. Facial Plast Surg Clin North Am 2006;14:301.
4. Sheen JH, Sheen AP. Aesthetic rhinoplasty. 2nd edition. St. Louis (MO): Mosby; 1987.
5. Daniel RK. Rhinoplasty: septal saddle nose deformity and composite reconstruction. Plast Reconstr Surg 2007;119:1029.
6. Lovice DB, Mingrone MD, Toriumi DM. Grafts and implants in rhinoplasty and nasal reconstruction. Otolaryngol Clin North Am 1999;32:113.
7. Gunter JP, Clark CP, Friedman RM. Internal stabilization of autogenous rib cartilage grafts in rhinoplasty: a barrier to cartilage warping. Plast Reconstr Surg 1997;100:162.
8. Daniel RK. Diced cartilage grafts in rhinoplasty surgery: current techniques and applications. Plast Reconstr Surg 2008;122:1883.
9. Guerrerosantos J. Temporoparietal free fascial grafts to the nose. Plast Reconstr Surg 1985;76:328.

10. Miller TA. Temporalis fascia grafts for facial and nasal contour augmentation. Plast Reconstr Surg 1988;81:524.
11. Kelly MH, Bulstrode NW, Waterhouse N. Versatility of diced cartilage-fascia grafts in dorsal augmentation. Plast Reconstr Surg 2007;120:1654.
12. Erdogan B, Tuncel A, Adanali G, et al. Augmentation rhinoplasty with dermal graft and review of the literature. Plast Reconstr Surg 2003;111:2060.
13. Calvert JW, Brenner KB, DaCosta-Iyer M, et al. Histological analysis of human diced cartilage grafts. Plast Reconstr Surg 2006;118:230.

Osteotomies

Eric J. Dobratz, MD[a,b,*], Peter A. Hilger, MD[a]

KEYWORDS

- Osteotomies • Lateral osteotomy
- Medial osteotomy • Intermediate osteotomy
- Nasal deformity • Nasal bones • Crooked nose

Rhinoplasty remains to be one of the most challenging facial plastic surgical procedures performed. The surgeon seeks to achieve the combination of aesthetic harmony with the surrounding facial features and preservation or development of nasal function and support. One of the most challenging and instrumental steps in achieving harmonious form and function during rhinoplasty is the successful completion of osteotomies. Osteotomies are performed to correct deformities of the bony nasal vault. Successful treatment of deformities of the bony vault is achieved through organized thinking, comprehensive knowledge of nasal anatomy, and thorough careful preoperative and intraoperative planning. In this review the authors discuss the pertinent anatomy, technical considerations, including selection of various osteotomy techniques, and complications that rhinoplasty surgeons should be aware of to optimize correction of deformities of the nasal bony vault.

ANATOMY

The bony framework of the external nose consists of the paired nasal bones and the ascending processes of the maxilla. The nasal bones are thick cephalically where they articulate with the frontal bone, and are thin as they extend inferolaterally where they articulate with the maxilla and the upper lateral cartilage.[1] This variability in thickness is important for consideration of placement of the osteotomies. For example, the lateral osteotomy should be placed in the thicker ascending process of the maxilla instead of the thin lateral nasal bone.

The nasal bones are supported by their articulation superiorly with the frontal bone at the nasofrontal suture line (nasion), laterally at the ascending process of the maxilla and in the posterior-midline where the bones are fused with the perpendicular plate of the ethmoid. It is important to consider the midline attachment to the perpendicular plate while treating the twisted nose deformity. In patients with this deformity, the nasal bones and ethmoid plate are deviated and the nasal bones may have variable symmetry, with one side being longer than the other. The surgeon must address the nasal bones and the deviated bony septum. If the deviation at the perpendicular plate is not treated, the patient will often have persisting deviation of the bony vault.

Inferiorly the nasal bones overlap the cephalic margins of the upper lateral cartilages, providing support to the cartilaginous middle vault. Thus, narrowing of the nose by infracture of the bony sidewall will also result in the narrowing of the middle third caused by this connection between the nasal bones and upper lateral cartilage. The surgeon should be aware of this especially after hump reduction, where the width of the broad native dorsal septum is significantly narrowed (**Fig. 1**). The resultant upper and middle vault narrowing may lead to profound obstruction in patients who already have a narrow bony base or when the base is significantly narrowed through lateral osteotomies with medial displacement of the bony base.

[a] Division of Facial Plastic and Reconstructive Surgery, Department of Otolaryngology Head and Neck Surgery, University of Minnesota, 420 Delaware Street, MMC 396, Minneapolis, MN 55455, USA
[b] Division of Facial Plastic and Reconstructive Surgery, Department of Otolaryngology Head and Neck Surgery, Eastern Virginia Medical School, River Pavilion, Suite 1100, 600 Gresham Drive, Norfolk, VA 23507, USA
* Corresponding author. Division of Facial Plastic and Reconstructive Surgery, Department of Otolaryngology Head and Neck Surgery, Eastern Virginia Medical School, River Pavilion, Suite 1100, 600 Gresham Drive, Norfolk, VA 23507.
E-mail address: dobratej@evms.edu

Clin Plastic Surg 37 (2010) 301–311
doi:10.1016/j.cps.2009.11.002
0094-1298/10/$ – see front matter

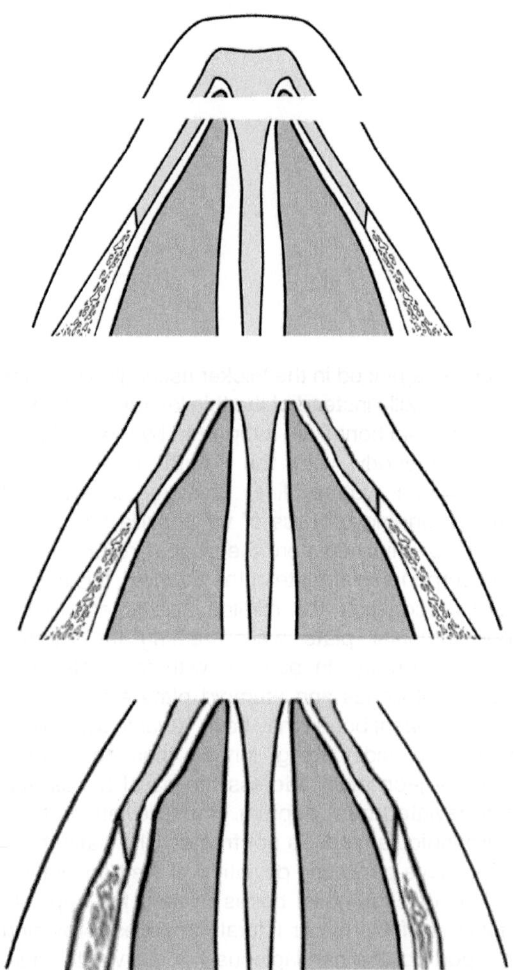

Fig. 1. The surgeon must beware of profound narrowing of the airway that may occur after hump reduction. The width of the dorsal septum is narrowed with excision of the hump. The overall narrowing of the nasal cavity can be profound when the bony base is narrow as well (*bottom panel*).

One must also take care to preserve the articulation of the nasal bones and upper lateral cartilage during dissection or rasping near the inferior edge of the nasal bones. Disruption of this junction will result in collapse of the upper lateral cartilage and a resulting depression of the middle vault that is difficult to correct. Rasping at the inferior medial edge of the nasal bone makes the superior medial edge of the upper lateral cartilage prominent; this is due to the flexible character of the cartilage, which may disarticulate and bend outward. This anomaly should be corrected as it may cause a persistent fullness after surgery.

The soft tissues overlying the bony framework include the skin, subcutaneous tissues, superficial musculoaponeurotic system, and periosteum. The relationship between the soft tissues and the underlying bony framework determines the overall contour of the nose, thus a comprehensive knowledge of these structures is required to achieve optimal results when altering the bony framework of the nose. The soft-tissue envelope varies in thickness over the dorsum of the nose (**Fig. 2**). The skin and subcutaneous tissues are thicker superiorly in the area of the nasion and inferiorly at the supratip. The soft tissue thins over the rhinion, the osseocartilaginous junction of the nasal bones, and the upper lateral cartilages. Thus, when altering the bony profile, a slight hump should remain at this junction to give an overall straight appearance of the profile. If the bony profile is straight there will be a small "saddle-nose" appearance when the soft tissues are redraped (see **Fig. 2**).

The periosteum represents the layer between the soft-tissue envelope and the underlying bony framework. It is important to use caution while raising the adherent periosteum from the nasal bones, because preserving the periosteum as an intact layer will provide a thicker flap, which provides better camouflage over the newly reconstructed bony framework. Raising the periosteum with the flap also decreases the risk for postoperative trophic changes. Minimal lateral elevation of the periosteum should be performed to preserve the periosteal attachments to the ascending process of the maxilla. This action will help stabilize the bony fragments after performing lateral osteotomies.

It is important to have a thorough understanding of the relationship between the bony/cartilaginous, and soft-tissue architecture of the nose. It is also important to understand the changes that occur in the bony framework with age. While performing osteotomies on young patients the nasal bones are soft and may result in greenstick fractures. These fractures are incomplete, making mobilization of the fragment difficult, therefore in younger patients continuous osteotomies are generally preferred to help avoid greenstick fractures and ensure proper mobilization. Older patients tend to have brittle bones or may have a history of previous fractures or surgeries that can lead to comminution while osteotomies are performed. In older patients one may preferably create greenstick fractures or incomplete osteotomies, with digital completion of the osteotomy in order to avoid comminution of the bony fragment.

It is also important to consider a patient's age when determining the degree of anatomic change that is to be created. Older patients have grown accustomed to their appearance and will be more affected by significant alterations in their

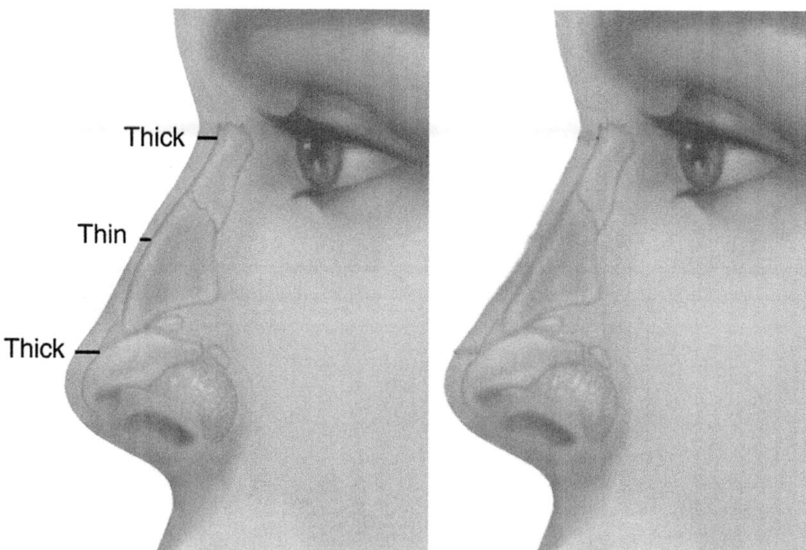

Fig. 2. The thickness of the skin over the nasal dorsum varies (*left*). A slight bony/cartilaginous hump should remain to allow for a straight profile. Completely removing the hump, creating a straight bony profile will result in a small "saddle-nose" appearance (*right*). (*Left diagram From* Hilger P. Nasal analysis. In: Papel I, Holt GR, Frodel JL, editors. Facial plastic and reconstructive surgery. Thieme; 2009; with permission.)

appearance. It is best to perform more conservative alterations to the bony framework in older patients. Younger patients tend to be more accepting of significant changes to their nasal appearance.

EVALUATION OF BONY VAULT

With all aspects of rhinoplasty, proper preoperative analysis is critical to obtaining optimal results. It is imperative to correctly determine the patient's deformities so that the most effective techniques for correction of these deformities may be performed. One should be able to visualize and palpate the external anatomy, and at the same time predict the underlying structure that determines the external appearance. Complete nasal and facial analysis is essential as the appearance of the bony vault must be in balance with the other aspects of the nose and the rest of the face. During nasal analysis, the nose is divided into vertical thirds with the upper one-third representing the bony nasal vault.

On anterior evaluation the overall alignment, length, and width of the bony vault should be determined. Alignment of the bony dorsum may be evaluated by determining a relative midline of the nose. A line defined by the mentum, upper incisors, philtrum, and glabella may be used to determine the midline. Deviation toward the right or the left should be determined in relation to this line and any continued deviation into the middle or lower one-thirds. Ideally the dorsum of the nose would be straight and symmetric on either side of this midline. Asymmetries may be caused by deviations of the bony vault toward one side of the nose or may be due to the width irregularities between the upper and middle one-thirds of the nose.

The width of the bony vault should be analyzed to include the width at the nasal facial sulcus or bony base and also at the dorsal ridge. The ideal width is influenced by features such as nasal length, projection, skin thickness, and other facial proportions, and will vary depending on the individual. The width of the nasal dorsum should be approximately two-thirds of the width of the alar base, which should approximate the intercanthal distance (**Fig. 3**).

The nasal bones and ascending process of the maxilla are palpated for irregularities. Previous fractures because of trauma or previous surgery with their associated inward or outward displacement may be palpated. The bones should be assessed for a concave or convex shape as this may require an intermediate osteotomy to correct the associated deformity. Significant differences in the height of the nasal bones should also be evaluated, as this will often occur in crooked nose deformities.

The profile evaluation of the bony dorsum determines the level of the radix, the nasofrontal angle, and dorsal alignment. The radix or root of the nose corresponds to the junction of the nasal and frontal bones, and this should be located at the level of

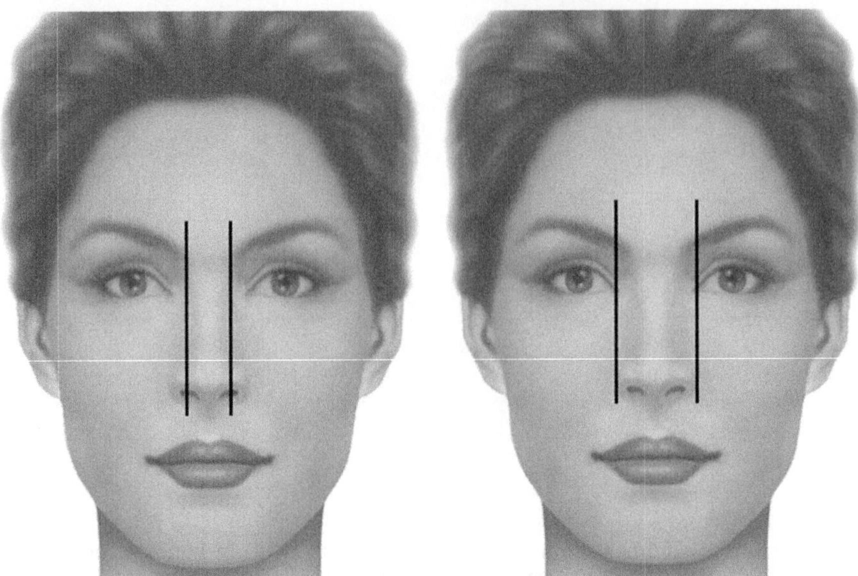

Fig. 3. The width of the bony dorsum should be approximately two-thirds the width of the alar base (*left*). The width of the alar base should approximate the intercanthal distance (*right*). (*From* Hilger P. Nasal analysis, In: Papel I, Holt GR, Frodel JL, editors. Facial plastic and reconstructive surgery. Thieme; 2009; with permission.)

the supratarsal crease. The nasofrontal angle, defined by glabella-to-nasion line intersecting with nasion-to-tip line, should be between 115° and 130°. A high radix or shallow nasofrontal angle may require rasping in order to improve the contour in this area. The desired change may be achieved through rasping; however, this change often becomes muted through healing, and long-term deepening of the radix is difficult to accomplish. Occasionally a transverse osteotomy at the nasal root may be performed to push down this area and deepen the radix. On the other hand, a low radix may accentuate the appearance of a dorsal hump, and this should be identified so that the surgeon may augment the radix with a graft, thus reducing the amount of hump to be removed. It is also important to determine the appropriate tip projection and rotation in evaluating the bony profile alignment. The tip and radix position will influence the dorsal height required to achieve an aesthetically pleasing profile.

It is important to include an intranasal evaluation for complete assessment of the bony vault. Collapsed nasal bones will be evident as they cause impingement of the airway and are often associated with the collapse of the attached upper lateral cartilage. This may contribute to decreased patency at the internal valve as the upper lateral cartilage collapses toward the septum. Patients who have had previous placed "low to low" osteotomies with medialization at pyriform aperture may present with nasal valve obstruction as well. The degree of airway impingement with this type of osteotomy will be accentuated in patients with preexisting narrow pyriform apertures, hypertrophied inferior turbinates, or long nasal bones.[2]

TYPES OF OSTEOTOMIES

Hump Reduction

The bony hump reduction is performed through an osteotomy. The techniques involved with hump reduction are described in detail in another article, so they are not repeated in this discussion. However, medial and lateral osteotomies are often performed to close an open roof that is created during a hump reduction. Here the authors discuss types of osteotomies by describing the medial, lateral, and intermediate osteotomies in further detail.

Medial Osteotomies

Medial osteotomies are generally performed along with lateral osteotomies to mobilize the nasal sidewall to close an open roof after hump reduction or to narrow the nasal base. Medial osteotomies may also be performed to straighten a deviated bony septum. Occasionally medial osteotomies will be performed without lateral osteotomies to place spreader grafts that extend beyond the medial bony/cartilaginous junction. This procedure may allow for greater lateral displacement of the nasal bone and upper lateral cartilage, allowing greater opening of the nasal airway.

Medial osteotomies may be performed as straight, fading, or perforating osteotomies (**Fig. 4**) and are generally not carried high into the root of the nose, as this may predispose the surgeon to create a rocker deformity (described later) during completion of the lateral osteotomy. However, when the septum is significantly deviated, the surgeon may carry the medial osteotomy high into the root to provide a fulcrum point for moving the septum to a more midline position. A lower fading osteotomy may then be performed to meet the lateral osteotomy. Other surgeons may perform the medial osteotomy and then mobilize and straighten the perpendicular plate of the ethmoid intranasally.

In the authors' practice, fading osteotomies are most often used because the root of the nose is solid bone and infrequently needs narrowing. These osteotomies also facilitate the precise completion of the lateral osteotomy without performing a percutaneous incision. The lateral osteotomy must communicate with the medial osteotomy to mobilize the nasal bone. If a fading medial osteotomy is not performed, a transverse osteotomy may be used to connect a straight medial osteotomy to the lateral osteotomy. This procedure may be performed percutaneously or under the skin envelope. Gryskiewicz[3] showed that percutaneous osteotomy incisions tend to heal well, with 94% of patients having imperceptible scars. The incision should be created as a stab incision with a number 11 blade. Occasionally a perforating transverse osteotomy will be used to complete the fading medial osteotomy that does not communicate completely with the lateral osteotomy. The transverse fracture connecting the medial and the lateral osteotomies may also be created through digital pressure.

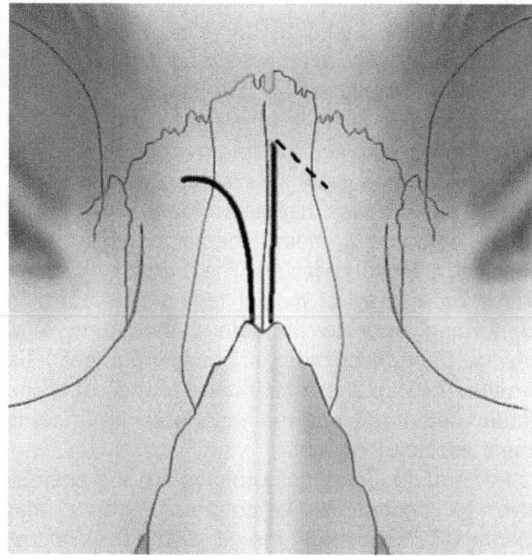

Fig. 4. Medial osteotomies may be performed as a fading osteotomy (*patient's right side*) or straight (*patient's left side*). A perforating transverse osteotomy is shown on the left side as well.

Medial osteotomies are performed through endonasal or external techniques. While performing endonasal rhinoplasty, an intercartilaginous incision is created and a pocket is raised in the supraperichondrial plane to an area just past the junction of the nasal bones and upper lateral cartilage. A Joseph elevator is then used to create a subperiosteal pocket over the nasal bones. A straight or curved guarded osteotome is passed through the incision, over the upper lateral cartilage, and is then articulated into the caudal edge of the nasal bone just lateral to the midline on the same side. The osteotomy is then performed and repeated on the opposite side in a similar fashion as indicated. During the external approach the caudal edge of the nasal bone is visualized after elevation of the soft-tissue envelope. The osteotome is articulated at the caudal edge of the nasal bone and the osteotomy is performed. If the upper lateral cartilage has been separated from the dorsal septum the osteotome is passed through this space to articulate with the caudal edge of the nasal bone, displacing the upper lateral cartilage laterally, and the osteotomy is then performed. In either approach, care must be taken to ensure that the attachment of the upper lateral cartilage to the nasal bone is not disrupted.

Occasionally in patients who undergo hump reduction with short nasal bones and a predominantly cartilaginous hump, the reduction will not create a significant open roof and osteotomies will not be performed. The surgeon should ensure that the patient has an adequate width at the nasal base and that there is a straight nasal bony vault before making a decision not to perform an osteotomy.

Lateral Osteotomies

Lateral osteotomies are traditionally described for closing an open roof after hump reduction, narrowing a wide nasal base, or straightening the deviated nose. The lateral osteotomy may also be used to increase the width of the nasal bones in patients who have had their nasal vault aggressively narrowed with previous surgery or trauma. These patients require lateral displacement of the nasal bone and attached upper lateral cartilage to provide an adequate airway.

The early techniques for lateral osteotomies, popularized by Joseph and those whom he trained, involved the use of a saw osteotomy technique.[4] A subperiosteal tunnel was created and the saw osteotomy began at the inferiormost aspect of the pyriform aperture, extending along the ascending processes of the maxilla ending at or beyond the nasofrontal suture (low to low). During saw osteotomies the curl of the saw causes a loss of height of the nasal bones. Surgeons began transitioning to the use of osteotomes instead of the saw to perform the lateral osteotomy. In time it became apparent that patients were experiencing postoperative nasal airway obstruction caused by the excessive narrowing of the lateral nasal walls with the "low to low" technique. Webster and colleagues[5] described the importance of leaving a triangular piece of bone at the pyriform aperture intact just superior to the level of the inferior turbinate. They described performing a curved osteotomy that started high, preserving the triangular bone at the pyriform, extending low onto the ascending process, and then curving back high to avoid extension into the frontal process (high to low to high). This pathway allowed for preservation of the airway by avoiding medial displacement of the inferior portions of the lateral nasal wall. By transitioning to a high position at the completion of the osteotomy, the frontal process is preserved. When the osteotomy is carried superiorly into the frontal process (low position) and the nasal bones are infractured, the radix acts as a fulcrum and the osteotomized segment beyond the radix lateralizes, creating a rocker deformity. By ending the osteotomy high the path can communicate with a transverse or fading medial osteotomy below the frontal bone, thus avoiding extension of the osteotomy into the frontal process and avoiding a rocker deformity.

Lateral osteotomies may be performed in a continuous or perforating fashion. For continuous lateral osteotomies a straight or curved guarded osteotome is generally used. The authors prefer to re-inject local anesthesia just before the osteotomy to hydrodissect the soft tissues overlying the bone and also to assist with hemostasis. Next, a subperiosteal tunnel is created before the osteotomy is performed. This protects the periosteum from injury, allowing for decreased bleeding and subsequent swelling and ecchymosis. The guard of the osteotome may be placed internally or externally. When the guard is placed internally, a submucosal tunnel is created along the nasal surface of the ascending process of the maxilla. The guard is placed beneath the mucosa, which is preserved, and the osteotomy is performed. This reduces swelling and provides increased stability of the fragment due to the reduced injury to the periosteum and mucosa.[6] When the guard is placed externally the osteotomy may be performed with or without a subperiosteal tunnel overlying the external surface of the ascending process. The guard is placed on the external surface just superior to the inferior turbinate and the osteotomy is performed. Advocates for this approach believe that they have superior control, as they are able to palpate the guard as it travels along the path of the osteotomy. As the unguarded edge passes on the mucosal surface, it can lead to extensive injury to the internal nasal mucosa. Becker and colleagues[7] described differences in intranasal mucosal injury with osteotomes of differing sizes. The 4-mm guarded osteotome caused mucosal tears 95% of the time and a 2.5-mm osteotome caused mucosal tears only 4% of the time. These investigators then evaluated computed tomography scans and noted that the average thickness of the lateral osteotomy site was 2.47 mm in men and 2.29 mm in women. Becker and colleagues concluded that the 2.5-mm osteotome was reliable and the least traumatic. The 2.5-mm osteotome also has a lower profile and causes less damage to the lateral soft tissues; however, palpation of the guard is more difficult and thus requires more skill to anticipate the path of the osteotomy. The 2- and 3-mm unguarded osteotomes are minimally traumatic to intranasal mucosa and lateral soft tissues during a continuous osteotomy; however, these tend to be reliable only in the hands of the most experienced surgeons.

At the completion of the lateral osteotomy, the osteotome is turned inward to complete the fracture and displace the fragment internally. The back-fracture that communicates the lateral and medial osteotomies may be performed as a transverse osteotomy, fading medial osteotomy, or facture by digital pressure. The medial and transverse osteotomy or medial fading osteotomy is performed prior to the lateral osteotomy and inward fracture of the nasal bone fragment. The fracture by digital pressure is performed after the lateral osteotomy and the nasal bone fragment is then displaced internally.

Perforating lateral osteotomies are the alternative to continuous osteotomies. Tardy and Denneny[8] described the use of the micro-osteotome to perform precise endonasal perforating osteotomies with minimal damage to the periosteum and intranasal mucosa. Murakami and Larrabee[4] compared a percutaneous perforating lateral osteotomy with continuous osteotomies. The perforating osteotomy resulted in a complete, irregular osteotomy with small comminutions along the path. There appeared to be equivalent narrowing with both techniques; however, the perforating osteotomy was noted to provide increased stability to the fragment. The investigators believed that this was a result of the preservation of the mucosa and periosteum.

Occasionally patients will present with an excessively collapsed bony vault caused by the aggressive narrowing of the nasal bones during a previous rhinoplasty (**Fig. 5**). Other patients present with a unilaterally narrowed bony vault as a result of trauma on the lateral surface of the nose with subsequent collapse of the fractured nasal bone. In these instances the patient will require lateral displacement of the osseous framework to widen the vault and open the airway. A transnasal percutaneous lateral osteotomy or "inside-out" lateral osteotomy allows for reliable mobilization of the previously traumatized nasal bone while preserving the periosteum to help support the new lateral position of the bone (**Fig. 6**). Byrne and Hilger[9] showed that mobilization of the nasal bone followed the medial to lateral vector of the osteotomy, allowing for lateralization of the segment several times without manipulation. At the conclusion of the case, a small piece of Merocel (Medtronic Inc, Minneapolis, MN, USA), is placed high in the nose and secured with externalized suture to stabilize the mobilized segments. However, this is often not required because of the stability provided by preservation of the lateral periosteum with this technique.

Intermediate Osteotomies

Intermediate osteotomies are generally performed to straighten nasal bones with significant convexity or concavity. These osteotomies may also be performed to correct a deviated nose with one nasal bone that is significantly longer than the other side. The osteotomy is performed in the midportion of the nasal bone, parallel to the lateral osteotomy. The exact location at which the osteotomy is performed within the midportion of the nasal bone depends on the anatomy of the nasal bone and the surgical goals. The osteotomy is often performed for convexity or concavity of the nasal bone, and in these cases the osteotomy is generally performed at the apex of the curvature of the bone.

Intermediate osteotomies may be performed as continuous or perforating osteotomies. The continuous intermediate osteotomy technique is similar to that of the medial osteotomy as described in earlier sections. The osteotome is placed at the caudal border of the nasal bone and the osteotomy is performed in a straight, continuous fashion. The periosteum is often not elevated this far laterally, allowing the soft-tissue attachments overlying the nasal bone to be left intact, which provides additional support to the fragments. The perforating osteotomy is performed as a postage stamp or interrupted osteotomy and is done percutaneously or

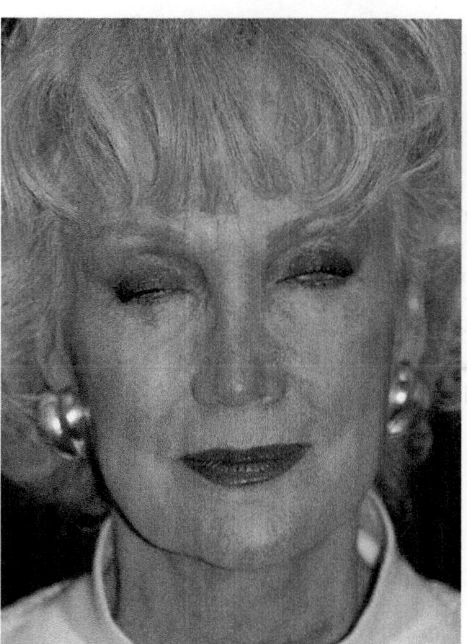

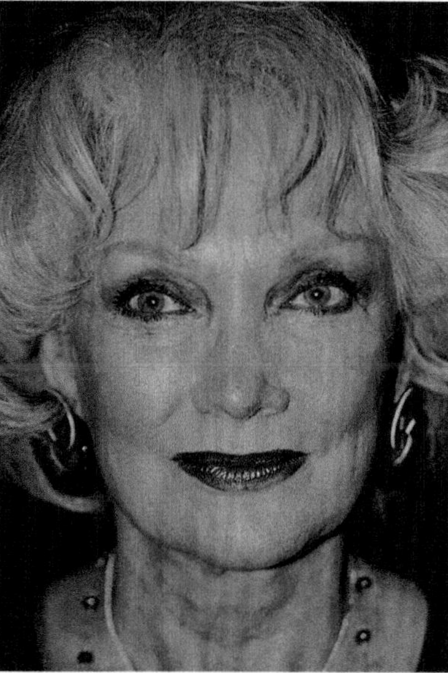

Fig. 5. A patient presents with collapse of the nasal bones due to excessive narrowing during previous rhinoplasty (*left*). She underwent "inside-out" lateral osteotomies with significant improvement of the nasal airway and appearance of the bony vault (*right*).

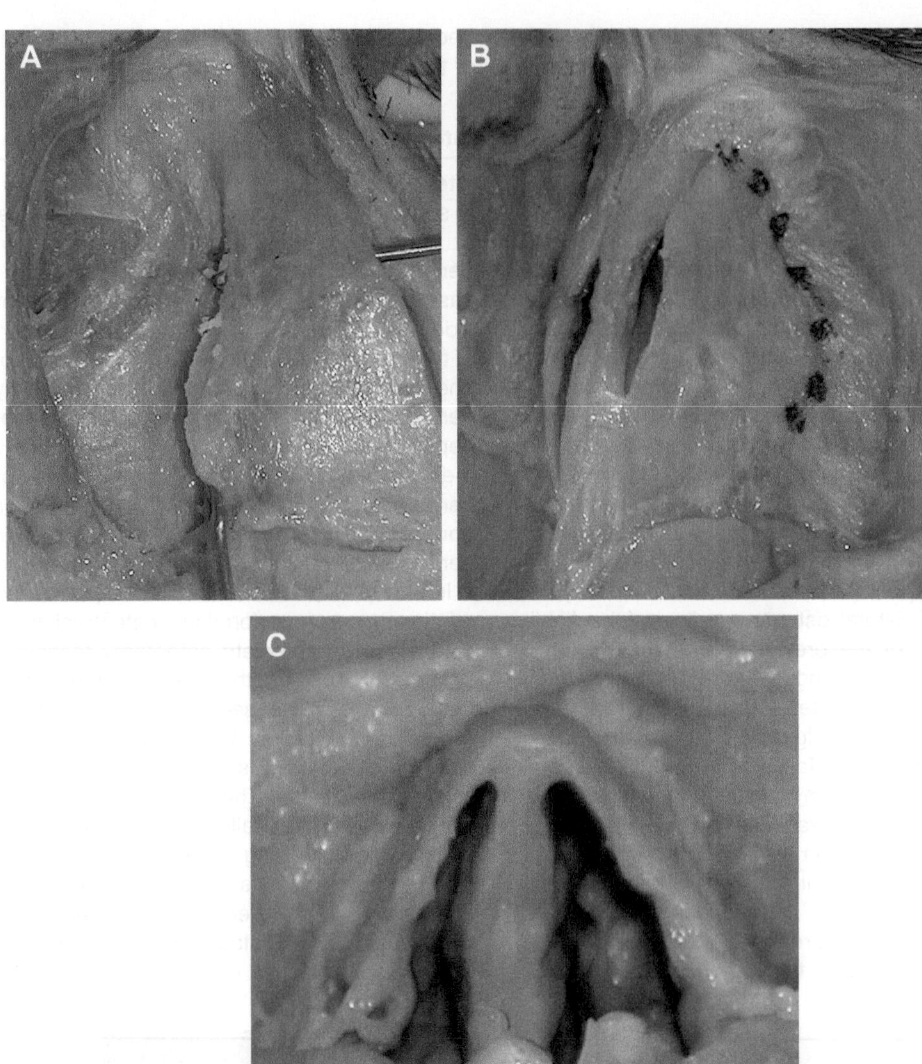

Fig. 6. A continuous osteotomy showing complete disruption of the periosteum (*A*). An "inside-out" perforating osteotomy showing preservation of the periosteum between the osteotomies (*B*). Photo (*C*) shows the difference in the stability of the osteotomized fragments. On the cadaver's right side the continuous osteotomy resulted in collapse of the nasal bone and a narrowed airway. On the cadaver's left side an "inside-out" perforating osteotomy was performed, resulting in increased stability of the fragment and a larger airway. (*From* Byrne PJ, Walsh WE, Hilger PA. The use of "inside-out" lateral osteotomies to improve outcome in rhinoplasty. Arch Facial Plast Surg 2003;5(3):251–25. Copyright 2003, American Medical Association. All rights reserved; with permission.)

intranasally, depending on the deformity. The percutaneous osteotomy is performed for a convex deformity, and the bone is pushed in as the osteotomy is performed. The intranasal perforating intermediate osteotomy is performed when there is a concave deformity, and the concave portion is pushed out as the osteotomy is performed.

The intermediate osteotomy is performed before the lateral osteotomy, which allows the stability to perform the osteotomy. The intermediate osteotomy cannot be easily performed after the lateral osteotomy because of the mobility of the nasal bone.

SEQUENCE OF OSTEOTOMIES

The sequence of the osteotomies will vary depending on the deformity that the surgeon wishes to correct. In general the medial osteotomy will be performed first as a straight or fading continuous osteotomy, depending on the surgeon's preferences and treatment goals. If an intermediate osteotomy is required, this is performed after the medial osteotomy but before the lateral osteotomy, to allow for stability of the nasal bone during the osteotomy. The lateral osteotomy is then performed and the mobilized segments are placed into the desired position.

The timing of the osteotomies within the time frame of the entire rhinoplasty procedure may vary depending on the surgeon's preference as well as the deformity being treated. In the case of a severely deviated nose, the surgeon may wish to perform the osteotomies first to allow for the midline positioning of the bony septum and nasal bones, thus allowing for the ultimate alignment of the middle and lower thirds from the now midline bony vault. In these cases sequence of osteotomies is performed in the following order (**Fig. 7**):

- The medialized nasal bone should be mobilized first with a medial, intermediate (if necessary), then lateral osteotomy.
- The medialized nasal bone is then displaced laterally to allow space for the midline repositioning of the deviated septum.
- A straight medial osteotomy is then performed on the opposite side into the nasal root, which is used as a fulcrum to reposition the septum in a midline position.
- The intermediate (if necessary) and lateral osteotomy is then performed on the opposite side and the nasal bone is placed into an appropriate position.

When the septum is not severely deviated and the osteotomies are being performed to narrow or widen the bony vault without reorientation in relation to the midline, the surgeon may wish to postpone the osteotomies until nearing the completion of the case. This postponement gives the surgeon the ability to hold pressure after the osteotomies, followed by immediate splinting of the nose to decrease the ultimate edema and bleeding associated with osteotomies. If the osteotomies are performed earlier in the case, the surgeon may still hold pressure to reduce the swelling and bleeding; however, the resultant edema is inevitable. The soft-tissue swelling may interfere with the surgeon's ability to evaluate the necessary structural changes that should be made to achieve the desired aesthetic result. Therefore it is often best to delay the osteotomies until the completion of the procedure whenever possible.

COMPLICATIONS

The correct execution of osteotomies requires a certain level of knowledge and skill. The

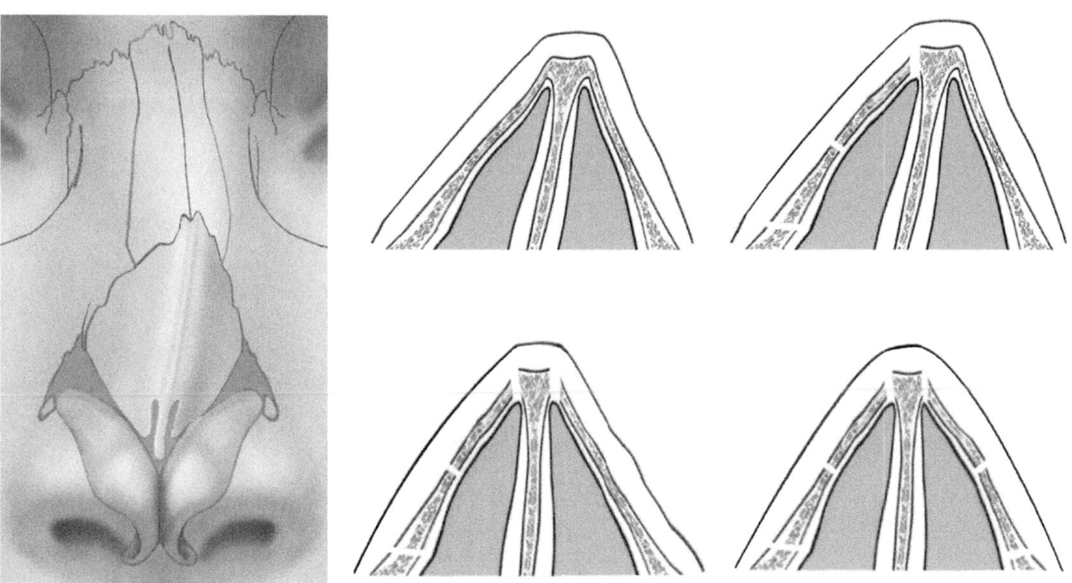

Fig. 7. Sequence of osteotomies for the deviated nose. First the medial, intermediate, and lateral osteotomy is created on the medialized nasal bone. This bone is then displaced laterally (*top right*). Next the medial osteotomy is created on the opposite side and the septum is repositioned to the midline (*bottom left*). Finally the intermediate and lateral osteotomy is created on the opposite side and the nasal bone is repositioned to straighten the bony vault (*bottom right*).

procedure is often performed under an envelope of soft tissue, and requires exceptional coordination based on tactile feedback. The surgeon should have knowledge of the bony vault anatomy and the consequences of inappropriately placed osteotomies. The authors have found cadaver dissection to be an invaluable experience, and have recommended this practice to all novice rhinoplasty surgeons. The surgeon may perform the various osteotomy techniques, then deglove the nose to compare the anticipated course of the osteotomies to the actual fracture pattern that occurs.

In practice it is important to carefully plan and execute the osteotomy to avoid complications. As stated in earlier sections, if the osteotomy is carried into the frontal process (low position) and the nasal bones are infractured, the osteotomized segment beyond the radix will lateralize, creating a rocker deformity. If this occurs, the surgeon should perform a percutaneous transverse osteotomy in a lower position to move the nasal bone independently of the nasal root. If the soft tissue and periosteum is excessively elevated beyond the osteotomy site, the fractured segment will lose support and may become a flail segment that is difficult to maintain in position. This situation may also occur if the segment becomes comminuted, which may happen if the patient has had multiple injuries in the past with previous fractures

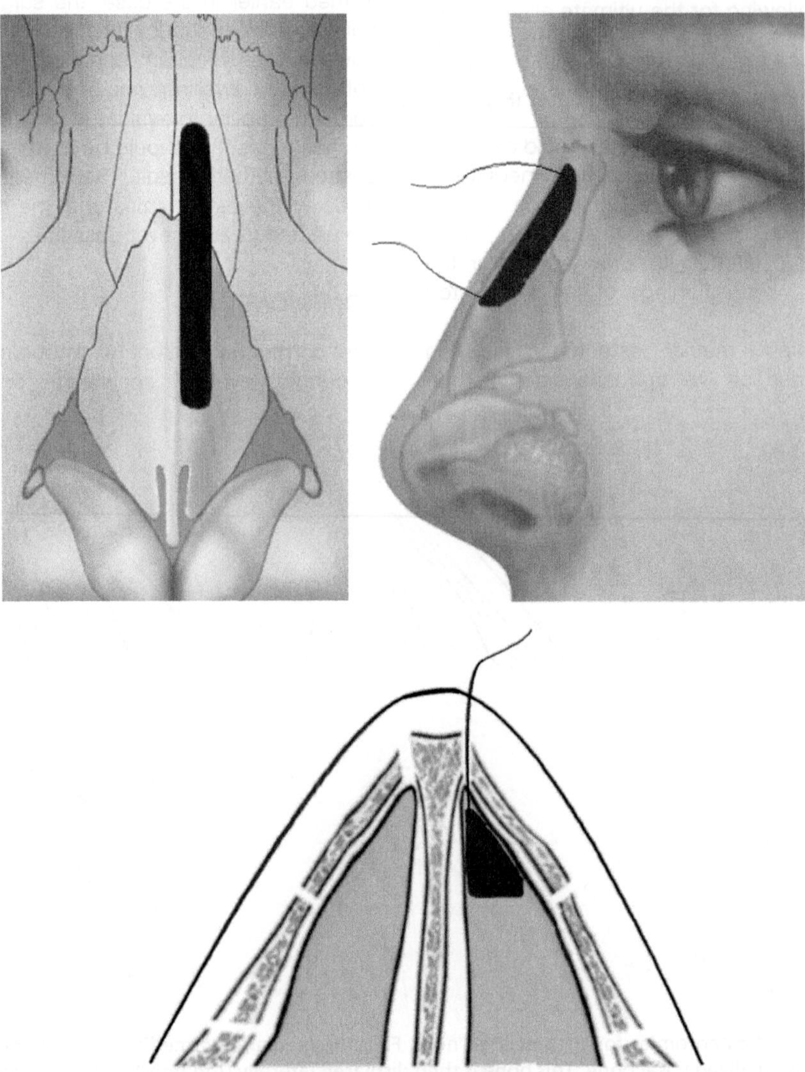

Fig. 8. In the case of a comminuted or flail segment, a Merocel sponge may be positioned high in the nasal vault to provide support. The sponge is secured with percutaneous sutures to hold the it in place, and is removed at 1 week postoperative. The superior suture is placed through the osteotomy site and then through the skin.

that have healed by a fibrous union. As the osteotomy is created comminution may occur, making it difficult to position the fragments. In these cases it may be necessary to place a piece of Merocel under the nasal bones and secure this with percutaneous sutures to help hold the flail segment or segments in place (**Fig. 8**). Extensive damage to the intranasal mucosa may result in synechiae between the lateral nasal wall and the septum. These adhesions may contribute to nasal airway obstruction and can be difficult to treat as they tend to reform after lysis of the adhesions. A piece of silastic sheeting may be placed for 2 to 3 weeks after surgery to try and discourage reformation of the adhesions. Epistaxis may also occur with significant mucosal injury. Bleeding is often temporary, and will resolve with expectant management and use of vasoconstrictant nasal spray such as oxymetazoline hydrochloride (Afrin). If packing is required, caution must be taken so as not to disrupt the position of the osteotomized bone because the packing may displace the bone laterally.

Improper placement of the osteotomy along the lateral nasal wall may lead to complications. An inappropriately low osteotomy may lead to nasal obstruction when the fragment is displaced medially into the airway in an effort to narrow the bony vault. A high osteotomy that is placed above the thick nasofacial sulcus will be easily palpable and visible under the thinner nasal skin that is located above the sulcus. The base will often remain too wide as well. Patients with thin skin may require the placement of perichondrium or a thin piece of crushed cartilage to disguise the osteotomies, especially with medial osteotomies. An incomplete osteotomy will result in incomplete movement of the nasal bones and persistent deviation of the bony vault.

Bony irregularities may form as well. Hyperostotic bone formation may occur, causing palpable or even visible irregularities. New and irregular bone formation may occur more frequently when the periosteum is not elevated in a continuous fashion and there is shearing or tearing of the periosteum. Aseptic necrosis may form in a comminuted fragment, which may result in an eventual palpable or visible dent. Either of these situations may require a revision procedure to rasp the hyperostotic bone, or to fill in or camouflage an area of missing bone. Occasionally a fragment of bone may become prominent after the back-fracture or communication between the medial and lateral osteotomies is performed. If this occurs the authors will often place a small 2-mm osteotome percutaneously over the spicule of bone and will push the fragment back into place with the osteotome. If this is not done, the fragment may move or degrade, leaving a palpable or visible dent.

SUMMARY

Nasal osteotomies may be used to treat various deformities of the bony nasal vault, including closing an open roof after hump reduction, straightening asymmetric or deviated nasal bones, narrowing a widened nasal base, or widening excessively narrowed nasal bones from prior trauma or rhinoplasty. To achieve optimal aesthetic and functional results one must have a comprehensive knowledge of the bony and cartilaginous framework of the nose and its relationship with the overlying soft tissues. A thorough understanding of the various osteotomy techniques will allow the surgeon to improve the overall contour and appearance of the nose, while ensuring preservation of or improvement on the functional internal anatomy of the nasal airway.

REFERENCES

1. Tardy ME. Surgical anatomy of the nose. New York (NY): Lippincott-Raven; 1990. p. 12.
2. Park SS, Becker SS. Repair of nasal airway obstruction in revision rhinoplasty. In: Becker DG, Park SS, editors. Revision rhinoplasty. New York (NY): Thieme; 2007. p. 52–68.
3. Gryskiewicz JM. Visible scars from percutaneous osteotomies. Plast Reconstr Surg 2005;116(6):1771–5.
4. Murakami CS, Larrabee WF. Comparison of osteotomy techniques in the treatment of nasal fractures. Facial Plast Surg 1992;8(4):209–19.
5. Webster RC, Davidson TM, Smith RC. Curved lateral osteotomy for airway protection in rhinoplasty. Arch Otolaryngol 1977;103(8):454–8.
6. Hilger JA. The internal lateral osteotomy in rhinoplasty. Arch Otolaryngol 1968;88(2):211–2.
7. Becker DG, McLaughlin RB Jr, Loevner LA, et al. The lateral osteotomy in rhinoplasty: clinical and radiographic rationale for osteotome selection. Plast Reconstr Surg 2000;105(5):1806–16 [discussion: 1817–9].
8. Tardy ME Jr, Denneny JC. Micro-ostoeotomies in rhinoplasty. Facial Plast Surg 1984;1:137–45.
9. Byrne PJ, Walsh WE, Hilger PA. The use of "inside-out" lateral osteotomies to improve outcome in rhinoplasty. Arch Facial Plast Surg 2003;5(3):251–5.

Surgical Treatment of the Crooked Nose

David Stepnick, MD, FACS[a,b,c,d,*], Bahman Guyuron, MD[a,b,e]

KEYWORDS

- Rhinoplasty • Septorhinoplasty • Crooked
- Deviated • Nose

Many surgeons consider mastery of septorhinoplasty to be one of the most difficult surgical challenges. Definitive predictable correction of the crooked nose is one of the most exigent (taxing) aspects of this operation; the literature is replete with references that describe how difficult it is to achieve long-term optimal results.[1–4] The surgeon must have the talent to methodically analyze the anatomy and aesthetics of a patient's nose as a unique structure and as part of the overall face, and must have an understanding of the interrelationships of the structural components of the nose and of the dynamics of change that result by altering these various structures. The surgeon must also have the surgical skill to appropriately change the structural framework and modify the soft tissue components of the nose to create the desired outcome, taking into consideration the forces of healing that can aid and work against the surgeon's goals.

An awareness of the historical development of the septorhinoplasty operation and the principles that drove changes in and refinement of techniques over the years allows the surgeon to apply these concepts to surgical treatment of the crooked nose, thereby increasing the chances of success. Up until 1890, surgeons attempted to correct deviations of the nasal septum by fracturing the septum and maintaining it in a midline position by intranasal tubes left in place over a period of months. Although this technique was generally successful for bony deviations, cartilaginous deflections were more resistant to the surgeon's efforts to restore their midline positions. The cartilage, being more elastic than the bone, was not easily fractured and tended to return to its original position. This tendency to return to its normal position persisted decades later, even when surgeons cross-hatched the cartilage, attempting to weaken its integrity and memory.

Morris Asch was a well-known pioneer nasal surgeon. He developed forceps specifically for the purpose of achieving reduction of the cartilaginous segment of the nasal septum. He described the technique and tools for closed septal redisplacement, a technique that relied on blunt force to disrupt the intrinsic memory and attachments of the cartilaginous septum. Asch recognized the danger of forceful and uncontrolled fracture of the perpendicular plate of the ethmoid or vomer, advocating his techniques for correction of cartilaginous deviations only; he did not address the factors responsible for the cartilaginous deformities and thus his patients did not have lasting

[a] Department of Plastic and Reconstructive Surgery, Case Western Reserve University, Cleveland, OH 44106, USA
[b] Department of Plastic and Reconstructive Surgery, University Hospitals Case Medical Center, Cleveland, OH 44106, USA
[c] Department of Otolaryngology–Head and Neck Surgery, Case Western Reserve University, Cleveland, OH 44106, USA
[d] Department of Plastic and Reconstructive Surgery, Center for Aesthetic Facial Surgery, University Hospitals, 29001 Cedar Road Suite 202, Lyndhurst, OH 44124, USA
[e] Department of Plastic and Reconstructive Surgery, Center for Aesthetic Facial Surgery, University Hospitals, 29017 Cedar Road, Lyndhurst, OH 44124, USA
* Corresponding author. Department of Plastic and Reconstructive Surgery, Center for Aesthetic Facial Surgery, University Hospitals, 29001 Cedar Road Suite 202, Lyndhurst, OH 44124.
E-mail address: David.Stepnick@uhhospitals.org

Clin Plastic Surg 37 (2010) 313–325
doi:10.1016/j.cps.2009.12.001
0094-1298/10/$ – see front matter. Published by Elsevier Inc.

improvement. Because of this lack of efficacy, his techniques were abandoned around the turn of the twentieth century.[5]

As there was no single technique that produced consistent results, various procedures were described by surgeons of the time, many of which seem to violate the fundamental surgical principles of present day surgery. Krieg[6] apparently understood that cartilage memory was often the cause of surgical failure, and described a technique in which the entire deflected cartilaginous segment along with the overlying mucosa was simply resected. This left a large perforation; the resultant crusting and bleeding could have been expected to produce more obstructive symptoms. Eventually, Krieg recommended removal of only the deviated portion of the cartilage with mucosal preservation, the precursor to the submucous resection procedure that became popular among surgeons decades later.[6]

In 1912, Otto Freer authored what can be considered a landmark paper of the times, *The Anatomy of Deflections of the Nasal Septum*, in which he painstakingly described various types of septal deformity. He wrote, "Of far more surgical consequence than the external form of deflections is their internal structure, my knowledge of which, taught me by my submucous resections by my open or flap method, virtual dissections on the living, is here set forth. The insight into the distorted anatomy of the deflected septum so gained has also shown me how deflections come to be and the propriety, denied by me in my earlier experience, of grouping them into traumatic deflections and those due to faulty growth."[7] It is evident that Freer recognized that the shape of the nose largely depends on the shape of the septum, but he advocated submucosal resection of the entire septal cartilage, seemingly not realizing the role that the septum played in the overall structural support of the nose. Many other surgeons such as Samuel Fomon and colleagues[8] felt that the only physiologically important structure in the nose was the mucosa, and when saddling occurred as a result of the removal of the entire septal cartilage, the blame was placed on cicatricial forces of healing rather than on the removal of the cartilage itself.

George Killian, a contemporary of Freer, recognized the structural importance of the dorsal and caudal portion of the septal cartilage, preserving it in his operations, thereby maintaining support. Other surgeons, such as Jacques Joseph, Maurice Cottle, and Jack Sheen, further refined surgical techniques, emphasizing preservation and realignment, which is now the basis of modern septorhinoplasty procedures. The 1 stage septorhinoplasty has become a surgical standard of care, because many surgeons in the mid-twentieth century recognized that septal surgery played an essential role in the management of the crooked nose and combined septoplasty and rhinoplasty into 1 operation.[9–17]

ETIOLOGY

Crooked noses are characterized by the deviation of the cartilaginous lower two-thirds of the nose in relationship to the bony upper one-third; the nose may take on a sinusoidal appearance. However, many variations can exist and asymmetry can result from any or all of the nasal thirds being off of the midline. Intrinsic and extrinsic forces produce nasal deviation.[2] There is almost always a major septal deformity in a patient with a severely deviated nose.[16,18–20]

An accurate diagnosis is requisite in the formulation of an appropriate surgical plan. Successful correction of the crooked nose requires an understanding of the developmental anatomy of the osseocartilaginous structures of the nose, the nasal function and physiology, and the surgical techniques, which can restore form, function, and achieve facial balance. The nasal bones, paired lateral cartilages, nasal septum, and turbinates must be addressed as an integrated whole, although arguably the key to successful repair (and the cause of most surgical failures) in most crooked noses is the nasal septum.

The nasal septum, seemingly a simple, unimportant structure, is actually complex. Studies have shown that in the ethmoideoseptal synchondrosis, postnatal endochondral ossification contributes to the growth of the ethmoid bone, the body of which is a derivative of the basicranial cartilage primordium. Unique in bone histology, there is a syndesmosis between the cartilaginous septum and the membranous vomer bone where new cartilage is formed in the perichondrium without endochondral ossification. Vertical growth depends on a complex interplay of resorption, new cartilage formation, and forces exerted on the apposing structures.[21]

In the absence of identified trauma, patients with a deviated septum or twisted nose often wonder when and how septal deformity developed; often the surgeon may not have a reliable answer. In a study by Gray, the incidence of septal deformity was investigated in 2380 Caucasian infants at birth, in 2112 adult skulls of 5 ethnic groups, and in 918 animals representing a variety of other mammalian species. Forty-two percent of infant septa were straight, 27% were deviated, and 31% were kinked. A similar ratio was found in the adult skulls. Gray observed that the varying degrees of septal deformity occur at a constant rate at birth and in adults, varying only slightly by ethnic group. Based on these observations, Gray concluded that septal deformity is of two kinds, which may occur independently or together: deformity of the quadrangular cartilage caused by direct trauma or pressure at any age; and combined septal deformity involving the cartilaginous and bony septum, caused by compression across the maxilla from pressures that occur during pregnancy or parturition.[22]

Evaluation of 93 consecutive patients who underwent septoplasty by one of the authors (BG) revealed 6 basic types of septal deformity: 40% of the patients had a septal tilt deformity, 32% had a C-shaped anteroposterior deviation, 14% had localized deviations or large spurs, 9% had S-shaped anteroposterior deformities, 4% had C-shaped cephalocaudal deformities, and 1% had an S-shaped anteroposterior deformity. Recognition of the type of deformity is important in surgical planning, because various surgical procedures are necessary to deal with the different types of septal deviation.[23]

In addition to the septum, the nasal bones can also contribute to a crooked nose deformity. The nasal bones are the most commonly fractured bones of the face and fractures of the nasal bones are one of the most frequent causes of a crooked nose. Progressive nasal obstruction after such an injury is not unusual, and loss of support and scarring can lead to decreased airflow and an asymmetric appearance. Internal and external valve collapse may occur.

The patient can sometimes can identify the specific injury that caused the crooked nose and, in these cases, knowledge about the mechanism of injury, force of impact, and vector of impact can be useful in understanding how the deformity developed and in surgical planning. When no specific injury is identified, childhood trauma, birth trauma, or intrauterine forces may be the cause of the crooked nose. Disturbance of the growth centers may result in asymmetric growth of the osseocartilaginous nose through childhood and especially during adolescence. Because in childhood the nose is composed primarily of cartilage, injuries to it may go unrecognized. The nasal bones are smaller and more compliant and tend to absorb energy applied as external trauma instead of fracturing.

When a nasal fracture occurs as a result of a low impact lateral force, 1 of the nasal bones may be depressed without harming the septum, resulting in a nose that appears deviated to the opposite side, but which in reality is not. Surgery that replaces the nasal bone in its native position corrects the asymmetry and illusion of crookedness, and restores baseline airflow. Likelihood of success in these cases is high.

As the magnitude of the force increases and the force vector becomes more oriented from a frontal direction, the nasal bones tend to splay and the nasal septum, acting as the shock absorber of the nose, can also fracture. The surgery becomes more difficult and the likelihood of success decreases.

Although developmental disturbance and trauma are the most common causes of a twisted nose, the surgeon must exclude other potential pathologies. Autoimmune, immunologic, and connective tissue diseases can result in damage and resorption of cartilage with resulting loss of structural support, scarring, and twisting. The use of drugs such as cocaine and nasal steroids, or mass lesions such as polyps or neoplasms can destroy normal structures, altering the appearance and symmetry of the nose. Although uncommon, a careful history and examination can exclude such unusual causes of a deviated nose.

If a patient has undergone previous surgery, whether done by a novice or an expert, and whether poorly done or executed extremely well, the process of healing, aging, and gravity can affect the appearance of the nose causing it to appear asymmetric and crooked.

EVALUATION OF THE PATIENT

A complete history and physical examination are necessary in any patient in whom surgical correction of the twisted nose is being considered. Although the nasal surgeon's primary focus is the nose and breathing, all other relevant data needs to be uncovered before offering surgery, including information about the patient's cardiovascular health, a personal or family history of diabetes or glucose intolerance, history of tobacco and alcohol use, history of easy bleeding or bruising, and history of the patient's psychological or psychiatric issues.

The surgeon should determine when the nose became crooked, and should know if gradual twisting occurred as the patient matured from a child to an adolescent and then to an adult, or if there was a more immediate and sudden cause of the deformity, such as with a facial or nasal trauma or from a previous surgery. The surgeon should understand if the patient's expectations are limited to improvement in breathing and straightening the nose, or if other aesthetic goals need to be addressed at the same time. The patient should be questioned about associated symptoms such as epistaxis, rhinitis, and congestion and their response to various pharmacologic interventions. The physician should ask whether there is a seasonal nature to the patient's complaints of congestion, whether it seems to be worse at various times of the day, and whether the patient routinely uses nasal steroid sprays or sympathomimetics (which can cause rebound). The patient should be asked whether breathing is more impaired during exertion or exercise and whether deep breathing through the nose exacerbates the symptoms.

The patient's general physical examination is usually performed by the primary care physician, however it is essential that the rhinoplasty surgeon examines not only the external and internal nose but also the nose in relation to the entire face. This skill must become second nature and the surgeon must be able to identify subtle nuances of facial form and symmetry. Even if the patient only desires surgical correction of a crooked nose, balance and symmetry of the facial aesthetic subunits must be evaluated separately and in relationship to the nose.

A systematic examination of the nose should occur in each patient contemplating rhinoplasty. Beginning with the upper third of the nose, the surgeon should examine the nose, the position and depth of the nasion, the position, length, and symmetry of the nasal bones, and the thickness of the skin overlying the bones. As the examination moves caudally, the surgeon determines whether there seems to be deficiency, collapse, or disarticulation of the upper lateral cartilages. Examination should determine if there is deviation of the entire nose or if it is primarily cartilaginous in nature.

Thereafter, the tip is examined and the surgeon notes whether it appears to be in the midline or not. Tip support, rotation, projection, bulbosity, symmetry, width of the lateral crura of the lower lateral cartilages, nostril shape, and the columella are assessed. The tip should be visualized at rest and with respiration, and should be palpated and visually examined. The caudal septum and the position of the anterior and posterior septal angles in relationship to the tip and the nasal spine should be assessed.

Intranasal examination includes a thorough examination of the septum and the turbinates before and after decongestion, and the response of the turbinates to the decongestion is noted. Anterior rhinoscopy alone is rarely sufficient to appreciate the subtle anatomy of the various forms that a septal deviation can assume, and in the case of a severely deviated septum, seeing beyond the crooked septum is often impossible without using a fiberoptic device for visualization. Spurs and alterations from midline should be identified, as should the presence of septal deviations, absence of cartilage from a previous nasal surgery, and the contribution of the dorsal septum to the outward appearance of the nasal dorsum. Examination should address whether or not the angle between the upper lateral cartilages and the septum approaches the ideal value of 9° to 15° degrees and if there is collapse on inspiration. Narrowing of the nasal valve can cause airway obstruction. The size and color of the turbinates should be noted and their potential role in obstruction must be determined. The Cottle maneuver, retracting the cheek skin laterally to see if airflow is improved, is often described as a way to determine whether valve collapse plays a role in airway obstruction; however, using a small curette or small cotton-tipped application to gently lift the nose in the area of the internal and external nasal valves is a much more precise technique for determining whether valve support is lacking. Deep inspiration with alar collapse indicates a weak external valve.

Photodocumention is essential and serves several functions. It allows the surgeon to precisely record visual abnormalities that can never be fully described in narrative fashion. It is a tool that aids in diagnosis and planning. With the help of digital manipulation, it may assist the patient in understanding what their nose may look like after the procedure and it may assist the surgeon in making sure the patient's expectations mirror the surgeon's plans. Photographs document the progress of healing and recovery and can be ultimately used as a tool for surgeon self-assessment and teaching. In cases of trauma or assault, photographs may play a medico-legal role.

Life-sized photographs are useful in surgical planning for any rhinoplasty, but can be particularly useful in the patient with a crooked nose (**Fig. 1**).[24] Standard rhinoplasty views are essential, but views from above can be useful in visualizing and recording the deformity in a patient with a twisted nose (**Fig. 2**). Furthermore, for the frontal view, an overhead light source is preferred to illumination by a flash from the camera or from flash umbrellas, because an overhead light source will accentuate the visibility of the deviation seen in the photographs, as it more closely duplicates the way sunlight or overhead lighting falls on the nose and casts shadows.

Radiographic imaging is usually not needed except when patients also suffer from allergy and/or paranasal sinus disease, computed tomography scanning can identify whether

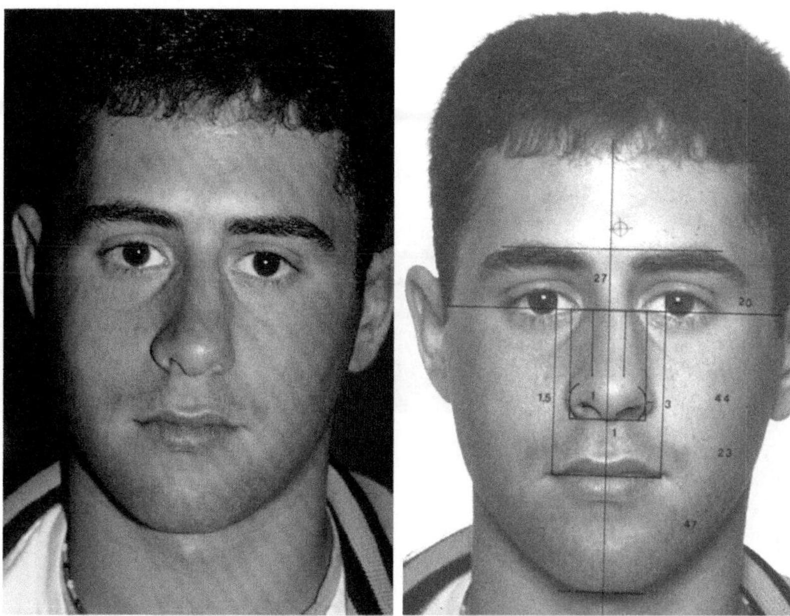

Fig. 1. Full-scale life-size photographs enable the surgeon, particularly in the case of the crooked nose, to draw a pleasing and proportionate profile and determine the difference between the patient's nasal outline and the surgical plan. This will help the surgeon to accurately define aesthetic goals.

inflammation of the mucosal lining of the sinuses is present or not. Furthermore, in patients with facies that seem to have some degree of abnormal growth and development, imaging can identify anatomic variations of the facial bones including variations of the nasal bones and turbinates (**Fig. 3**).

TREATMENT

Symmetry, balance, proportion, and nasal function must be considered when a surgeon develops a therapeutic plan to repair a crooked nose. For decades, surgeons have described 2 primary techniques by which the twisted nose can be straightened: endonasal and external approach techniques.[25] Even though there is some argument about the best approach to affect the desired changes both these approaches have a role in the surgeons' hands and the choice of technique depends on whether the surgeon attempts to deconstruct and reconstruct the nose or create the illusion of symmetry by techniques that camouflage asymmetry such as the placement of strategically positioned cartilaginous onlay grafts. The camouflaging technique can be particularly effective in combination with the deconstruction and reconstruction technique, but it does not address the functional complaints related to airflow in patients in whom airway compromise is an issue. When nasal obstruction is not an issue and when a patient has an insolated deformity, camouflaging techniques have the most value. In general, techniques that primarily employ camouflage are technically less demanding than techniques that deconstruct and reconstruct the nose, and some may thus consider these methods to be more reliable because the underlying structural integrity of the nose is not altered. However, the surgeon must be aware that the grafts can be visible or become visible, and the result is primarily an aesthetic improvement and not a functional enhancement. When used in combination with the techniques described later in the article, an isolated graft to camouflage deformity or to

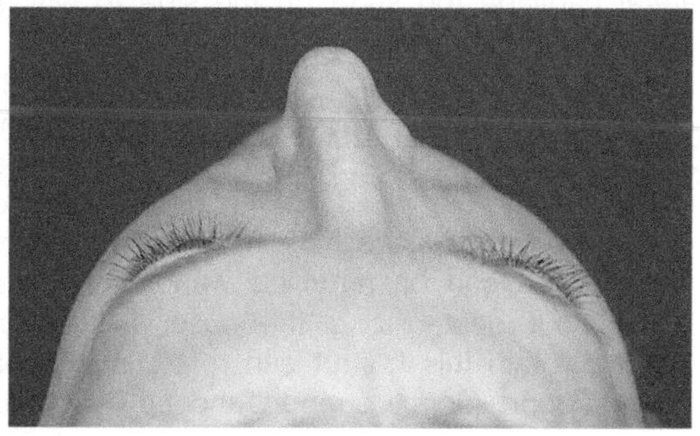

Fig. 2. Although not typically part of the standard series of views obtained for photo documentation of septorhinoplasty, the view from above is useful as it readily shows how the nose deviates from the midline.

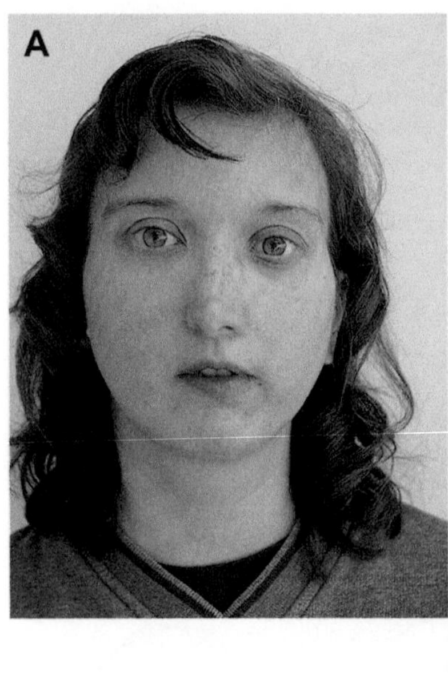

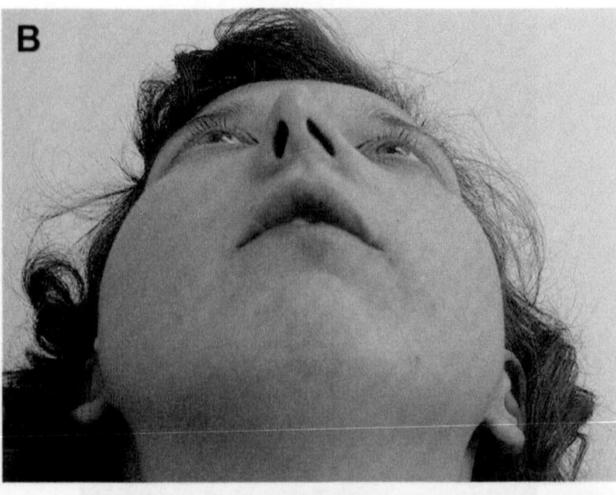

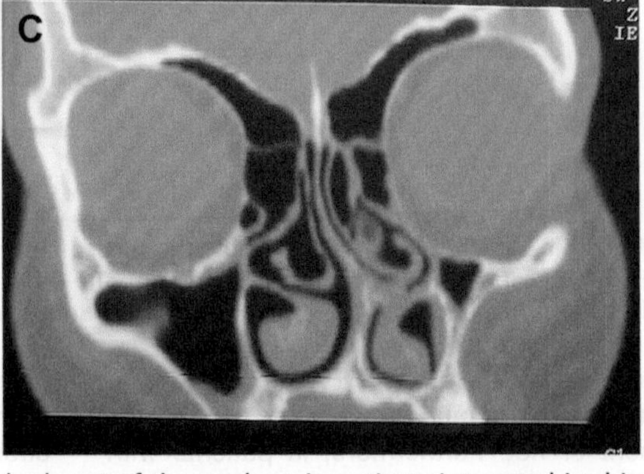

Fig. 3. (*A–C*) Radiographic imaging is not a standard part of the work-up in patients interested in rhinoplasty. However, it can be helpful in patients who may benefit from concurrent sinus surgery, in patients with rhinogenic migraines, or in patients with abnormal growth and development.

correct an imperfect surgical result can be extremely valuable. The primary focus of this discussion is related to correction of the visual asymmetry and restoration of optimal airway function.

In the same manner that a modern skyscraper is constructed of I-beams assembled in a well established three-dimensional grid with supporting beams, cross beams, and other features familiar to the civil engineer, the nose is constructed of interlocking and joined cartilages and bones that provide analogous structural support. Although this framework creates a stable structure that provides a patent airway and houses the functionally important turbinates, it can thwart surgical attempts to correct the twisted nose when the surgeon incompletely dismantles and rebuilds the interlocking osseocartilaginous framework. As previously mentioned, a twisted nose almost always has an associated crooked septum and a crooked nose treated without addressing the deviated septum is doomed to failure. A well-executed septoplasty is thus the key to successful long-term correction of a twisted nose. It is important to separate the upper lateral cartilages from the septum to correct the anterior nasal deviation. However, it is crucial not to trim the upper lateral cartilages until the septoplasty and nasal bone osteotomy are completed. Often correction of the anterior nasal deviation mandates differential upper lateral cartilage trimming which, if done before straightening the nasal frame, leaves the lateral cartilage too short on the side to which the anterior nose deviates.

CORRECTING THE DEVIATED SEPTUM: GENERAL PRINCIPLES

- Deviated cartilage that is not part of the 1-cm L-strut can be removed without concern about destabilizing the nose. Failure to maintain this L-strut can result in loss of support (dorsal support and tip support), saddling, columellar retraction, and tip ptosis.
- Spurs and crooked cartilage at the center of the septum may result in nasal obstruction, sinus, and migraine headaches caused by

contact with the turbinates but they do not, in general, contribute to support of the midvault.

- Scoring the concave side of the septal cartilage may be necessary to release the memory/spring of the cartilage. Scoring alone may produce unpredictable outcomes. The cartilage's response to the scoring has to be controlled by the use of spreader grafts or internal nasal splints.
- Unilateral or bilateral spreader grafts, typically fashioned from the resected cartilaginous nasal septum, are important components of the reconstructed nose, as they reinforce the septum and support it in a midline position. Graft sources also include the bony perpendicular plate.
- Permanent sutures anchored in positions such as the midline maxillary crest may be needed to keep the septum in the intended midline position.

SURGICAL DETAILS

A twisted nose can result from intrinsic and extrinsic forces acting on the bony, cartilaginous, and soft-tissue components of the nose.[1] Extrinsic force is created by scar contractures or congenitally asymmetric attachments of the osseocartilaginous skeleton, whereas intrinsic forces are inherent or acquired septal cartilaginous abnormalities.[1]

The authors believe that the most reliable way to correct the crooked nose is via the wide exposure provided by the external rhinoplasty approach, discussed in later sections and correction of all the deviated components of the nose, the nasal bones, the septum, and the tip structures. The intrinsic and extrinsic forces that lead to septal deviation and a crooked nose must then be identified and released, thereby straightening the septum and bony-cartilaginous pyramid while maintaining structural support of the dorsum and the tip so that dependable long-term results can be achieved. Structure and function go hand-in-hand and the surgeon must understand airflow dynamics and the role of the turbinates. These important structures need to be managed appropriately as part of any procedure designed to correct the twisted nose.

External rhinoplasty is an approach rather than a procedure. Although the terminology differs, with some surgeons describing this procedure as an open rhinoplasty or an open structure rhinoplasty, all terms refer to the process by which the supporting framework of the nose is visualized, altered, and the desired changes in the relationship of these structures to each other is changed to achieve the desired functional and aesthetic outcome. The external approach offers the student and the accomplished surgeon unparalleled visualization of the paired upper and lower lateral cartilages, the nasal bones, and the nasal septum. It is imperative that surgeons have a thorough understanding of the three-dimensional spatial relationships of the skin and the nasal substructure, and understand how alterations in these various anatomic structures affect the ultimate function and appearance of the nose. In patients with a crooked nose, the external approach is unsurpassed in providing exposure to this complex three-dimensional anatomy and provides a high degree of accuracy and the best level of control.

A discussion of incision placement is beyond the scope of this article but is critical in providing necessary exposure for an external approach rhinoplasty. Dissection in the proper plane (just superficial to the mucoperichondrium of the lower and upper lateral cartilages) is vital in maintaining hemostasis. As dissection proceeds cephalically, the nasal bones are identified. Their periosteum is incised about 2 mm above and parallel to their caudal border and a Woodson, Cottle or similar elevator is used to elevate the periosteum of the nasal bones, staying medial to the intended areas of lateral osteotomies.

Once the osseocartilaginous skeleton has been widely exposed, attention is turned toward exposure and release of the septum. The lower lateral cartilages are retracted inferiorly and laterally, and the dorsal septum is identified just caudal to the upper lateral cartilages. Sharp dissection allows identification of the septal mucoperichondrium, which is then elevated off the septum. Once the correct plane is established, cephalad dissection under the upper lateral cartilages should precede dissection toward the bony septum, as visualization improves once the upper lateral cartilages are released from the septum. Division of the upper laterals from the nasal septum begins the systematic release of the extrinsic forces, which may contribute to nasal deviation. If interlocking scrolls between the upper and lower lateral cartilages are present, cephalic trim of the lower lateral cartilages also helps to eliminate these deforming forces. Occasionally, when asymmetric upper lateral cartilages cause twisting of the septum, the releasing maneuver alone is sufficient to straighten the nose. Continued dissection releases the mucoperichondrial and mucoperiosteal attachments from the septum and after release of these extrinsic forces, the septum is reassessed.

Making sure to maintain adequate support, the intrinsic forces responsible for a deviated nasal septum must then be identified and addressed. After analysis of 1224 septal surgeries, one of the authors (BG) previously described 6 different categories of septal deviation. Differentiation of these classes of deviation is important, as the procedures necessary to correct the deformities differ. Because correction of the contributing septal deformity is essential for achieving symmetry of the crooked nose, it is useful to review these deviations and their treatment.

Posterocaudal resection of the septum leaving an L-shaped strut is a maneuver common to the correction of all 6 types of septal deformities. Resected septum can include portions of the quadrangular cartilage, maxillary crest, perpendicular plate of the ethmoid and/or the vomer. It is important to preserve an L-strut consisting of at least 10 mm of dorsal and caudal septum left attached to the nasal spine and the perpendicular plate (the keystone area to avoid delayed nasal collapse and resultant deformity).

In this classification of deformity, a Class I septal deviation is designated as a septal tilt (**Fig. 4**A). The quadrangular cartilage is frequently displaced to one side of the maxillary crest. Straightening is achieved by separating the posterocaudal septum from the vomer and partially mobilizing the quadrangular cartilage at its junction with the perpendicular plate. In addition to posterocaudal resection of the septum, correction of this deformity requires removal of the overlapping portion at the maxillary crest, repositioning the septum in the midline, and anchoring the septum in the midline with a figure-of-eight suture.

For a C-shaped anteroposterior deformity (Class II) (**Fig. 4**B), straightening is accomplished by posterocaudal resection of the septum, osteotomies of the nasal spine and residual vomer, partial disjunction of the quadrangular cartilage from the perpendicular plate, if necessary, and cephalocaudal scoring of the cartilage only if needed. To help ensure that the cartilage remains in its new position in the midline, bilateral (extramucosal) stents are placed at the end of the procedure and kept in position for at least 2 and preferably 3 weeks.

C-shaped cephalocaudal septal deviation (Class III) (**Fig. 4**C) is corrected by completely releasing the cartilaginous septum from the maxillary crest, partially releasing the cephalic portion of the quadrangular cartilage from the perpendicular plate, performing an osteotomy of the nasal spine, posterocaudal resection of the septum, and anteroposterior scoring of the concave cartilage. Spreader grafts are placed anteriorly (after osteotomies have been performed) to secure the cartilage in a midline position. Placement of spreader grafts on the concave side of the septal deformity is of utmost importance. As with the Class II deformity, extramucosal stents are applied posteriorly.

Posterocaudal resection of the septum, repositioning of the nasal spine and vomer bone, osteotomies, and bilateral cephalocaudal scoring of the concave areas of the septal cartilage is necessary to correct an S-shaped anteroposterior deviation (Class IV) (**Fig. 4**D). Cartilage position is directed by spreader grafts, and extramucosal stents are placed if necessary. The externally visible twisted nose is eliminated as the septal deformity is corrected.

Class V septal deviation, an S-shaped cephalocaudal deviation, is corrected by releasing the septum from the maxillary crest, partially releasing the cartilaginous septum from the perpendicular plate, posterocaudal resection of the septum, and bilateral anteroposterior scoring of the concave portion of the cartilage (**Fig. 4**E). The anterior portion of the septum is supported with bilateral spreader grafts; bilateral extramucosal stents are placed posteriorly. Localized deviation of the septum (Class VI) is corrected by removal of the deviated portion of the cartilage and bone and application of stents (**Fig. 4**F).

Sometimes an isolated or independent deformity of the caudal septum exists, resulting in deviation of the nasal tip. In extreme cases, the caudal septum can twist at an angle of 90° or even more from the plane of the midline. Sometimes, this portion of the septum can be redundant and simple excision of the twisted septum will suffice; however, the surgeon must carefully assess the effect that resection of this portion of the septum will have on the nasal form in relation to tip support, vertical position of the columella and so forth. When this portion of the septum needs to be preserved but is found to be displaced off of the maxillary crest, a small triangular wedge of cartilage from the inferior septum at the posterior septal angle is removed and the septum is brought into a midline position. A permanent suture is used to secure this portion of the septum to the periosteum of the maxillary crest. Pastorek and colleagues[26] describe a similar maneuver intended to secure the caudal septum in the midline in which the septal cartilage along the maxillary crest is dissected free but not excised. In this modified swinging door technique, the caudal septum is flipped over the nasal spine, which acts as a doorstep, thereby securing this portion of the septum in a straighter position. Regardless of the specific nuances of the technique, the suture used to anchor the septum to the maxillary crest is key.

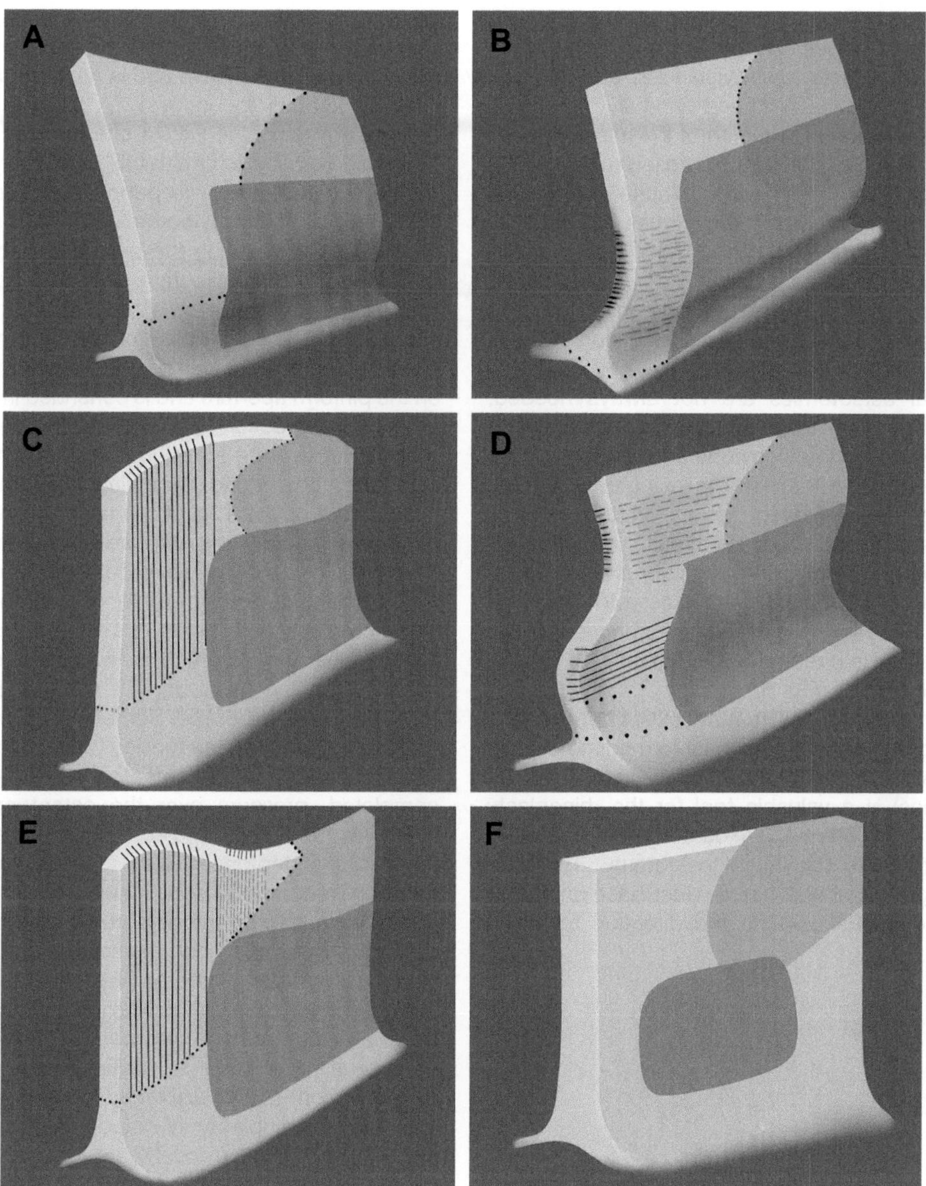

Fig. 4. (*A*) Class I septal deviation, designated as a septal tilt. (*B*) Class II septal deviation, a C-shaped anteroposterior deformity. (*C*) Class III septal deviation, a C-shaped cephalocaudal septal deviation. (*D*) Class IV septal deviation, an S-shaped anteroposterior deviation. (*E*) Class V septal deviation, an S-shaped cephalocaudal deviation. (*F*) Class VI septal deviation, a localized deviation of the septum.

Once the septum has been straightened, the nose is carefully reassessed for any remaining cartilaginous asymmetries and these are addressed by appropriate trimming of the upper lateral cartilages. Cephalic trim of the lower lateral cartilages may also be indicated.

Careful analysis of the nasal deformity leads the rhinoplasty surgeon to the most appropriate maneuver to achieve correction. Some surgeons prefer to correct the severely deviated bony dorsum first, thereby providing a base on which the middle vault can be set, whereas other surgeons, particularly in cases of a more mildly deviated middle-third region, first address the lower two-thirds of the nose and the septum.

At times, a deviated upper third of the nose is the only factor contributing to a crooked dorsum, whereas by virtue of their attachment to the upper lateral cartilages, the nasal bones can direct the middle vault away from the midline.

The number and location of osteotomies is chosen based on whether or not dorsal reduction is desired and on the specific position and length of the nasal bones. With the external approach, the nasal bones are easily visualized, and the periosteum can be elevated and carefully preserved. The periosteum in the region of the nasal process of the maxilla is important to preserve, because it helps to prevent the inward collapse of the nasal bones. Many osteotomy techniques are used by various surgeons with similarly good results, but certain principles such as using sharp instruments and making careful directed movements help to maximize the safe atraumatic application of these techniques.

Medial osteotomies are not always needed, particularly when dorsal reduction results in a large open roof, but should be done before intermediate and lateral osteotomies. The osteotomy can be performed under direct vision via the external rhinoplasty approach. Various osteotomes, including a 6-mm curved guarded osteotome, may be used to complete this osteotomy, which begins at the junction of the nasal bones and the septum and is directed approximately 15° lateral from the midline (**Fig. 5**).

When significant asymmetry exists between the length of the nasal bones, an intermediate osteotomy (in combination with medial and lateral osteotomies) is a valuable tool for the rhinoplasty surgeon. The intermediate osteotomy runs parallel but anterior to the lateral osteotomy. Typically, the longer nasal wall has a wider base and is on the side contralateral to the direction to which the dorsum is deviated. Intermediate osteotomies may also be used for nasal bones that are excessively convex or concave and is typically done on the side that is too convex. A transcutaneous perforating technique with a sharp 2-mm osteotome can be used to create this osteotomy.

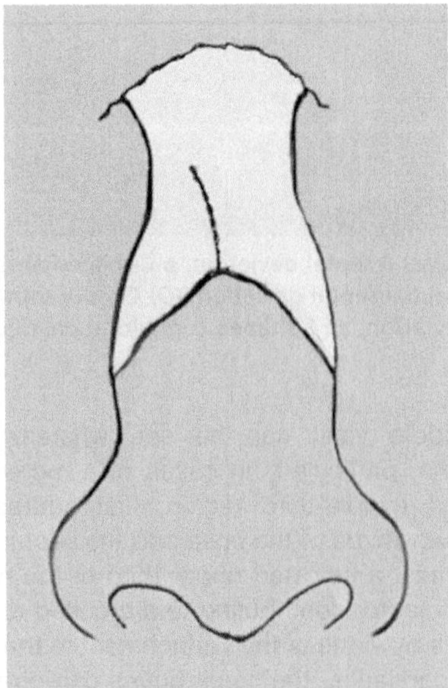

Fig. 5. Course of the medial osteotomy, beginning paramedian adjacent to the septum and directed approximately 15° from the midline.

Lateral osteotomies are performed as transcutaneous perforating osteotomies or endonasally, after carefully elevating the periosteum, typically in a high-low-high direction, thereby protecting the nasal airway at the nasal base, leaving a small triangle of bone at the base of the piriform aperture. This osteotomy begins 3 to 4 mm anteriorly on the piriform aperture and is continued in a posterocephalic direction up to the level of the medial canthus. The path is low in the middle third of the nose, maximizing narrowing, and then high again in the upper third of the nose to meet with the medial osteotomy and to prevent over narrowing. When the nasal base is wide and over narrowing is not a concern, the inferior portion of the osteotomy can be initiated in a low position, and similarly the upper portion of the osteotomy can be lower on the nasal bone if narrowing of the root of the nose is desired. Sometimes, a unilateral osteotomy may be performed in cases of the crooked nose. Once osteotomies have been completed, pressure over the osteotomy sites can minimize bruising and ecchymosis. In addition to precise osteotomies with minimal periosteal trauma, Tardy and Denney[27] use an assistant to apply pressure over the osteotomy sites until the procedure has been completed. Precise, atraumatic, complete osteotomies help ensure a successful outcome. Rarely is it necessary to remove a wedge of bone between the septum and the lateral nasal bone to facilitate repositioning the nasal bone that is displaced too far laterally.

Following completion of osteotomies, spreader grafts (discussed previously) are placed, as indicated. These grafts are ideally harvested from septal cartilage and are approximately 5 mm high and can be up to 30 mm long. They are secured to the upper lateral cartilages and the dorsal septum with at least 2 mattress sutures, reinforcing the cartilaginous septum, restoring support, and maximizing internal valve integrity. If mid-vault widening is undesirable, these grafts are placed 1 mm below the septal plane. Spreader grafts may be used bilaterally, but unilateral spreader grafts can be used effectively particularly in the crooked nose for restoration of dorsal aesthetic lines or to camouflage residual deformity. Septal batten grafts may also be used in the caudal septal region if structural integrity of the cartilage itself is insufficient to maintain a long-term midline position.

Suture placement need not and should not be the same in every patient, and various techniques have been described as adjuncts toward achieving symmetry of the middle nasal vault. Dayan and Shah[28] describe a suture placed between the nasal bones and the upper lateral cartilage with a unilateral spreader graft for patients with dorsal septal asymmetry. Pontius and Leach[29] use a sidewall spreading suture whose action is to lift a depressed upper lateral cartilage by pulling on the opposite nasal bone. Differential suturing of the upper lateral cartilages to the spreader grafts and septum can be performed to create force vectors that pull the middle

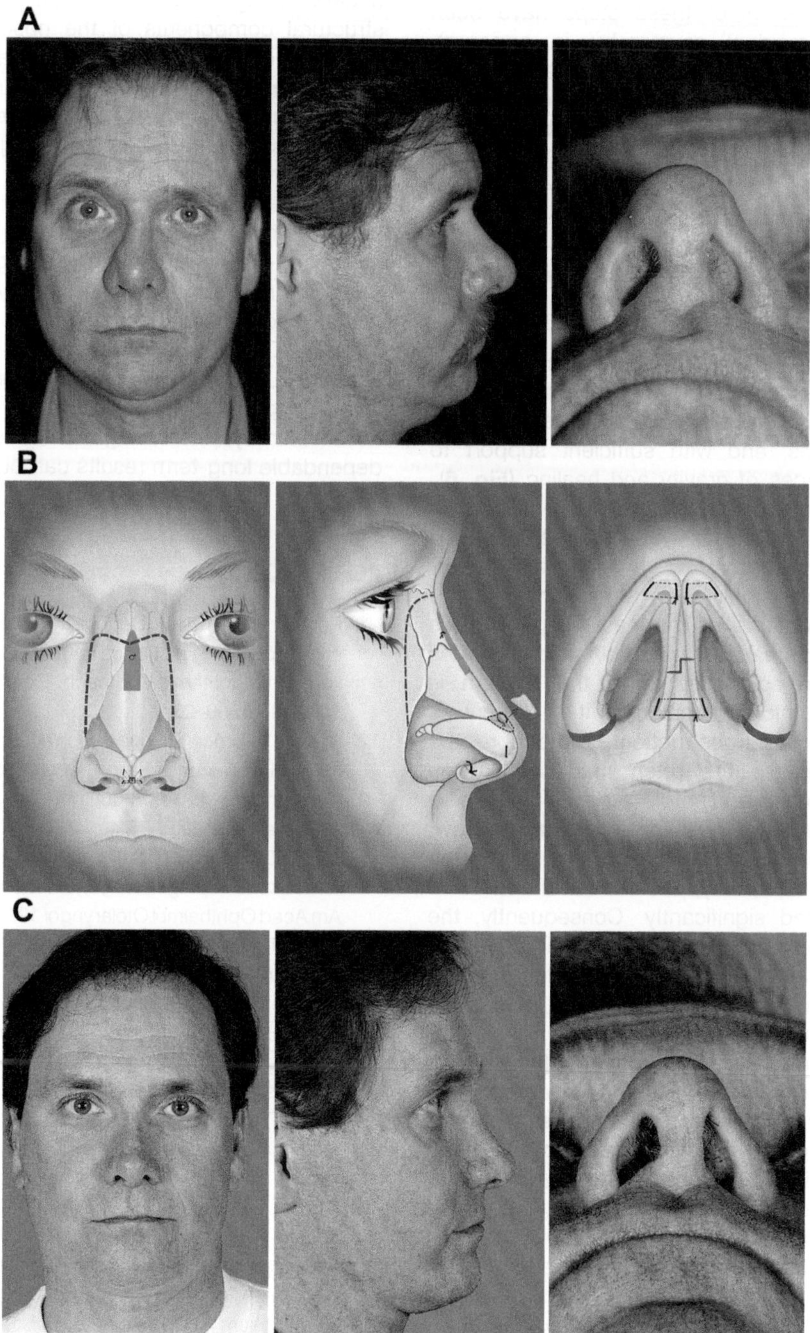

Fig. 6. (*A*) Preoperative views of patient with a crooked nose: frontal, lateral, and base views. (*B*) Diagrammatic details of surgery showing placement of sutures, osteotomies, cartilage graft, and management of the alar base and supratip. (*C*) Postoperative views of patient (4 years, 4 months) who had a crooked nose: frontal, lateral, and base views.

vault in the desired direction to rectify minor deformities.[30,31]

The final step in correction of a deviated nose is assurance that tip structures are symmetric. Any unilateral deficiency is corrected by advancement of the lower lateral cartilage on that side and the excess is eliminated by reduction to align the domes in the midline. Occasionally, even after all of these steps have been completed, residual asymmetry is apparent. Particularly in these cases, camouflaging onlay grafts is a valuable technique. These grafts, either fashioned from sculpted cartilage placed and sutured in a precise position, or as crushed or morselized cartilage, can balance dorsal irregularities and produce the desired appearance of a straight nose. The skin–soft-tissue envelope is closed once the surgeon's goals have been achieved. A nose that does not meet the aesthetic ideal on the operating room table will not achieve the optimal result once the nose has healed. The final result should be a nose and tip that is straight, sculpted to follow aesthetic lines, and with sufficient support to withstand forces of gravity and healing (**Fig. 6**).

Whereas inferior turbinate hypertrophy is not always seen in patients with a recently acquired nasal deformity, anatomic variations and hypertrophy are commonly seen particularly in longstanding deviations of the nasal septum. This compensatory change in the turbinate or tubinates needs to be addressed once the septum is restored to a midline position, as it will otherwise contribute to nasal obstruction. Furthermore, the inferior turbinates are often medialized when a nasal osteotomy and medial repositioning is performed, especially if the osteotomy is initiated low, if the inferior turbinates extend anterior to the plane of the osteotomy, or if the nasal bones are long or shifted significantly. Consequently, the position of the inferior turbinates should be examined subsequent to the completion of the osteotomy, and if a medial transposition is noted, the inferior turbinates should be reduced.

In addition to simple resection of the anterior portion of the turbinate, a submucosal resection may be performed in cases of compensatory turbinate hypertrophy, removing the turbinate bone and preserving the mucosa. This removes the obstruction and creates controlled scarring, which leads to decreased turbinate size but preserves functional turbinate mucosa. The submucosal resection can either be performed by incising along the anterior and inferior portion of the turbinate, dissecting the bone from the mucosa, then removing the bone, or with an inferior turbinate blade of a microdebrider.

SUMMARY

Successful surgical correction of the crooked nose can be a daunting task even for the most experienced rhinoplasty surgeon. Careful analysis of the anatomy, function, and aesthetics of a patient's nose and face precedes the formulation of a surgical plan and necessarily involves an understanding of the interrelationships of the structural components of the nose and of the dynamics of change that result by altering these various structures. Symmetry, balance, proportion, and nasal function must all be considered when a surgeon develops a surgical plan to repair a crooked nose.

The intrinsic and extrinsic forces that lead to septal deviation and a crooked nose must be identified and released, thereby straightening the septum and bony-cartilaginous pyramid while maintaining structural support of the dorsum and the tip. Camouflaging techniques act as an adjunct. Following these principles ensures definitive and predictable correction of the crooked nose thereby increasing the likelihood that dependable long-term results can be achieved.

REFERENCES

1. Rohrich R, Gunter J, Deuber M, et al. The deviated nose: optimizing results using a simplified classification and algorithmic approach. Plast Reconstr Surg 2002;110:1509–23.
2. Byrd H, Salomon J, Flood J. Correction of the crooked nose. Plast Reconstr Surg 1998;102:2148–57.
3. Constantian M. An algorithm for correcting the asymmetrical nose. Plast Reconstr Surg 1989; 83(5):801–11.
4. Anderson J. Straightening the crooked nose. Trans Am Acad Ophthalmol Otolaryngol 1972;76(4):938–45.
5. Asch M. Treatment of nasal stenosis due to deflective septum with and without thickening of the convex side. Laryngoscope 1899;6:340–61.
6. Krieg R. [Resection der cartilago quadrangularis septi nasem sur heilung der scoliosis septi]. Medicinishes Cocrespondenz blatt Wurtenburgishen Artzlicken Verein Stuttgart 1886;56:201 [in German].
7. Freer O. The anatomy of deflections of the nasal septum. Trans 34th Annual Meeting Amer Laryngol Assoc. Atlantic City, NJ, May 9–11, 1912. p. 71–87.
8. Fomon S, Gilbert J, Silver G, et al. Plastic repair of the obstructing nasal septum. Arch Otolaryngol 1948;47:7–20.
9. Metzenbaum M. Replacement of the lower end of the dislocated septal cartilage versus submucous resection of the dislocated end of the septal cartilage. Arch Otolaryngol 1929;9:282–96.

10. Salinger S. Deviation of the septum in relation to the twisted nose. Arch Otolaryngol 1939;29:520–32.
11. Seltzer A. The nasal septum: plastic repair of the deviated septum associated with a deflected tip. Arch Otolaryngol 1944;40:433–44.
12. Maliniac J. Role of the septum in rhinoplasty. Arch Otolaryngol 1948;48:189–201.
13. Converse J. Corrective surgery of nasal deviations. Arch Otolaryngol 1950;52:671–708.
14. Becker OJ. Problems of the septum in rhinoplastic surgery. Arch Otolaryngol 1951;53:622–39.
15. King E, Ashley F. The correction of the internally and externally deviated nose. Plast Reconstr Surg 1952; 10:116–20.
16. Dingman R. Correction of nasal deformities due to defects of the septum. Plast Reconstr Surg 1956; 18:291–304.
17. Wright W. Principles of nasal septal reconstruction. Trans Am Acad Ophthalmol Otolaryngol 1969;73: 252–5.
18. Gorney M. The septum in rhinoplasty: form and function. In: Millard D, editor. Symposium on Corrective Rhinoplasty, vol. 13. Miami, FL, January 15–18, 1975. St. Louis: Mosby; 1976. p. 180.
19. Killian G. The submucous window resection of the nasal septum. Ann Otol Rhinol Laryngol 1905;14: 363–93.
20. Spector M. Partial resection of the inferior turbinates. Ear Nose Throat J 1982;61:200.
21. Baume L. The nasal septum: an endochondral growth center. J Dent Res 1961;40:625.
22. Gray L. Deviated nasal septum: incidence and etiology. Ann Otol Rhinol Laryngol Suppl 1978;87 (3 Pt 3 Suppl 50):3–20.
23. Guyuron B, Uzzo C, Scull H. A practical classification of septonasal deviation and an effective guide to septal surgery. Plast Reconstr Surg 1999;104: 2202–9.
24. Guyuron B. Precision rhinoplasty. Part I: the role of life-size photographs and soft-tissue cephalometric analysis. Plast Reconstr Surg 1988;81:489–99.
25. McKinney P, Shively R. Straightening the twisted nose. Plast Reconstr Surg 1979;64:176–9.
26. Pastorek N, Becker D. Treating the caudal septal deflection. Arch Facial Plast Surg 2000;2:217–20.
27. Tardy M, Denney J. Micro-osteotomies in rhinoplasty. Facial Plast Surg 1984;1:137–45.
28. Dayan S, Shah A. A suture suspension technique for improved repair of a crooked nose deformity. Ear Nose Throat J 2004;83:743–4.
29. Pontius AT, Leach JL Jr. New techniques for management of the crooked nose. Arch Facial Plast Surg 2004;6:263–6.
30. Toriumi DM, Ries WR. Innovative surgical management of the crooked nose. Facial Plast Clin North Am 1997;1:63–77.
31. Guyuron B, Behmand R. Caudal nasal deviation. Plast Reconstr Surg 2003;111(7):2449–57.

Lengthening the Short Nose

P. Craig Hobar, MD, FRCS[a,b,*], William P. Adams, MD[a],
C. Alejandra Mitchell, MD[a,b]

KEYWORDS

- Short nose • Nasal lengthening
- Secondary rhinoplasty • Facial balance

The short nose is a challenging problem in rhinoplasty.[1] The short nose is characterized by 1 or more of the following:

1. Disproportion with the midface and other areas of the face
2. An excessively obtuse nasolabial angle
3. Excessive nostril show.

The short nose can be a naturally occurring aesthetic disproportion, the result of a congenital abnormality, or traumatic deformity. The surgical approach depends mostly on the quality of the lining, skeleton, overlying skin, and the amount of correction desired.

ANALYSIS

Although the diagnosis is usually obvious, precise soft-tissue analysis is beneficial for surgical planning. The method the authors use is a simple soft-tissue cephalometric analysis that can be performed in less than a minute.[2] Six measurements are taken:

1. Midfacial height: the distance from the glabella to the bottom of the ala.
2. Lower facial height: the distance from the subnasale to the menton.
3. Nasal length: the distance from the root of the nose at the level of the supratarsal fold to the tip projecting point.
4. Chin vertical: the distance from the stomion to the menton.
5. Tip projection: the distance from the junction of the cheek and the ala to the tip of the nose.
6. Chin projection: the distance from the anterior projecting point of the chin to a line drawn from the half-way point of nasal length and extending through and beyond the anterior projecting point of the upper lip.

This analysis allows for determination of ideal nasal length with respect to the midface and chin vertical portion of the lower face. In the face with ideal proportions, nasal length should be two-thirds of the midfacial height and approximately equal to chin vertical. In a face where either the midface or chin vertical is abnormal, the most aesthetically ideal subunit should be used as the reference. The goal is not to blindly match a set of numbers, but to quickly and precisely obtain a useful and practical guide for surgical planning.

SURGICAL APPROACH

There have been several techniques described to lengthen the nose. The techniques that we have found most useful and effective are described here.

Technique 1: Septal Extension Graft

In the patient with no lining restriction, good overlying skin quality, and abundant septal cartilage of

[a] Department of Plastic Surgery, UT Southwestern Medical Center, 1801 Inwood Drive, Dallas, TX 75390, USA
[b] 9101 North Central Expressway, Suite 600, Dallas, TX 75231, USA
* Corresponding author. Department of Plastic Surgery, UT Southwestern Medical Center, 1801 Inwood Drive, Dallas, TX 75390.
E-mail address: phobar@gmail.com (P.C. Hobar).

Clin Plastic Surg 37 (2010) 327–333
doi:10.1016/j.cps.2009.11.004
0094-1298/10/$ – see front matter

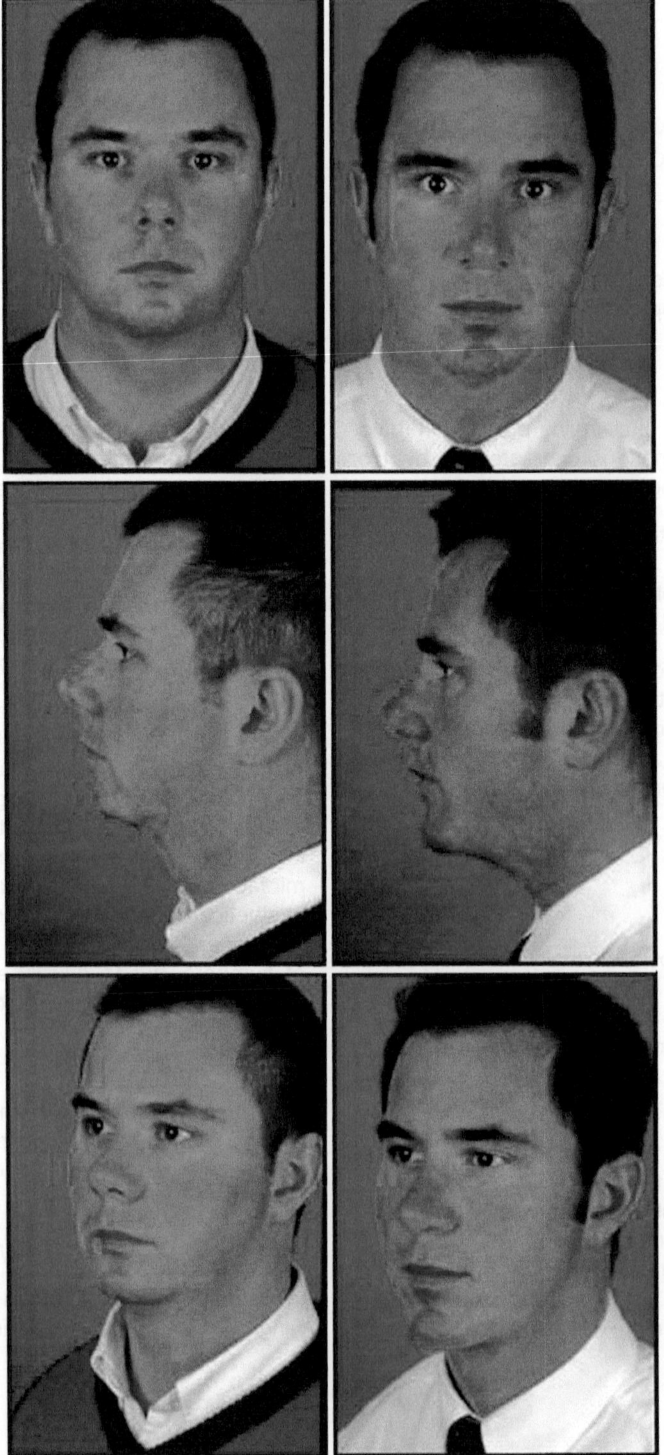

Fig. 1. Case 1. Septal extension graft technique used in a primary rhinoplasty to lengthen the short nose before (*left*) and after (*right*) the procedure. A genioplasty was also performed.

adequate strength, this is a powerful and straightforward way of lengthening the nose and controlling tip projection at the same time. The technique and its applications have been well described by Byrd and colleagues,[3,4] and the reader is referred to these references for an excellent description of the technique.

Case 1: Primary rhinoplasty

A 27-year-old man sought surgical correction of a shortened over-rotated nose and improvement of what he perceived as a weak chin. Midfacial height was used as the reference unit for desired nasal length and chin vertical. An open approach was used. Adequate septal cartilage was harvested for graft material. The lower lateral cartilages were freed from the upper lateral cartilages. A septal extension graft was placed along the dorsal septum to allow 5 mm of nasal lengthening and control of tip projection. A sliding genioplasty was performed to gain 5 mm of increase in chin vertical and 8 mm of increase in anterioposterior projection (**Fig. 1**).

Case 2: Secondary rhinoplasty

A 28-year-old woman underwent a rhinoplasty as a teenager and had been living with a shortened, severely over-rotated nose since that time. She had good skin quality and a large amount of good quality septum. Facial analysis showed her

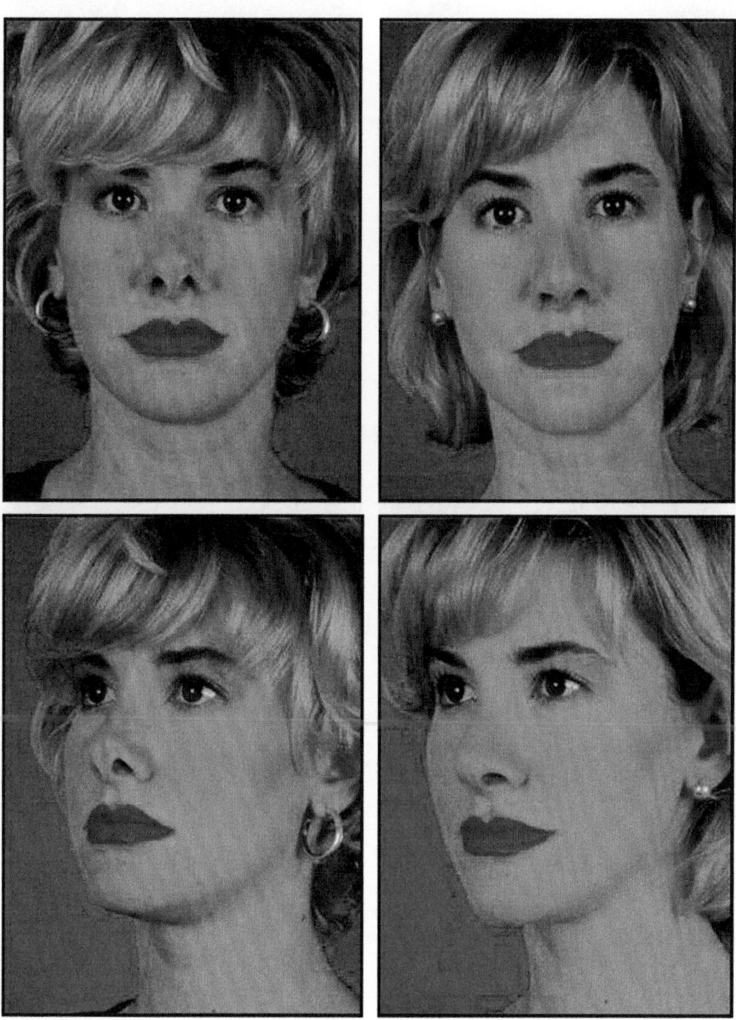

Fig. 2. Case 2. Septal extension graft technique used in a secondary rhinoplasty to lengthen the short over-rotated nose before (*left*) and after (*right*) the procedure.

nose to be approximately 6 mm short in relation to her midface height and chin vertical. An open approach was used. The lower lateral cartilages were mobilized and using a septal extension graft; 6 mm of lengthening was achieved (**Fig. 2**).

Technique 2: Rib Graft

The use of a rib graft is an excellent technique when more strength, than can be provided with a septal extension graft, is needed to overcome the soft tissue forces. Rib graft is also the preferred technique when septum has been previously harvested or is inadequate. When there is deficiency of the dorsum, the rib graft can be used as a cantilever graft, with the distal extension serving in a similar manner as the spreader graft. The author prefers a straight segment of the 10th rib. The 11th rib is naturally straight but frequently of inadequate length. Many prefer a rib located higher and

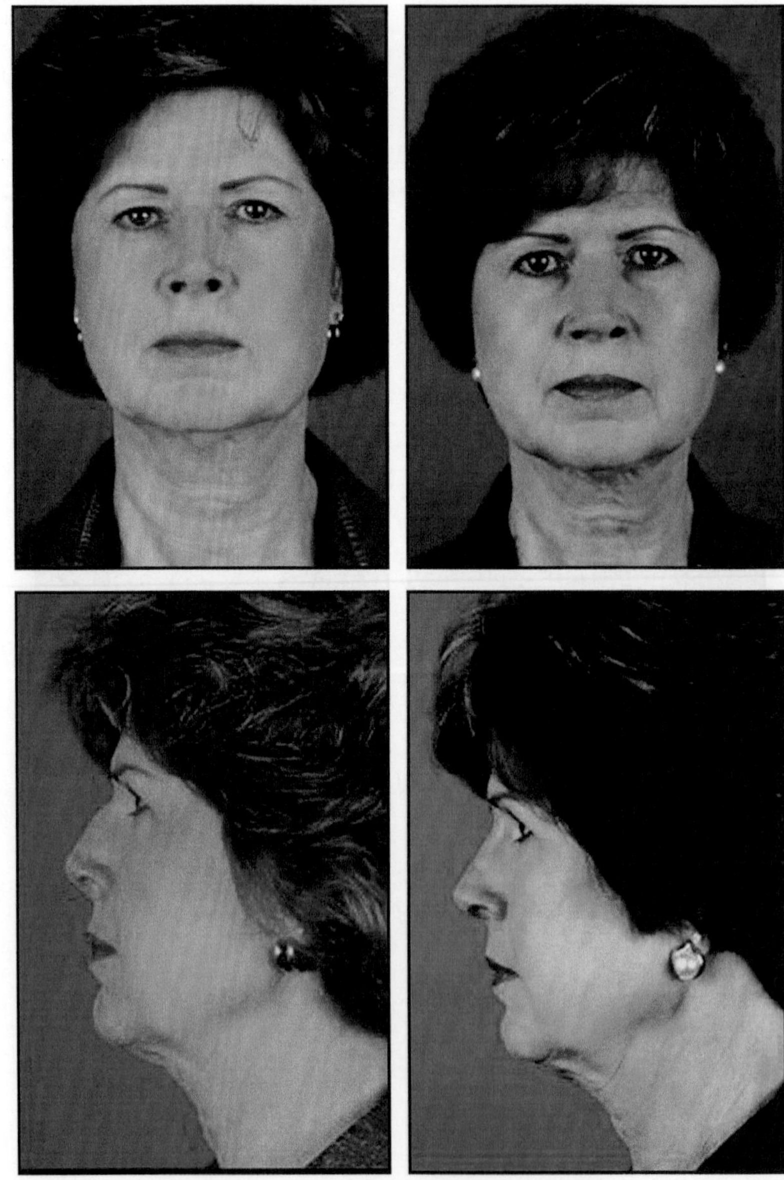

Fig. 3. Case 3. Rib graft technique used in a secondary rhinoplasty to lengthen the short over-rotated nose, and repair the step-off deformity before (*left*) and after (*right*) the procedure.

supported with a K-wire as has been popularized by Marin and Gunter.[5] When the dorsum is adequate and a dorsal extension graft would interfere with an already adequate dorsum, a columellar graft using the 10th rib is a good alternative. The rib is placed just distal to the caudal septum and fixed to the anterior nasal spine of the maxilla with a threaded K-wire. If this produces excessive columellar show, an adequate adjacent portion of the caudal septum is resected. By controlling the length and angle off the maxilla, another powerful and precise method is available for controlling nasal length and tip projection. The anterior aspects of the lower lateral cartilages are fixed either to the tip or over the tip of the precisely positioned rib.

Case 3: Secondary rhinoplasty

A 44-year-old woman who had a previous attempt at correction of a posttraumatic nasal deformity with a rib graft presented for secondary rhinoplasty. She presented with a visible step-off at the superior edge of her rib graft and a shortened over-rotated nose. Facial analysis showed her nasal length to be short in relation to her midface by 5 mm and short in relation to her chin vertical by 6 mm. Through an open rhinoplasty, the rib was removed and replaced with another rib graft contoured at the superior aspect to blend in with the normal bone at the radix. This new graft was also of adequate length to allow de-rotation of her lower lateral cartilages after separation from the upper lateral cartilages. The nose was lengthened by 5 mm (**Fig. 3**).

Technique 3: Complex Osteotomy Nasal Lengthening

This technique is reserved for the most complex type of nasal lengthening, usually related to posttraumatic or congenital causes. There is usually a lining deficiency that cannot be overcome with the 2 previously described methods. Grafts or lining flaps are of limited usefulness and usually not rewarding for these difficult situations. If the lining is released high in the nasal cavity where the healing is quick and contracture is prevented by the bony surroundings, a powerful advancement of the lining can be achieved. We know this based on our experience with LeFort 3 osteotomies.

Wolfe[6] described a technique to achieve powerful nasal lengthening using cranial nasal separation based on techniques routinely used in craniofacial surgery, particularly the LeFort 3 osteotomy. The senior author prefers a similar techinique but has modified it to allow the osteotomies to pass anterior to the nasolacrimal apparatus and medial orbit (**Fig. 4**).

As long as the osteotomy passes anterior to the turbinates, separation from the skull base and remainder of the face can be achieved safely. As the nose is lengthened, the caudal septum is impacted and distorted. This is a similar phenomenon, but from a reverse direction, that occurs in maxillary impaction for vertical maxillary excess. This is easily overcome by resecting an adequate amount of caudal septum. Rigid fixation with a small titanium plate and interposition bone graft at the nasal route keeps the nose where it is positioned.

Case 4: Secondary posttraumatic rhinoplasty

A 48-year-old woman presented with a posttraumatic nasal deformity. She had undergone multiple surgeries and previous attempts at nasal correction but had a persistent severely shortened nose with excess rotation. Examination suggested she had a significant lining restriction and her overlying soft-tissue envelope was scarred and suboptimal. A complex nasal osteotomy was performed with an 11-m interposition graft and titanium plate fixation. External nasal lengthening of 7 mm was achieved (**Fig. 5**).

Case 5: Posttraumatic rhinoplasty

A 26-year-old woman was involved in a motor vehicle accident. She presented with severe secondary posttraumatic facial deformities including a significantly shortened nose and contracted nasal lining. She underwent a complex

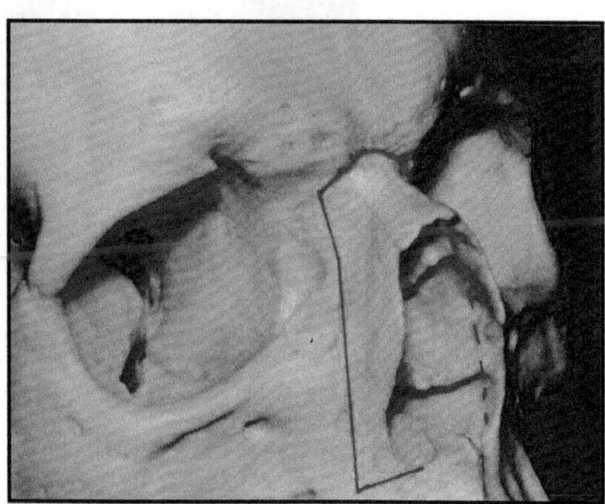

Fig. 4. Senior author's technique of complex nasal osteotomies for nasal elongation. This is indicated in particularly difficult posttraumatic or congenital deformities with a severe lining deficiency.

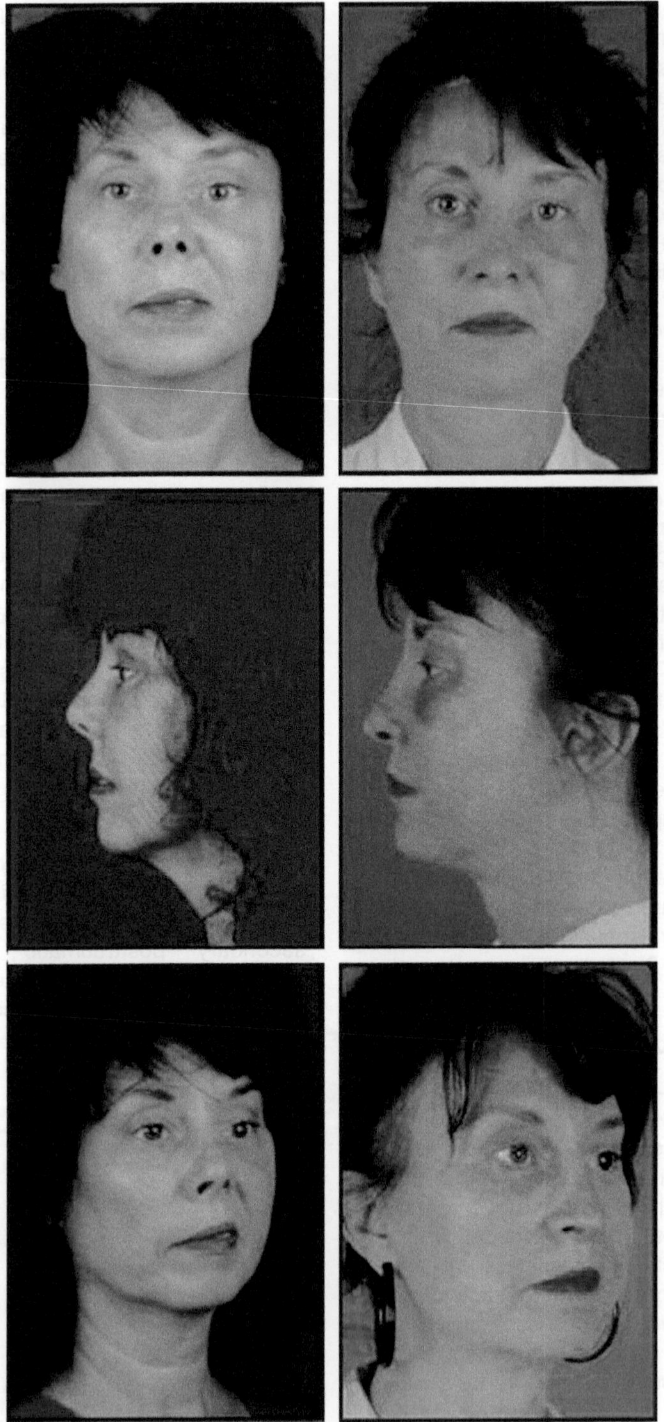

Fig. 5. Case 4. Complex nasal osteotomy technique used in a secondary posttraumatic rhinoplasty before (*left*) and after (*right*) the procedure.

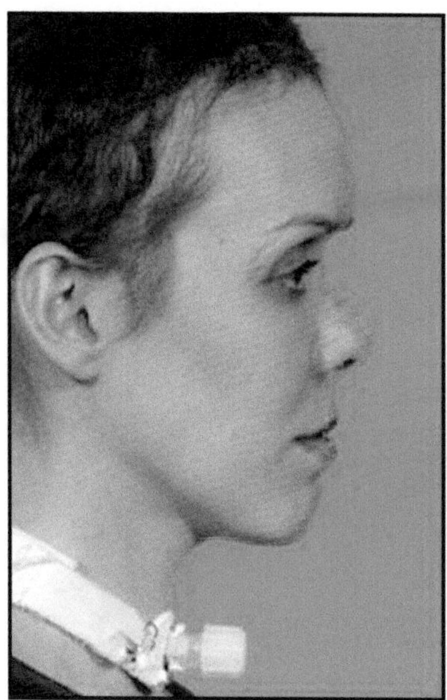
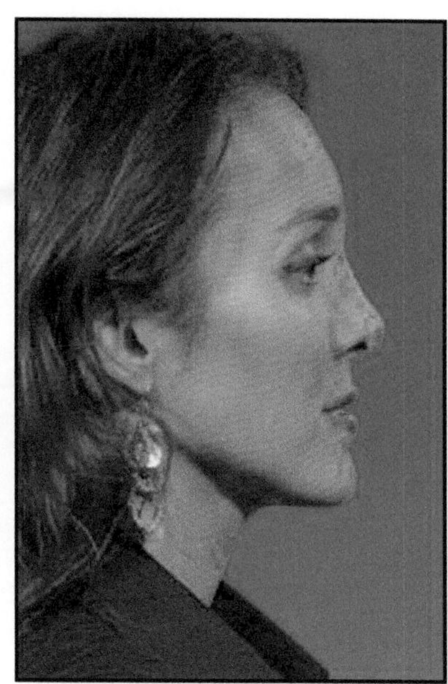

Fig. 6. Case 5. The complex nasal osteotomy technique used in a secondary posttraumatic rhinoplasty before (*left*) and after (*right*) the procedure.

osteotomy nasal reconstruction as described earlier (**Fig. 6**).

REFERENCES

1. Gunter JP, Rohrich RJ. Lengthening the aesthetically short nose. Plast Reconstr Surg 1989;83:793–800.
2. Byrd HS, Hobar PC. Rhinoplasty: a practical guide for surgical planning. Plast Reconstr Surg 1993;91: 642–54.
3. Byrd HS, Andochick S, Copit S, et al. Septal extension grafts: a method of controlling tip projection shape. Plast Reconstr Surg 1997; 100(4):999–1010.
4. Ha RY, Byrd HS. Septal extension grafts revisited: 6-year experience in controlling nasal tip projection and shape. Plast Reconstr Surg 2003;112(7):1929–35.
5. Marin VP, Landecker A, Gunter JP. Harvesting rib cartilage grafts for secondary rhinoplasty. Plast Reconstr Surg 2008;121(4):1442–8.
6. Wolfe SA. Lengthening the nose: a lesson from craniofacial surgery applied to post-traumatic and congenital deformities. Plast Reconstr Surg 1994; 94(1):78–87.

Asian Rhinoplasty

Dean M. Toriumi, MD[a,*], Colin D. Pero, MD[b,c]

KEYWORDS

- Asian rhinoplasty • Revision rhinoplasty
- Augmentation rhinoplasty

Cosmetic rhinoplasty in the Asian patient population differs from traditional rhinoplasty approaches in many aspects, including preoperative analysis, patient expectations, nasal anatomy, and surgical techniques used. Platyrrhine nasal characteristics are common, with low dorsum, weak lower lateral cartilages, and thick sebaceous skin often noted. Typically, patients seek augmentation of these existing structures rather than reductive procedures. Patient desires and expectations are unique to this population, with patients often seeking improvement and refinement of their Asian features, not radical changes toward more characteristic White features. Use of alloplastic or autologous materials is necessary to achieve the desired results; the use of each material carries inherent risks and benefits that should be discussed with the patient. Autologous cartilage, in particular use of costal cartilage, has shown to be a reliable, low-risk technique, which, when executed properly, produces excellent long-term results. An understanding of cultural perspectives, knowledge of the nasal anatomy unique to Asian patients, and proficiency with augmentation techniques are prerequisites in attaining the desired results for patient and surgeon.

PREOPERATIVE EVALUATION

Preoperative counseling of the Asian rhinoplasty patient demands attention to cultural concerns in addition to cosmetic concerns and functional complaints. Commonly, patients describe their desire to achieve elevation of the nasal dorsum, refinement of the nasal tip, narrowing of the nasal base and correction of their columellar or premaxillary retraction.

Characteristics of the Asian nose include: low nasal dorsum with caudally placed nasal starting point, thick, sebaceous skin overlying the nasal tip and supratip, weak lower lateral cartilages, small amount of cartilaginous septum, foreshortened nose, retracted columella, and thickened alar lobules (**Fig. 1**).

Each patient's desire to balance augmenting their Asian nasal features with maintenance of the appearance of an Asian nose is unique for each individual and should be elucidated during the initial consultation and preoperative visits. Demonstration of the proposed changes to the patient with a computer-imaging program can aid communication between patient and surgeon of the proposed changes (**Fig. 2**A, C). Fulfillment of the patient's stated wishes may produce a modification of the patient's ethnic identity, and computer imaging helps the patient to better understand the possible outcome. When available, preoperative and postoperative results of previous patients may help demonstrate the spectrum of changes possible and aid the patient in deciding on the desired postoperative result.

Discussion of incision placement (including base reduction and auricular and rib cartilage harvest), possible complications, postoperative care, and follow-up schedule are discussed at the initial consultation and preoperative visit. If rib cartilage is likely to be used, the patients are instructed to expect their nose to be stiffer initially and to soften with time. If a significant amount of nasal lengthening or premaxillary augmentation is expected, the patient is counseled that there may be an initial tightness or fullness to the upper lip. Occasionally, a crease in the lip may be seen.

[a] Division of Facial Plastic and Reconstructive Surgery, Department of Otolaryngology-Head and Neck Surgery, University of Illinois at Chicago Medical School, 1855 W. Taylor Street Rm 2.42 MC 648, Chicago, IL 60611, USA
[b] Division of Facial Plastic and Reconstructive Surgery, Department of Otolaryngology-Head and Neck Surgery, University of Texas-Southwestern Medical School, Dallas, TX, USA
[c] Private Practice, 5425 W. Spring Creek Parkway, Suite 170, Plano, TX 75024, USA
* Corresponding author.
E-mail address: dtoriumi@uic.edu (D.M. Toriumi).

Clin Plastic Surg 37 (2010) 335–352
doi:10.1016/j.cps.2009.12.008
0094-1298/10/$ – see front matter

plasticsurgery.theclinics.com

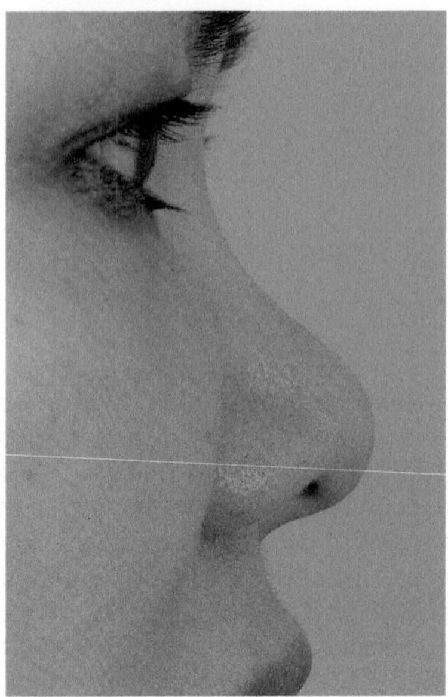

Fig. 1. Preoperative photograph of patient seeking primary rhinoplasty. Note low dorsum, thick skin, inadequate projection of nasal tip, and suboptimal alar-columellar relationship.

The risk of this sequela must be balanced against the desire for lengthening and premaxillary augmentation.

SURGICAL PLANNING

The senior author (DMT) performs the procedure on patients under a general anesthetic on an outpatient basis. Preoperative photography includes full face and close-up frontal, both lateral, and three-quarter oblique views, and a close-up base view with and without inspiration to demonstrate dynamic collapse. Computerized imaging is performed on every preoperative rhinoplasty patient. The preoperative photographs and the computer imaging are displayed during surgery and referred to throughout the operation to help achieve the desired results. Preoperative injections of the nose and donor cartilage site(s) are made with 1% lidocaine with 1:100,000 epinephrine. Infiltration of the columella, area between the intermediate crura, the subperichondrial planes over the upper and lower lateral cartilages, and the subperiosteal plane over the nasal bones along the nasal dorsum and sidewalls is performed. The nasal septum is injected in a subperichondrial plane using hydrostatic dissection to elevate the mucoperichondrial flap from the underlying cartilage. A preliminary assessment of the relative size of the cartilaginous septum can be made by probing with the injection needle to identify the boundaries of the septal cartilage. Most Asian patients have a small cartilaginous component to their septum and frequently require additional cartilage for augmentation.

If additional cartilage is needed, the appropriate donor site(s) are also injected. If auricular cartilage is to be used, the planned incision is marked on the posterior auricular surface 3 to 4 mm lateral to the postauricular sulcus and infiltrated with local anesthetic. One or both ears may be used. The authors rarely use auricular cartilage as it is not a good option for augmenting the nasal dorsum because the ends of the cartilage can curl and deform over time.

If costal cartilage harvest is planned, a 1.1- to 1.5-cm incision is marked overlying the right sixth rib and injected with local anesthetic. The right chest is chosen because of ease of access for the right-handed surgeon and to avoid confusion with cardiac pain postoperatively. Neurosurgical pledgets saturated with 0.05% oxymetazoline are placed in the nose and a sterile preparation and drape are performed. Separate instruments for auricular or costal cartilage harvest are segregated from those for the nasal surgery. In addition to traditional rhinoplasty instrumentation, a Castro-Viejo caliper is used intraoperatively to document parameters, which aid in assessing likely outcomes (eg, graft dimensions, supratip break, middle vault, and dorsal graft width).

Surgical Technique

The procedure is initiated with a midcolumellar inverted-V incision made with a number 11 blade scalpel. A number 15 blade scalpel is used to make bilateral marginal incisions with extensions in the vestibular skin 2 to 3 mm posterior to the columellar incision and extending toward the soft-tissue facet. Sharp Converse scissors are used to carefully dissect the tissue over the medial crura and extend the medial aspect of the marginal incisions into the soft-tissue triangle area, connecting with the remaining marginal incision laterally, thereby exposing the lower lateral cartilages. Sharp dissection, with minimal spreading, limits tissue damage, aids in hemostasis, and minimizes postoperative edema. Dissection is carried over the nasal dorsum to expose the dorsal cartilaginous septum to the level of the nasal bones. A Joseph elevator is used to elevate the periosteum over the nasal bones in the midline. It is imperative that the periosteum is elevated laterally only to the extent that will allow the dorsal graft to fit snugly over the dorsum. Failure to maintain this tight pocket is a major contributor to postoperative migration of the dorsal graft. If changes to nasal

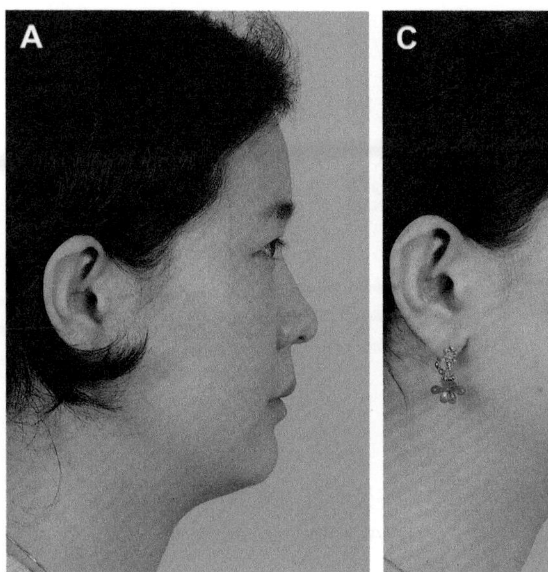

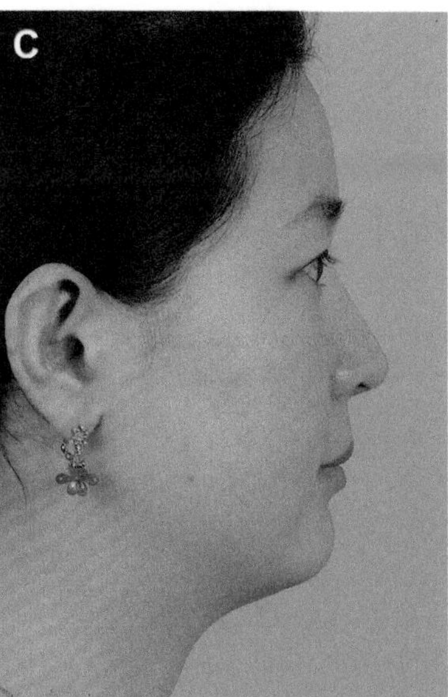

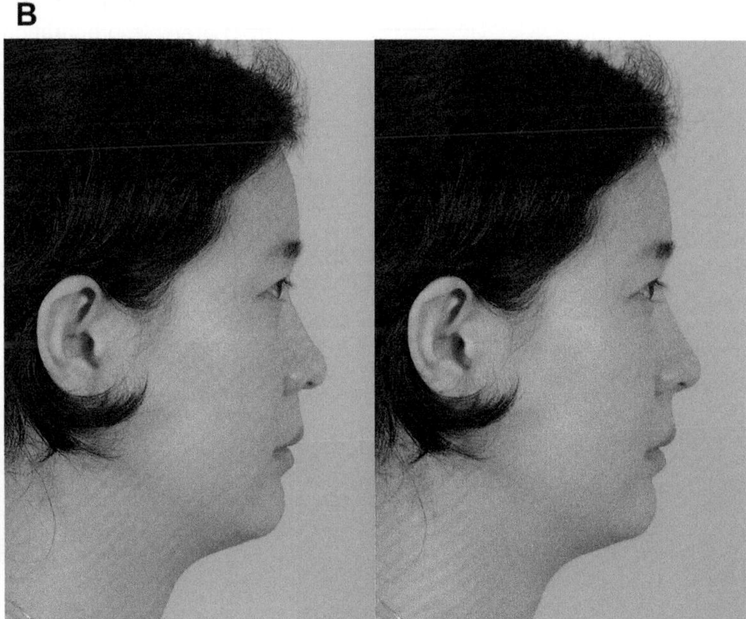

Fig. 2. Preoperative images. (*A*) Clinical photograph, preoperative lateral view. (*B*) Computer imaging showing proposed outcome. (*C*) One-year postoperative lateral view.

length, projection, or premaxillary augmentation are planned, or the caudal septum is deviated, the lower lateral cartilages are dissected apart in the midline to expose the anterior septal angle and the caudal septum. Care is taken to elevate the mucoperichondrial layer from the septum in the appropriate bloodless plane, thereby minimizing the risk of postoperative septal perforation. Harvesting of the septal cartilage involves preservation of 1.5-cm caudal and dorsal struts to allow for adequate support postoperatively.

In rare cases the caudal septum may have been resected, damaged, or deviated and requires replacement. In these patients, a 1.5-cm dorsal strut may be left and the caudal strut is replaced with a caudal septal replacement graft (**Fig. 3**A, B). The caudal septal strut is notched to allow the graft to fit into a notch in the nasal spine without slipping cephalically (**Fig. 4**). This maneuver aids in nasal lengthening and correction of columellar retraction and allows for rotational changes to the nasal tip. It can also be used for correction of the deviated caudal septum. The caudal septum is dissected posteriorly to the anterior nasal spine and the entire caudal septum is exposed. In the situations mentioned earlier, the excess septal

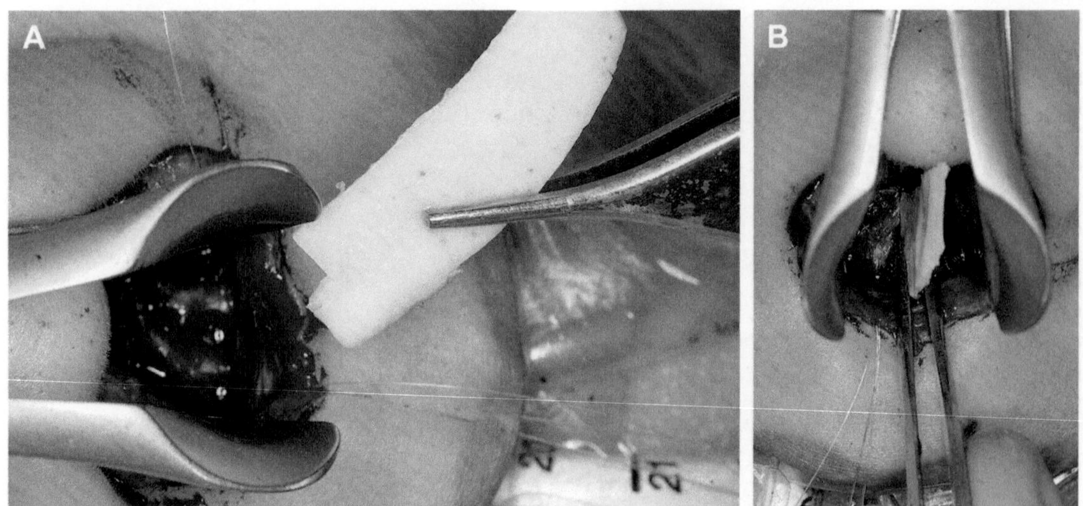

Fig. 3. Intraoperative photograph of caudal septal replacement graft (*A*) before insertion and (*B*) graft positioned before stabilization.

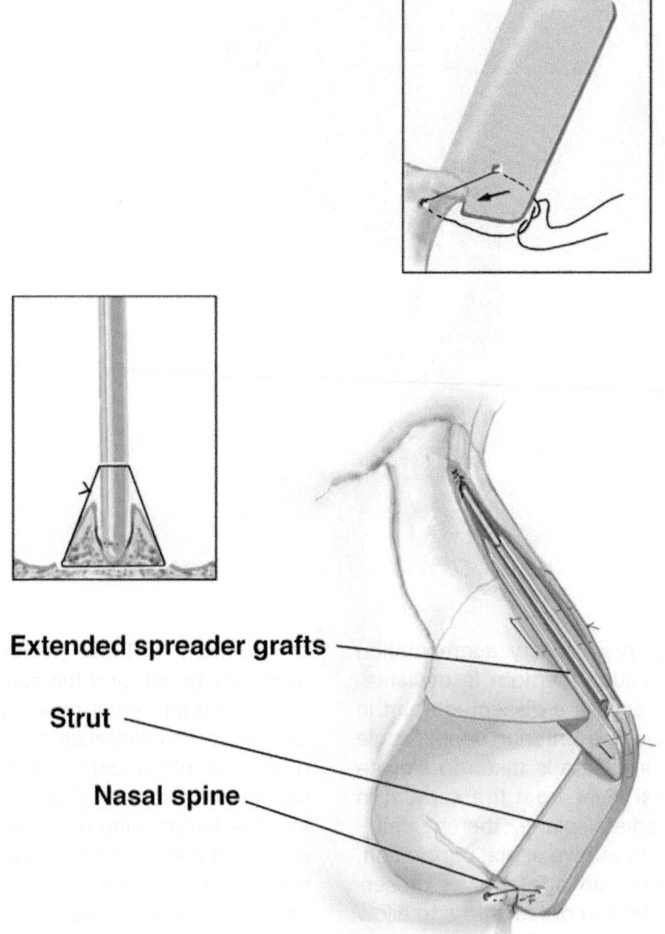

Fig. 4. Caudal septal replacement graft with notch sutured and fixated into notch in nasal spine. The graft is stabilized with extended spreader grafts.

cartilage is removed in continuity with the caudal strut. Any deviated bony septum or septal spurs are also removed, with care taken to preserve the mucoperichondrial flaps. Following resection of the septal cartilage, the need for further cartilage material for grafting is assessed. If a significant dorsal augmentation is planned (>5 mm), the authors' preference is to harvest costal cartilage at this time. If minimal extra cartilage is deemed necessary following septal cartilage harvest, auricular cartilage may be harvested at this time. The authors rarely use auricular cartilage in Asian patients as most patients require significant cartilage grafting to augment their nose.

COSTAL CARTILAGE HARVEST

When performing costal cartilage harvest, the authors typically use the lateral aspect of the sixth rib that abuts the bony/cartilaginous junction. The chest wall is palpated to determine the shape of each rib and the 3.75-cm (1.5-in) 27-gauge needle used during local anesthetic injection is used to locate the bony-cartilaginous junction and any sites of calcification. The sixth rib is more commonly used as it lies at the inferior aspect of the breast. This allows placing the incision in the region of the inframammary crease to allow better camouflage of the incision. Asian women patients typically have small breasts and do not have a well-defined inframammary crease. The authors use a small incision measuring 1.2 cm to minimize scarring. If the authors need to perform dorsal augmentation and premaxillary augmentation 2 costal cartilage segments may be needed. In this case the authors may harvest the seventh rib in addition to the sixth rib. Selection of the rib depends on which rib has the best contour for the desired grafts.

The incision is initially 1.2 cm in length and is planned over the inferior aspect of the right breast; it is usually stretched to approximately 1.6 cm with the retraction. Sharp dissection is performed through the dermal and subcutaneous tissues. The muscle fascia is incised in a cruciate fashion and blunt dissection is used to expose the perichondrium over the cartilage. Troublesome bleeding is uncommon and judicious use of bipolar cautery is used to minimize postoperative pain. A rectangular strip of perichondrium is incised with a number 15c scalpel and dissection carried lateral to medial to elevate the perichondrium from the anterior surface of the cartilage. The incision is manipulated laterally and medially as needed to maximize exposure with a minimum incision length. Wider exposure is important for the occasional or novice rib graft surgeon and a 3.0- to 5.0-cm incision is advised in these circumstances. Following removal, the perichondrium is placed in saline impregnated with antibiotic (400 mg ciprofloxacin/500 mL normal saline). The perichondrium along the superior and inferior aspects of the cartilage is then elevated with a Freer elevator to the deep aspect of the rib (**Fig. 5**). Following adequate elevation, a number 15c scalpel is used to incise the cartilage halfway through the thickness laterally, then medially. Typically the authors harvest 3 cm to 4 cm of costal cartilage depending on what is needed. There is commonly a significant connection between the sixth and seventh ribs that is also partially incised with a number 15c scalpel. A Freer elevator is used to complete the incisions carefully without disrupting the deep perichondrial layer. The cartilage is then elevated off the underlying perichondrium. Adequate severing of the connections to the seventh rib and complete transection of the medial and lateral aspects of the rib will aid elevation of the rib without fracturing the rib cartilage. Following removal, the cut edges of the remaining rib cartilage are trimmed using Takahashi forceps to minimize palpability. The wound is irrigated and a Valsalva maneuver performed to verify that the pleura has not been violated. The procedure is performed on an outpatient basis, although overnight observation with postoperative radiographs is advised for the surgeon less experienced with costal cartilage grafting. Closure is performed at the end of the operation to maintain accessibility should further material be required. Closure is performed in a layered fashion, closing the muscle and its fascia with 3-0 polydioxanone suture (PDS), the breast tissue and deeper subcutaneous tissue with 4-0 PDS, the superficial subcutaneous tissue and deep dermal sutures with 5-0 PDS and a running, locking vertical mattress 6-0 nylon suture for the skin.

RIB CARVING

Success with the use of costal cartilage depends on the method of carving the cartilage and decisions made in use of the grafting material. The cartilage is carved into 3 segments with a number 10 blade scalpel. The outer layers represent the anterior (superficial) and posterior (deep) surfaces of the rib in anatomic position (**Fig. 6**). If a large dorsal graft is anticipated, care must be taken to leave the central portion of the graft an appropriate thickness for augmentation with possible sacrifice of 1 or more of the outer layers. The rib cartilage is carved throughout the operation and kept in antibiotic-impregnated saline. It is observed throughout the operation for any tendency for

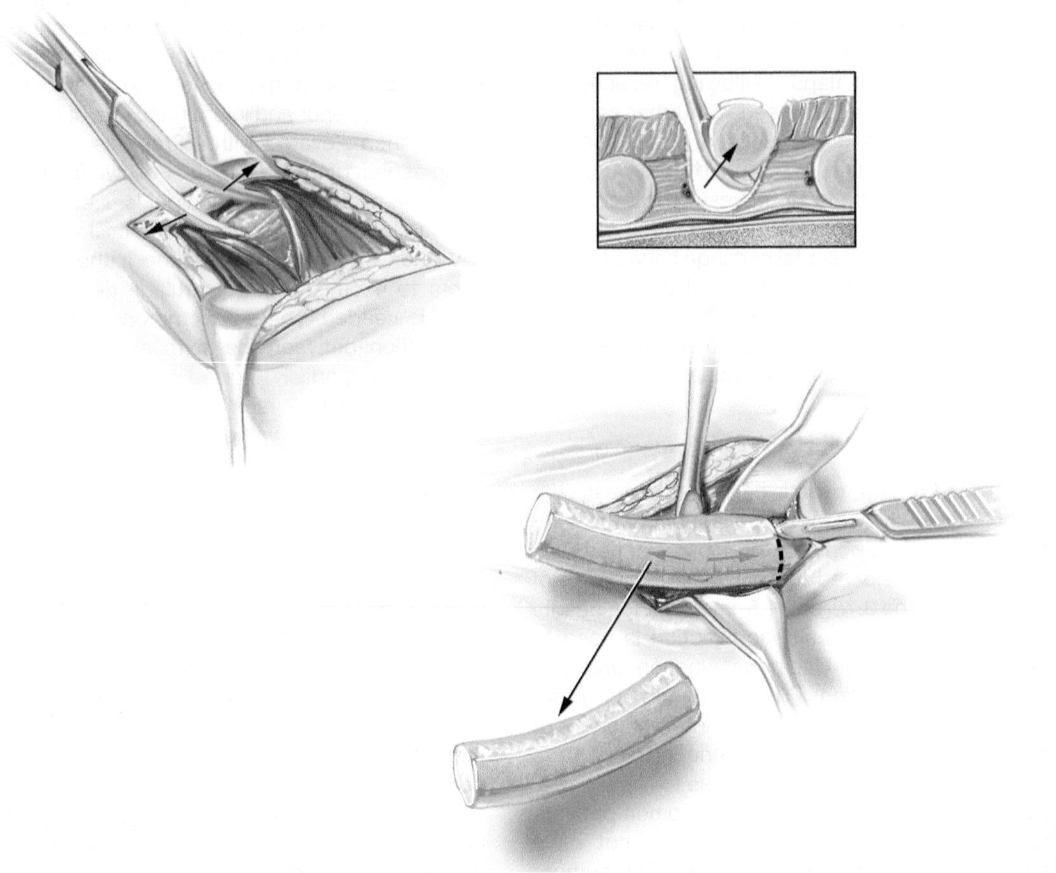

Fig. 5. Rib cartilage harvest. (*A*) Blunt dissection to separate muscle fibers and expose anterior perichondrium. (*B*) Elevation of rib from underlying (deep) perichondrium using Freer elevator. (*C*) Continuing elevation of rib and incision of medial portion of rib (half-thickness with scalpel and remainder with Freer elevator to avoid damaging underlying structures) allows removal.

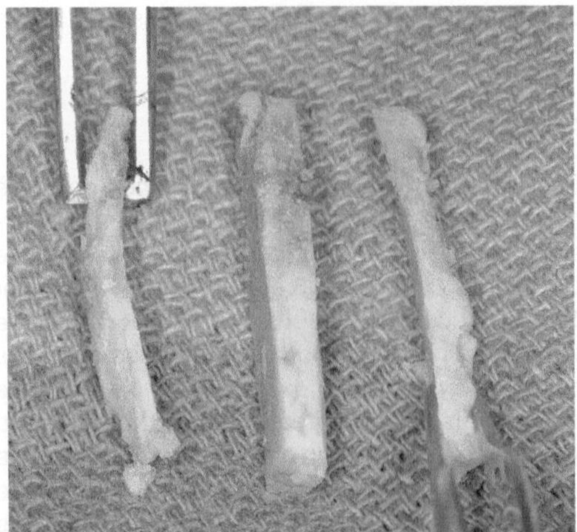

Fig. 6. Careful carving of rib cartilage produces anterior, middle, and posterior segments, which demonstrate differing degrees of warping intraoperatively.

warping. This tendency can be determined within 30 minutes and can be used in selecting the appropriate pieces for grafts and orientation so that the curvature is advantageous for the graft purpose.

Rarely, a second rib harvest may be needed to obtain sufficient grafting material, more commonly in revision operations with a need for implant removal/replacement and previous septal cartilage harvest.

BONY VAULT MANAGEMENT

In most Asian patients who are undergoing dorsal augmentation, medial and lateral osteotomies are not necessary. When augmenting the nasal dorsum it is desirable that the platform for the dorsal graft (bony dorsum) is wider than the actual dorsal graft itself to create the proper pyramidal contour of the dorsum, with the base being wider and the dorsal graft being narrower (**Fig. 7**). This

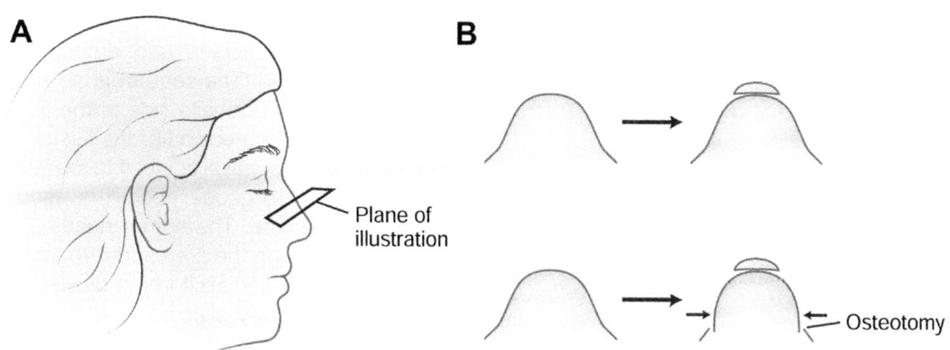

Fig. 7. Dorsal augmentation using costal cartilage graft. (*A*) Plane of illustration. (*B*) Ideally the dorsal graft is applied to a wider base to create a smooth transition from nasal bones to the dorsal graft. In most Asian patients osteotomies are not needed when performing dorsal augmentation. Previous incorrectly performed lateral osteotomies can cause an unnatural vertical transition from nasal dorsum and sidewalls to the maxilla.

contour creates a natural look to the nasal dorsum, with the leading edge of the dorsal graft creating symmetric brow tip aesthetic lines. If the bony dorsum is narrowed with osteotomies then the bony dorsum may be too narrow and create a tubular appearance to the nasal dorsum with vertically oriented sidewalls. The surgeon may choose to perform lateral osteotomies if the nasal dorsum is excessively wide and no dorsal augmentation is necessary. If the bony dorsum is deviated then osteotomies may be necessary to straighten the dorsum. In some patients if a nasal bone is in-fractured because of previous trauma it may be advisable to out-fracture the abnormally positioned nasal bone. If the lower third of the nose is wide, narrowing the upper third of the nose may create imbalance between the upper and lower segments of the nose. If significant deviation or inappropriate width exists, manipulation of the bones is performed before addressing the nasal base. However, the nasal base should be assessed before any bony vault manipulation.

If there is no deviation, nasal width is then assessed. Most primary Asian rhinoplasty patients have a wide nasal dorsum but may not need narrowing because of planned dorsal augmentation. The surgeon should take care not to narrow the nasal bones near the ascending process of the maxilla excessively as this may lead to an unnatural appearance characterized by lack of a smooth transition from the nasal dorsum to the sidewalls and cheek (**Fig. 8**). The transition from the maxilla to the nasal sidewalls and dorsum should be pyramidal in shape, not rectangular. Commonly seen in revision patients, asymmetries from previously poorly performed osteotomies or excessive narrowing from previous surgery must be corrected by widening of the bony nasal vault. For this reason, many Asian patients undergoing revision rhinoplasty may require out-fracture of the nasal bones with use of a Boies elevator to achieve sufficient width to allow for a smooth transition following placement of the dorsal graft. This transition provides for an aesthetically appropriate shadow along the nasal sidewall and avoids the unnatural appearance caused by excessive medialization of the nasal bones.

Correction of bony nasal deviation or excessive width can be accomplished with the judicious use of medial and lateral osteotomies, which must often be combined with out-fracture of 1 nasal bone to achieve straightening in crooked noses. Medial osteotomies are best avoided to prevent instability of the nasal bones, but may be required if thick cortical bone is present in the midline, preventing appropriate back-fracture from the lateral osteotomy sites. The medial osteotomies are performed first, with a 3-mm straight osteotome placed at the junction of the cartilaginous and bony septum and performed with a 10° to 15° laterally fading movement. Lateral osteotomies are then performed as needed. A number 15 scalpel is used to make a stab incision above the inferior turbinate insertion onto the piriform aperture. Local anesthetic is used to infiltrate and hydrodissect the planned osteotomy site. A 3-mm straight osteotome is used to perform the lateral osteotomy in a high-low-high fashion.

Care should be taken to evaluate the three-dimensional orientation of the nasal bone. Often, medialization of the entire bony segment above the osteotomy site is inappropriate. Commonly, the bony segment nearest the dorsum requires a different degree of medialization than does the base of the segment near the maxilla. In-fracture is performed with the osteotome, with attention

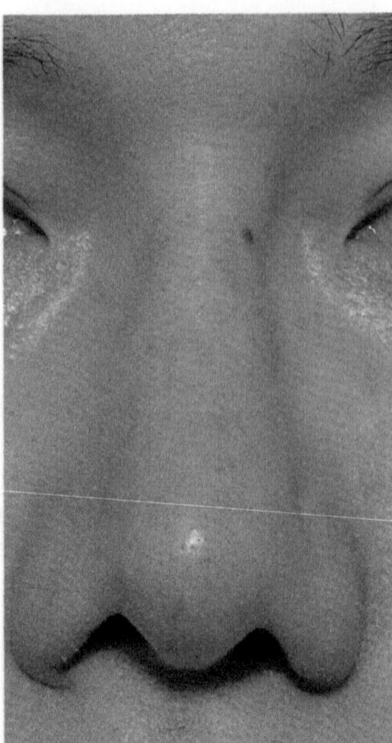

Fig. 8. Preoperative photograph of patient seeking revision rhinoplasty with previously performed inappropriate osteotomies with poor transition of dorsum to nasal sidewalls and maxilla.

to this three-dimensional aspect of the bone movement.

NASAL BASE

Following correction of any bony deformities, attention is turned to the nasal base. An assessment of any problems with deviation of the caudal septum, facial asymmetry, or anterior nasal spine positioning is performed by photographic analysis and intraoperative diagnosis. Viewing the nose from above the patient's head is invaluable to assess for deviations and asymmetries.

If the nasal base is midline, augmentation, lengthening, and strengthening may be obtained using a columellar strut, extended columellar strut, or caudal septal extension graft. If the nasal base is deviated, a swinging-door maneuver, caudal septal extension graft, or caudal septal replacement graft may be required to achieve correction. The anterior nasal spine may need to be shifted to set the base in the midline. Premaxillary augmentation may be performed by a separate premaxillary graft with possible incorporation of an extended columellar strut or by augmentation with a caudal septal extension or caudal replacement graft.

If significant caudal septal deflection exists, the caudal septum may need to be moved or resected and replaced. For minor caudal septal deflections off the spine, a swinging-door maneuver may be performed. Dissection of the caudal septum from the anterior nasal spine and anterior maxillary crest is performed. The septum is secured in the midline or on the opposite side of the nasal spine using 4-0 PDS secured to fibrous tissue on either side of the anterior nasal spine. If this is inadequate for stability, a 16-gauge needle is used to drill a hole in the spine. The suture needle may then be passed through the area and through the relocated septum to secure it in the desired position. Splinting grafts may also be used to secure the base of the graft to soft tissue around the spine.

Commonly, lengthening or blunting of the nasolabial angle is desired in Asian rhinoplasty. Changing the nasolabial angle in the Asian patient can change the upper lip position and create stiffness in the upper lip. This change must be discussed with the patient beforehand to ensure the patient understands the potential consequences of changing the nasolabial angle. The caudal septum must also be strong enough to support the large dorsal graft without collapse. The weaker cartilage found in Asian patients may not withstand collapse over time, which may lead to tip ptosis, loss of projection, and polly-beak deformity. In these patients, a caudal septal extension graft or caudal septal replacement graft is indicated. The caudal septal extension graft is used if the caudal septum and anterior nasal spine are located in the midline or for minor deviations of these areas. The caudal septal extension graft is secured to the existing caudal septum by an overlapping technique, which may correct minor caudal deviations, or by an end-to-end configuration with the use of extended spreader grafts and splinting grafts to secure the graft to the caudal septum (**Fig. 9**). Using a noted curvature of the donor cartilage in a manner to combat any tendency toward deviation of the columella and tip aids correction of the deformity.

On rare occasions when the caudal septum is severely deviated or damaged from previous surgery or trauma, the caudal septum may need to be resected and replaced with a caudal septal replacement graft. In these patients, the caudal septum is resected, leaving a dorsal strut of 1.5 cm extending from the nasal bones and bony septum. The native tip deviation and position of the anterior nasal spine are noted. On rare occasions, the nasal spine is off midline and contributes to the deviation. In these patients, a 5-mm straight osteotome placed on the spine is used to determine the optimum position of the spine to align it with the nasal bones while observing from the head of the bed. The osteotome is then driven into the spine at a slight angle toward the desired position. The osteotome is then used as a lever to move the

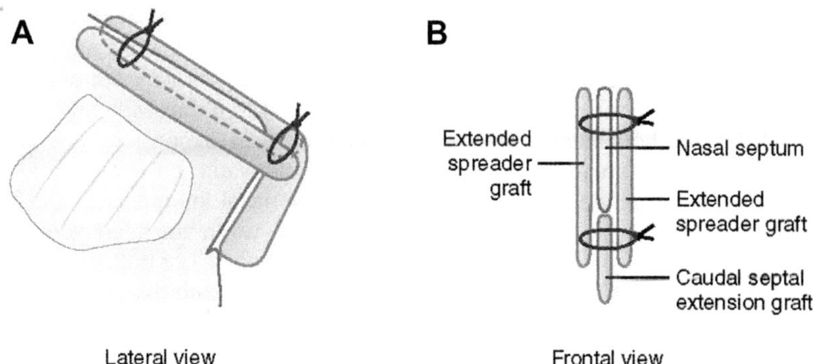

Fig. 9. Caudal septal extension graft, bilateral spreader grafts, and splinting grafts. (*A*) Lateral view. (*B*) Cross section.

spine to the desired position, thereby widening and displacing the notch toward the midline (**Fig. 10**A, B). Two 4-0 PDS are secured to fibrous tissue on either side of the anterior nasal spine or into holes drilled in the spine using a 16-gauge needle.

The caudal septal replacement graft is carved with care to note any subtle deviation of the graft, which can be used to combat the native tip deviation. One of the lateral pieces of costal cartilage with a straight orientation should be selected. If a sufficiently straight piece is unavailable, thin pieces of curved costal cartilage can be used to splint and counteract any deviation of the caudal septal replacement graft. The graft should be kept longer at this stage (often 35–40 mm) to allow for setting adequate tip projection following application of the spreader grafts and reapproximation of the lower lateral cartilages. The graft may be trimmed before the final tip work is completed. A notch is carved in the graft to allow for appropriate premaxillary augmentation. The size of the premaxillary portion of the notched segment must be carefully considered. A larger premaxillary segment aids lengthening and blunting of a retracted nasolabial angle, but risks the production of tension and creasing of the upper lip. The graft is placed in the notch and sutured securely in place.

If more significant premaxillary augmentation is required, a separate premaxillary graft can be incorporated into the nasal base stabilization. An extended columellar strut or caudal septal

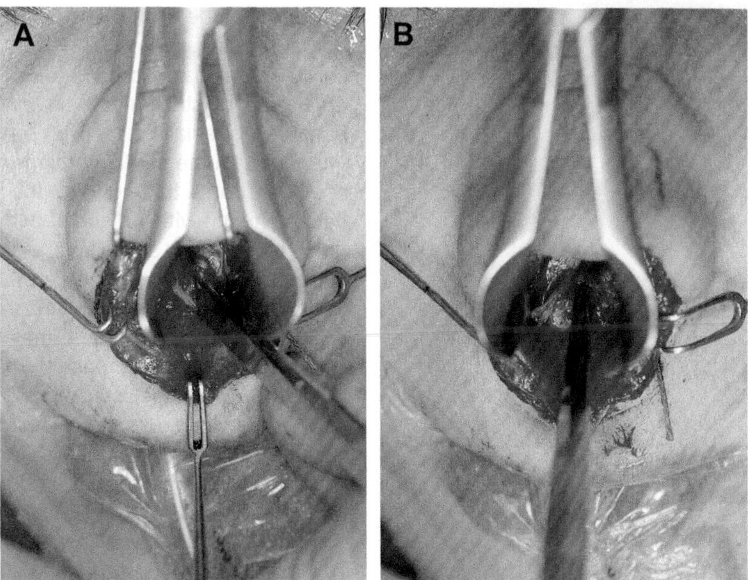

Fig. 10. Repositioning of the nasal base. (*A*) Osteotome placed in anterior nasal spine at an angle. (*B*) Osteotome manipulated to partially fracture anterior nasal spine laterally. This relocates notch to the midline and allows placement of caudal septal replacement graft (as in **Fig. 4**).

replacement graft can be carved to fit into the notch created in the anterior nasal spine, as described earlier. The notched portion of the graft extending anterior to the anterior nasal spine is then incorporated into a horizontally oriented premaxillary graft. This graft is carved to fit anterior to the spine in a carefully dissected pocket along the premaxilla.

SPREADER GRAFT PLACEMENT

Following nasal base stabilization, attention is turned to placement of spreader grafts. In Asian rhinoplasty, the use of spreader grafts serves several purposes. The incorporation of the grafts with a strong nasal base provides a firm structural foundation for dorsal grafting, aids in setting and preserving nasal length and projection, and helps to open the nasal valve. In addition, the strength of the grafts resists the cephalic movement of the tip complex, thereby preventing the overrotation and nasal shortening that may be seen as tip projection is increased (**Fig. 11**).

Typically, spreader grafts are carved from the central portion of the previously carved costal cartilage. They are tapered at each end and the caudalmost portion should be trimmed along its inferior margin slightly so as not to block the nasal valve. Any deviations of the grafts should be noted and used appropriately to combat any native dorsal septal or tip deviation. Opposing curvatures may be used to minimize any deflection. Dimensions of the grafts vary but are typically 20 to 40 mm long, 4 to 6 mm wide and 1.5 to 3 mm thick. Differences in dimensions are used to account for middle vault collapse, middle vault width, need for nasal lengthening, and so forth. If the nasal bony width has been increased by out-fracture, a portion of 1 or both spreader grafts may be placed underneath the caudal nasal bones to prevent the bone from collapsing medially. The grafts are sutured to the remaining dorsal septum or dorsal septal strut. They are then sutured to the caudal septal extension graft or caudal septal replacement graft (**Fig. 12**A, C). Manipulation of this complex in multiple dimensions enables the surgeon to alter tip projection, nasal length, dorsal height, and tip rotation. These parameters must be set with great care otherwise one can easily create deformity such as overprojection, excess length, or short or overrotated tip. Once the proper position and middle nasal vault width have been obtained, the upper lateral cartilages are sutured to the spreader grafts and nasal septum. Care must be taken to prevent entrapping the nasal mucosa when suturing the spreader grafts in place. Also, sagging mucosa into the nasal valve area may produce blunting of valve and impaired airflow. Prevention of this is accomplished with careful mattress approximation of the septal mucoperichondrial flaps in this area.

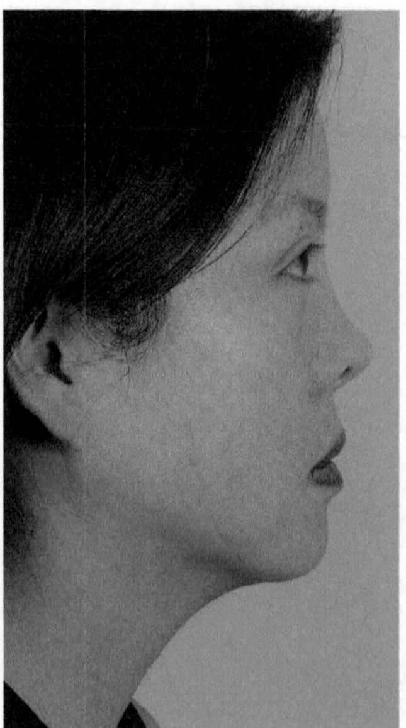

Fig. 11. Preoperative photograph of patient seeking revision rhinoplasty. Note overrotated tip and short nose deformity, caused by an L-shaped Silastic implant that projected the nasal tip. As tip projection is increased rotation must be restricted to avoid the overrotation as seen in this patient.

DORSAL GRAFT

Septal cartilage is the first choice of material for dorsal grafting, followed by costal and auricular cartilage, in that order. The senior author does not use alloplastic materials in rhinoplasty. In Asian patients, especially in revision operations, there is often inadequate septal cartilage (in length, thickness, or both) to augment the dorsum to the desired height with 1 piece. If only minor augmentation is desired, a single layer of septal cartilage is carved into a canoe-shaped graft, with care taken to taper all sides to maximize camouflage. If needed, the septal cartilage may be stacked and sutured together to increase dorsal height.

Auricular cartilage, stacked or in single layers, can be used as a dorsal graft but can be problematic because of its inherent irregular contour tendency to curl or deform, and potential resorption if stacked.

Costal cartilage dorsal grafts should be carved in similar fashion as the septal cartilage, with care taken to note any tendency toward warping. The bending of the cartilage tends to be in an anterior/posterior direction with respect to its

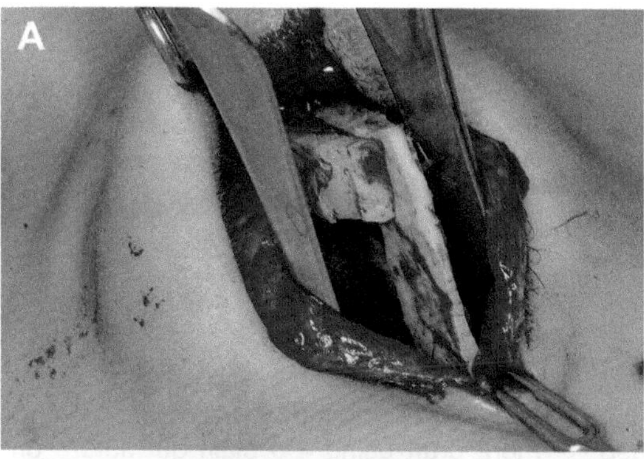

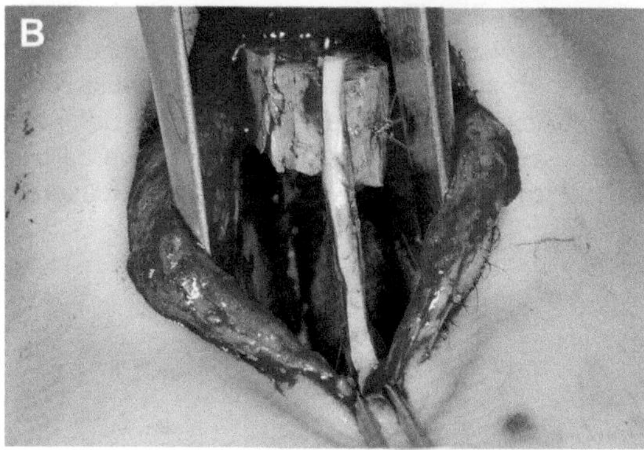

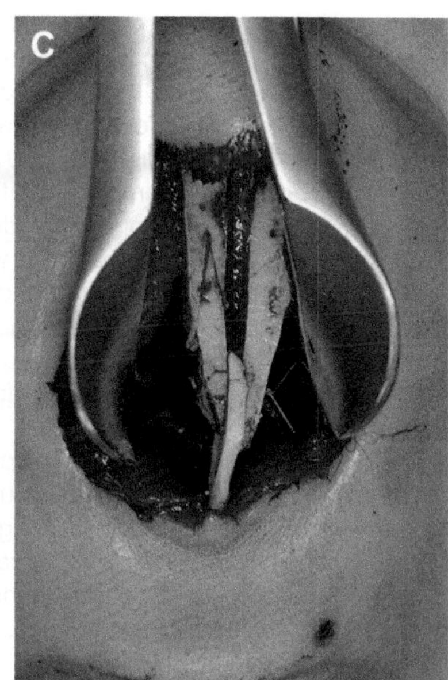

Fig. 12. Intraoperative photograph demonstrating placement of bilateral extended spreader grafts to secure caudal septal replacement graft. (*A*) Surgeon's view. (*B*) Base view. (*C*) Frontal view.

native position in the chest (before harvest).[1] It is uncommon to see warping in a lateral direction when carved as described and fixated properly. The cartilage is generally carved into a canoe-shaped graft, with tapered edges to aid camouflage. It is imperative that any native curvature of the graft be noted. It is recommended that the graft have some curvature so the tendency of the cartilage to bend is known. The concave side should be placed against the nasal dorsum to avoid unsightly irregularity from the cephalic and caudal ends becoming visible with minor warping (**Fig. 13**). By positioning the dorsal graft with the concave surface oriented downward against the dorsum, suturing the graft to the upper lateral cartilages will resist any additional curvature. The subtle convexity produced from the properly placed dorsal graft following minor warping may be barely detectable and may be corrected by nasal compression exercises performed by the patient.

Proper fixation of the graft begins with the initial elevation of the skin and soft-tissue envelope. Care to restrict the elevation of the periosteum over the nasal bones to preserve a tight pocket enables the surgeon to securely fixate the cephalic end of the dorsal graft into a tight pocket over the upper bony dorsum. The tight pocket helps to minimize any displacement of the upper aspect of the dorsal graft.

Following stabilization of the nasal base and spreader grafts, the dorsal graft is placed along the dorsum to assess for appropriate augmentation. The graft is removed and refined as needed to achieve the appropriate effect. The dorsal graft is carved sequentially for hours to allow close monitoring of the tendency of the costal cartilage

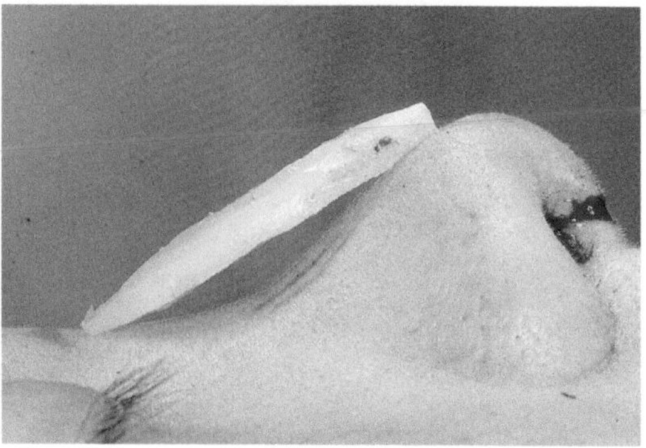

Fig. 13. Dorsal graft before refinement and camouflage. Note slight curvature of graft. The concave surface is placed in contact with the dorsum.

dorsal graft to warp. Final placement and fixation are delayed until tip manipulation is complete.

Perichondrium is used around the edges of the graft to camouflage the transition from graft to dorsum and prevent graft visibility (**Fig. 14**A, C). This technique produces 1 mm of additional augmentation when placed along the dorsal surface and should be taken into account when carving the graft. A small piece of perichondrium is also sutured in place to the undersurface of the graft, which prevents postoperative graft migration. Before final placement of the graft, the nasal dorsum is roughened with a fine rasp (**Fig. 15**). The graft is then placed into the cephalic subperiosteal pocket and sutured to the upper lateral cartilages or underlying spreader grafts using 5-0 PDS along both sides of the caudal aspect of the graft. If needed, a transcutaneous suture may be placed through the cephalic end of the dorsal graft to further prevent graft migration. Rarely, if the dorsal graft is noted to be mobile following attempts to secure it, a transcutaneous threaded Kirschner wire is placed through the graft into the nasal bones. The wire is removed on postoperative day 7, with care taken to prevent elevation of the graft on removal.

TIP WORK

The medial crura are reapproximated to the columellar strut or caudal septal extension or replacement graft using 4-0 plain gut suture on a Keith needle. This maneuver preliminarily sets tip projection and rotation. A 5-0 PDS is used to reapproximate the medial and intermediate crura to the level of the domes. The native tip deformity is then assessed by examining the native cartilages and the preoperative photographs. Measurements of

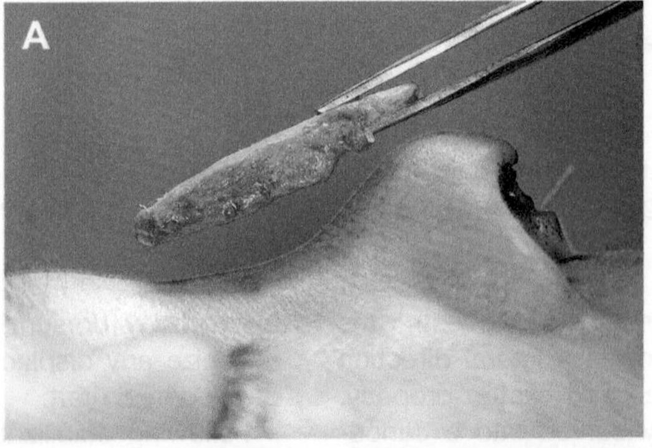

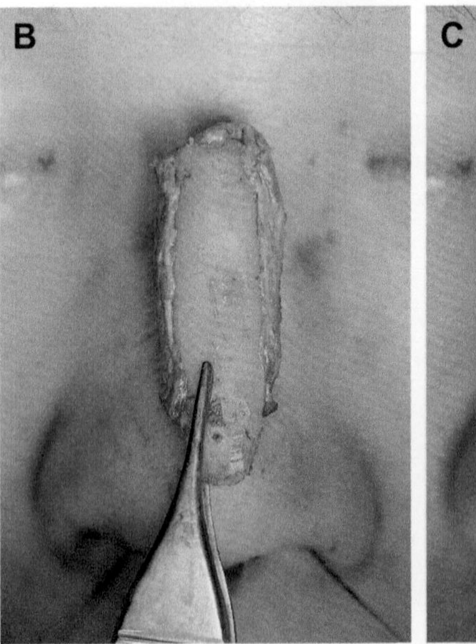

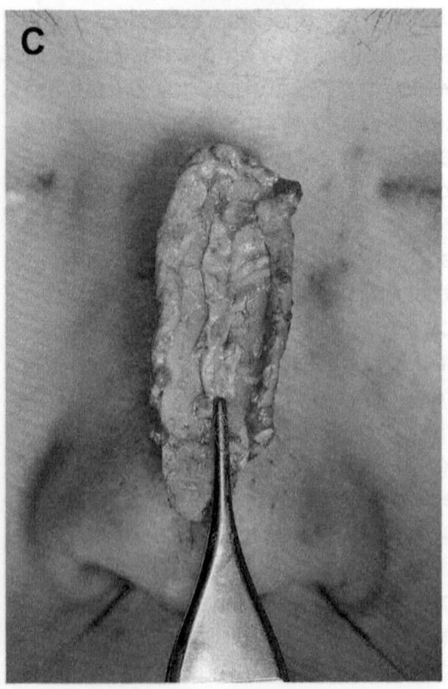

Fig. 14. Dorsal graft following final carving and camouflage with perichondrium. (*A*) Lateral view. (*B*) Frontal view of graft. (*C*) Undersurface of graft. Note perichondrium used for camouflage along lateral edges and undersurface of graft to aid in graft fixation.

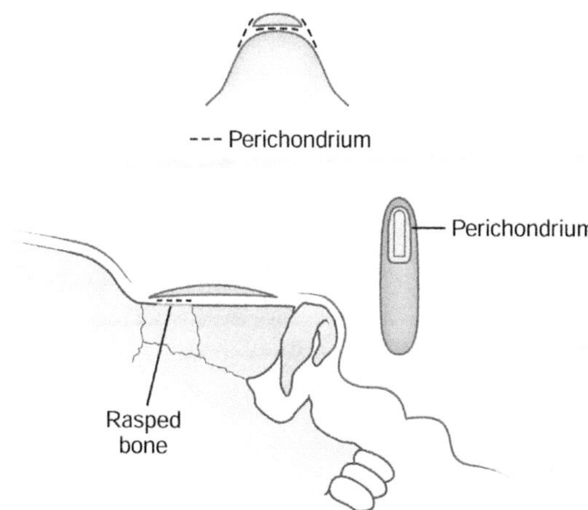

Fig. 15. Correct placement of costal cartilage graft with perichondrium used for camouflage along lateral edges of graft, and for improved adherence along undersurface of graft with perichondrium abutting previously rasped bone.

cephalic positioning, supratip break, and tip width are made using a finger goniometer and Castro-Viejo calipers.

Commonly, some degree of tip narrowing is required. Conservative bilateral cephalic trims are performed. Even if the lateral crura are cephalically positioned, repositioning with lateral strut grafting is rarely necessary in Asian patients as their skin is thick and the tip cartilage orientation does not affect tip shape to the same extent as patients with thinner skin. If the ala are retracted or arched cephalically, repositioning of the lateral crura into a more caudal position can be performed to bring the alae down and correct the alar notching. If repositioning is necessary the lateral crura are dissected carefully from the underlying vestibular skin. Lateral crural strut grafts are carved and sutured to the undersurface of the lateral crura. Depending on the amount of projection desired and inherent strength of the lateral crura, typical lateral crural strut grafts measure 30 mm × 4 mm × 1.5 mm. Care is taken to place the grafts with the concavity facing the vestibular skin to aid stenting of the external nasal valve. They are sutured to the remaining lateral crura with 5-0 PDS with the knot placed on top of the lateral crura to avoid extrusion through the vestibular skin. The grafts are then placed in a carefully dissected pocket oriented in a vector paralleling the nostril margin toward, but not reaching, the piriform aperture. These pockets should not be positioned too far caudally as this can result in accentuation of a hanging alar lobule, which is frequently a problem with Asian patients. Asymmetric pockets may be dissected to account for asymmetric alar positions. Correction of asymmetrically retracted or arched nasal ala can be accounted for by appropriately positioned pockets.

Tip bulbosity is corrected with the flattening of the lateral crus produced by lateral crural strut graft placement. If repositioning is not performed, bulbosity can be addressed by lateral strut grafting without repositioning or simply by placing bilateral dome binding sutures. If lateral crural strut grafts are placed, the vestibular skin is dissected from the undersurface of the lateral crura, with the lateral end of the lateral crus maintained in the soft tissue near the piriform aperture. Smaller lateral strut grafts 20 mm to 25 mm long are used and sutured to the undersurface of the lateral crura. In many Asian patients placement of a simple dome binding suture is adequate to decrease nasal tip bulbosity. After placing the dome sutures additional tip projection can be achieved using either onlay tip grafts or shield tip grafts.

Patients with thick, sebaceous skin or those in need of a more significant increase in tip projection require significant grafting to project and achieve refinement in the tip. A shield graft combined with lateral crural grafts may be used in this situation. The graft is carved in the shape of a shield and sutured in place to provide increased tip projection and augmentation of the infratip lobule. Lateral crural grafts are sutured to the posterior surface of the shield graft set at approximately a 45° angle and then fixated to the existing lateral crura. The lateral crural grafts act to stabilize the tip graft, provide graft camouflage and prevent unwanted rotation of the shield graft caused by cephalically oriented force applied by the thick skin envelope (**Fig. 16**A, B). Before closure crushed cartilage or soft tissue (perichondrium or temporalis fascia) are used to camouflage the leading edge of the shield graft.

If shield grafting is not used, tip grafting using softer pieces of rectangular cartilage and soft tissue can be used. In these patients such grafts are positioned horizontally over the domes and sutured with 6-0 Monacryl sutures (**Fig. 17**A, B). Manipulation of these grafts helps to set the supratip break, projection, and overall refinement to the nasal tip.

The dorsal graft is removed and replaced repeatedly to assess the relationship between the projection and dorsal height during the process of tip refinement. Following the achievement of appropriate projection, the dorsal graft is positioned and fixated to the upper lateral cartilages with at least 2 6-0 Monacryl sutures.

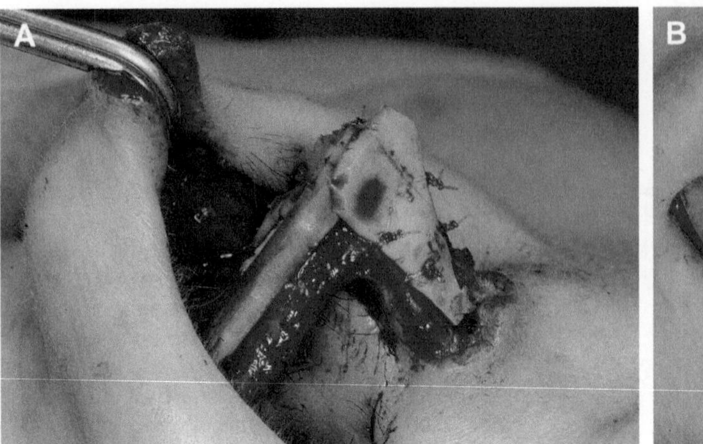
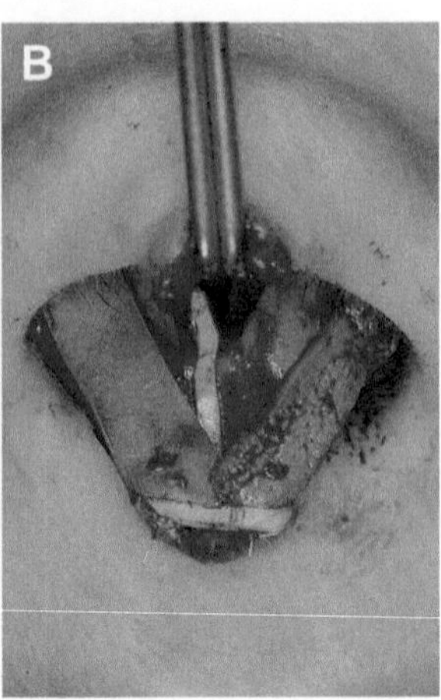

Fig. 16. Shield-shaped tip graft with lateral crural grafts. Intraoperative view of tip graft with lateral crural grafts. (*A*) Surgeon's view. (*B*) Frontal view.

The skin and soft-tissue envelope is then redraped and the nose assessed for any other deficiencies or persistent abnormalities. Onlay grafts to the columellar and plumping grafts to the premaxilla are placed as needed. Observation and palpation from the head of the bed are performed to determine the need for onlay grafting along the dorsal graft or middle vault to prevent future asymmetries.

ALAR BATTEN AND ALAR RIM GRAFTS

The need for alar batten grafts is determined by the nasal bone length, skin thickness, repositioning of the lateral crura, and preoperative valve collapse.[2] These grafts are rarely needed in Asian patients as their airway tends to be wider, with thicker lateral sidewalls. Alar battens are placed in precisely dissected pockets in the lateral soft tissue or sutured to the existing cartilaginous framework.

The need for alar rim grafts is assessed by the degree of bulbosity, pinching of the tip, external nasal valve collapse, and need to smooth the transition from the tip lobule to the alar lobule. Alar rim grafts are placed along the nostril margin in a carefully dissected pocket and should end medially behind the tip complex. Alar rim grafts are rarely needed in Asian patients as their alar lobules

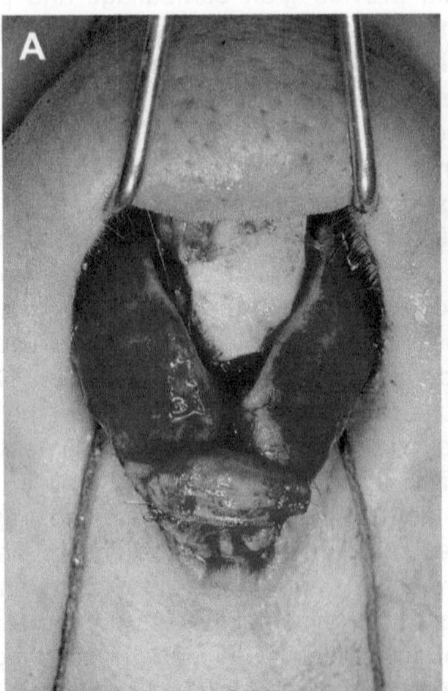
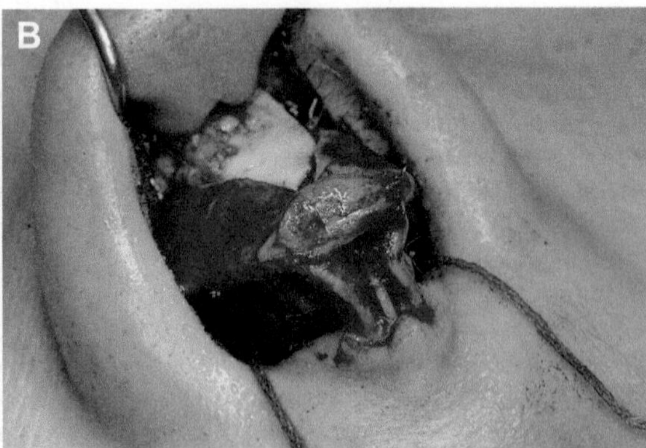

Fig. 17. Horizontally oriented onlay tip graft using soft cartilage. (*A*) View from above. (*B*) Surgeon's view.

tend to be thicker and are rarely pinched or collapsed.

CLOSURE

Closure is accomplished using a single 6-0 PDS in the midline to reapproximate the skin envelope. A 4-0 plain gut suture on a Keith needle is used to reapproximate the mucoperichondrial flaps in a mattress fashion. A 5-0 chromic gut suture is used to close the marginal incisions. 7-0 black nylon interrupted vertical mattress sutures are used for the columellar skin closure. A 6-0 fast-absorbing gut suture is used to close the medial extent of the marginal incision near the soft-tissue triangle.

Folded pieces of nonadherent gauze coated with a thin layer of bacitracin are used as nasal packing. Lateral wall splints are used if lateral crural strut grafts have been used. These are radioopaque 0.25-mm-thick nasal splints trimmed to fit over the supra alar groove. They are sewn into place over and through the lateral crural strut grafts to aid healing in the immediate postoperative period. They are removed on postoperative day 7. Vestibular splints are used if the nostrils are asymmetric or the internal diameter of the airway is compromised. Bacitracin is applied to the suture lines and a drip pad is placed.

BASE REDUCTIONS

Nasal base width is assessed following closure of the marginal and midcolumellar incisions. Asian rhinoplasty patients occasionally require nasal base reductions, although the need for these should be balanced against the tendency for Asian patients to form hyperpigmented scars. The need for base reduction is increased because of the flare produced from lateral crural repositioning and alar rim grafting. The internal versus external component of flare is assessed and marked with a marking pen (**Fig. 18**A). Alar base reduction is performed with a number 11 blade with a diamond-shaped excision to promote eversion of the skin edges. A single 5-0 PDS is used to approximate the deep tissues and 7-0 nylon sutures in an interrupted vertical mattress fashion used to close the skin (**Fig. 18**B, C).

Postoperative Care

Patients are seen on the first postoperative day, the packing is removed, the nose is cleansed with hydrogen peroxide, and bacitracin ointment

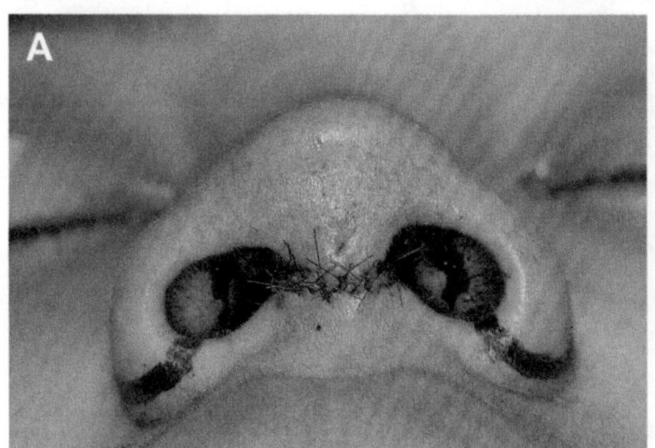

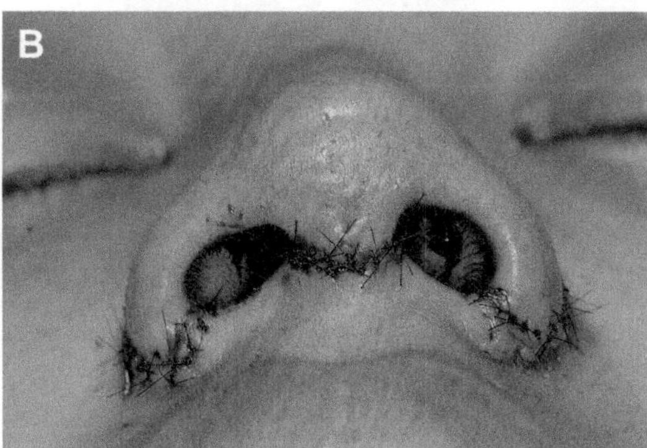

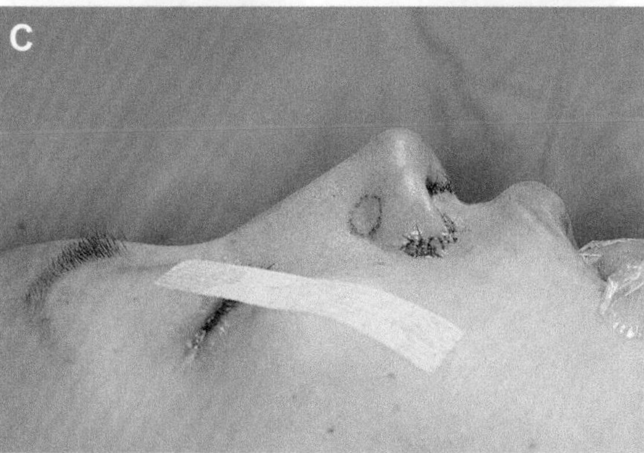

Fig. 18. Intraoperative view of base reduction (internal and external). (*A*) Markings before excision. (*B*) Following excision and closure, base view. (*C*) Lateral view.

is placed. The cast and midcolumellar sutures are removed on postoperative day 7. The base reduction sutures are removed on postoperative day 14. Patients are given a second-generation cephalosporin and mild narcotic postoperatively. Revision rhinoplasty patients are also given an oral fluoroquinolone and antibiotic rinses to perform postoperatively.

Complications

Complications with Asian rhinoplasty are similar to conventional rhinoplasty and include bleeding, infection, scarring, visible cartilage grafts, dorsal graft visibility, asymmetries, asymmetric nostrils, and nasal obstruction. Auricular cartilage can result in pain, bleeding, infection, hypertrophic scars, keloids, deformation of auricle, scar bands, and necrosis of anterior conchal skin. Risks associated with costal cartilage harvest include pain, bleeding, infection, hyperpigmented scarring, hypertrophic scarring, pneumothorax, and cartilage warping. Patients rarely complain of significant pain and are able to return home on the day of surgery.

Discussion

Asian rhinoplasty differs from traditional rhinoplasty in preoperative counseling and in operative technique. Augmentation of the existing nasal structural framework is the primary goal of the operation, in contrast to traditionally reductive techniques. In Asian rhinoplasty 1 of the most common goals is to increase projection of the nasal dorsum. Creating a natural nasal dorsum requires great attention to detail and proper grafting materials (**Fig. 19**).

The need for augmentation dictates the need for grafting material. Many surgeons use alloplastic materials for augmentation because of ease of use, minimal operative time required, and lack of donor site morbidity. Alloplastic graft materials include silicone, Gore-Tex (WL Gore and Associates, Newark, DE, USA), and porous polyethylene.[3,4] Opponents of alloplastic materials cite increased rates of infection, extrusion, thinning of skin over Silastic implants, displacement, translucency of the implant, and pain with alloplasts.[5,6] Autologous materials include nasal septal cartilage,

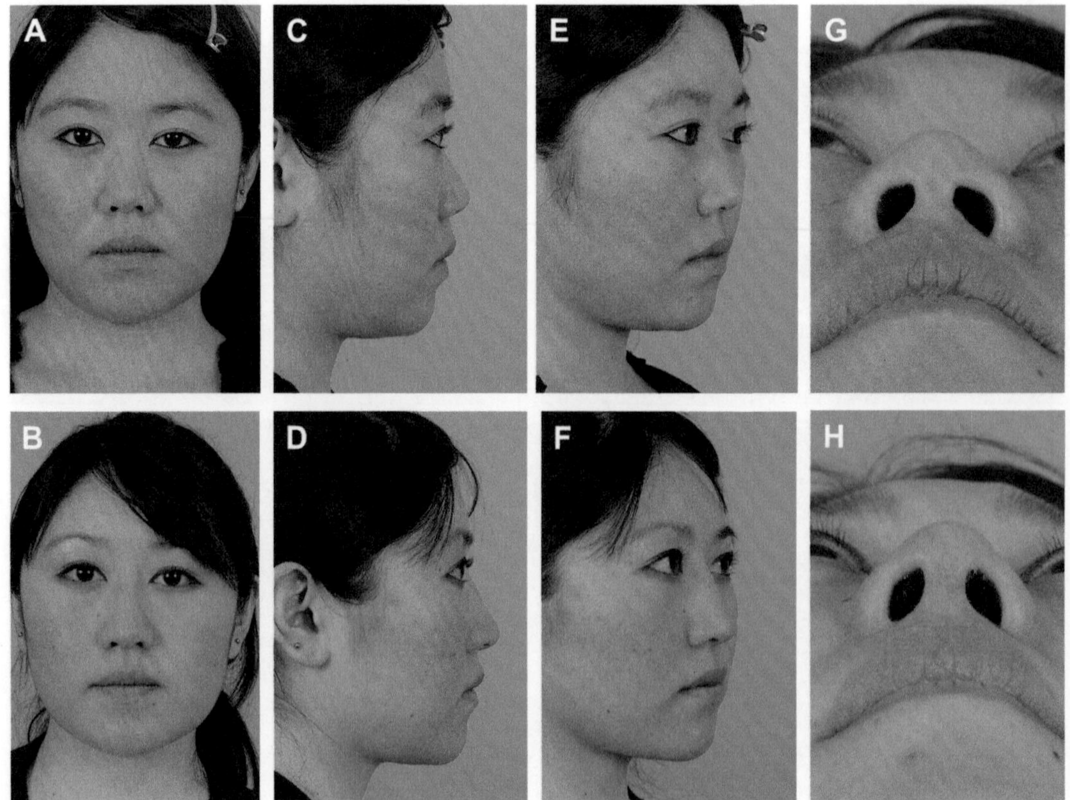

Fig. 19. Asian patient who underwent dorsal augmentation using costal cartilage. (*A, C, E, G*) Preoperative views. (*B, D, F, H*) One-year postoperative views.

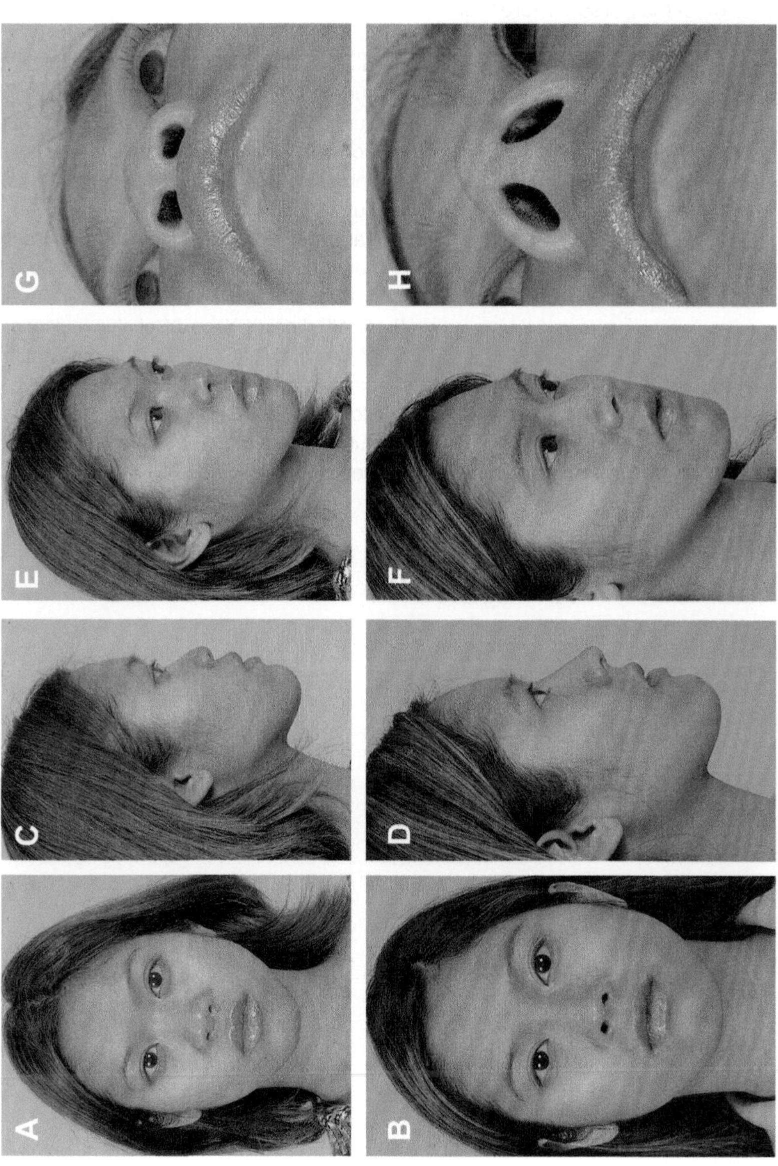

Fig. 20. Patient underwent previous augmentation with Silastic implant that extruded through her nasal tip, leaving a scar on her nasal tip. She underwent reconstruction with costal cartilage with placement of a dorsal graft, septal replacement graft, and shield tip graft with lateral crural grafts. (*A, C, E, G*) Preoperative views. (*B, D, F, H*) Two-year postoperative views.

auricular cartilage, costal cartilage, iliac bone, and split calvarial bone grafts. Autologous materials are preferred because of their decreased rates of infection, extrusion, foreign body reaction, and preferred handling characteristics. Septal cartilage is preferred for dorsal augmentation up to 3 mm in thickness because of ease of harvest and carving and favorable shape. Costal cartilage is the material of choice for augmentation of the dorsum more than 3 mm in thickness (**Fig. 20**). It does not demonstrate resorption,[7] and produces predictable results in experienced hands, with low incidence of warping or visibility of the grafts. A significant learning curve is associated with use of costal cartilage; special care should be taken when starting to use this material as there are many potential pitfalls if it is not used properly.

SUMMARY

Asian rhinoplasty requires knowledge of the anatomy and aesthetic ideals unique to the Asian rhinoplasty patient. Use of autologous cartilage in a structured approach is the preferred grafting method to achieve the desired long-term results in this patient population.

REFERENCES

1. Kim DW, Shah AR, Toriumi DM. Concentric and eccentric carved costal cartilage: a comparison of warping. Arch Facial Plast Surg 2006;8(1):42–6.
2. Toriumi DM. New concepts in nasal tip contouring. Arch Facial Plast Surg 2006;8:156–85.
3. Godin MS, Waldman SR, Johnson CM. Nasal augmentation using Gore-Tex. Arch Facial Plast Surg 1999;1(2):118–21 [discussion: 122].
4. Romo T III, Sclafani AP, Jacono AA. Nasal reconstruction using porous polyethylene implants. Facial Plast Surg 2000;16(1):55–61.
5. Parker PJ. Grafts in rhinoplasty: alloplastic vs autogenous. Arch Otolaryngol Head Neck Surg 2000;126(4): 558–61.
6. Jin HR, Lee JY, Yeon JY, et al. A multicenter evaluation of the safety of Gore-Tex as an implant in Asian rhinoplasty. Am J Rhinol 2006;20(6):615–9.
7. Horton CE, Matthews MS. Nasal reconstruction with autologous rib cartilage: a 43-year follow-up. Plast Reconstr Surg 1992;89(1):131–5.

Ethnic Rhinoplasty

Rod J. Rohrich, MD*, Kelly Bolden, MD

KEYWORDS

- Ethnic • Non-Caucasian • African American • Hispanic
- Middle Eastern • Rhinoplasty

The United States has become more racially and ethnically diverse over the past century, and this trend is expected to continue over the next 50 years. According to the US Census Bureau,[1] minorities (or non-Caucasians) compose roughly one-third of the United States population and are expected to become the majority by 2042. In 2050, the US Census Bureau projects the nation to be 54% minority. The Hispanic population is projected to increase nearly 300% between 2008 and 2050, from 46.7 million to 132.8 million. The African American population is projected to increase from 46.7 million to 65.7 million.[1]

A similar trend is occurring in plastic surgery. According to statistics by the American Society of Plastic Surgery,[2] cosmetic plastic surgery procedures for "ethnic" patients increased by 13% between 2006 and 2007, comprising nearly a quarter of the cosmetic plastic surgery procedures performed in 2007. Since 2000, cosmetic plastic surgery procedures increased 173% in Hispanics and 129% in African Americans. Within these demographics, nose reshaping is among the top 3 most commonly requested surgical cosmetic procedures.[3]

With this dramatic paradigm shift, it is imperative that rhinoplasty surgeons have an appreciation for the various concepts of aesthetic beauty among different races and ethnicities, as well as the unique anatomic characteristics of each population. The successful rhinoplasty surgeon must possess in his or her armamentarium the techniques to consistently modify the "ethnic" nose while maintaining facial harmony, balance, and cultural aesthetics.

Although the basic tenets of plastic surgery hold true for patients of any ethnicity, there are several important differences that distinguish rhinoplasty in the "ethnic," or non-Caucasian patient, from Caucasian patients. This article reviews the unique anatomic characteristics of "ethnic" noses, specifically African American, Hispanic, Indian, and Middle Eastern noses. In addition, the article addresses the aesthetic objectives and reviews specific techniques to achieve consistent, harmonious, and racially congruent results.

DEFINING THE ETHNIC RHINOPLASTY

The term "ethnic" rhinoplasty is peppered throughout the literature and is somewhat misleading, as it infers that rhinoplasty in the non-Caucasian patient is a singularly defined entity. In reality, "ethnic" rhinoplasty is a generic term that harbors a multitude of complexities. This terminology typically refers to rhinoplasty in African American, Hispanic, Indian, Middle Eastern, and Asian patients. However, even defining these specific ethnic groups is difficult as they are multiracial mixtures defined by cultural, geographic, and historical factors.

In an effort to bring order to the broad anatomic and morphologic variations among these patients, several investigators have developed subcategories within each ethnicity.[4–9] The concern for lumping these ethnicities into a single category, or even multiple subcategories, is the tendency of the surgeon to adapt the patient to a prespecified treatment algorithm, rather than adapting an individualized treatment algorithm for each specific patient. While subcategories can be helpful adjuncts, it is critical that the surgeon has a command of the common yet variable anatomic features within specific races and cultures. Equally important, the surgeon must understand and respect various cultural aesthetics and be

Department of Plastic Surgery, University of Texas Southwestern Medical Center, 1801 Inwood Road, Dallas, TX 75390-9132, USA
* Corresponding author.
E-mail address: rod.rohrich@utsouthwestern.edu (R.J. Rohrich).

Clin Plastic Surg 37 (2010) 353–370
doi:10.1016/j.cps.2009.11.006

plasticsurgery.theclinics.com

equipped with the appropriate operative techniques to achieve a successful and racially congruent result.

For the purposes of this article, the term "ethnic" (albeit a drastic generalization) refers to African American, Arabic, Indian, and Hispanic patients. These populations have several common anatomic features, as well as frequent geographic and cultural overlap. The Asian patient is discussed in a separate article elsewhere in this issue.

NASAL AESTHETICS IN THE ETHNIC PATIENT

Harmony and symmetry are essential elements of beauty, and are the ultimate goals of any surgical plan regardless of a patient's race or ethnicity.[10,11] Standards of beauty in Western society have been largely influenced by Northern European characteristics.[12,13] Millard[14] described the aesthetic Caucasian female face as having clear, pale, smooth skin; large, widely spaced, soft eyes with long lashes; high cheekbones; and a medium-sized mouth with gentle lips that are not too thick. Aesthetics specific to the nose included a straight, narrow bridge; well-defined projecting tip; refined alae; and a nasolabial angle of approximately 90° to 95° in men and 95° to 100° in women.[12,13] In strong contrast, the African American nose is generally characterized by a wide, low dorsum; less tip projection and definition; increased alar flaring or increased interalar width; a shorter nasal length; an acute columellar-labial angle; and a low radix.[4–7,15–20] It must be borne in mind that there will be considerable variability in these characteristics from one patient to the next, given the history of the African diaspora and the multiple ethnic backgrounds of most African Americans. Each patient's nose and his or her overall appearance will reflect this multicultural history, and this variation contributes to the complexity of rhinoplasty in this community, as well as the Indian, Hispanic, and Arabic communities that share similar features.

Given such tremendous variability within these ethnicities, it is inappropriate for the surgeon to use the aesthetic standards and techniques commonly used in Caucasian rhinoplasty patients

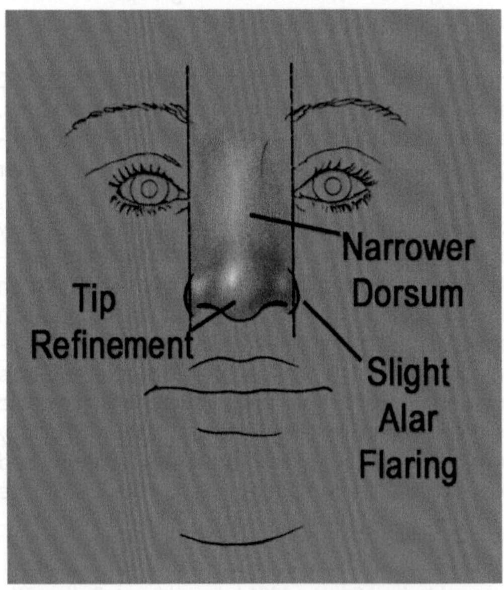

Fig. 1. Aesthetic goals of ethnic rhinoplasty. (*From* Gunter JP, Rohrich RJ, Adams Jr WP. Dallas rhinoplasty: nasal surgery by the masters. 2nd edition. St Louis (MO): Quality Medical Publishing Inc; 2007. p. 1112; with permission.)

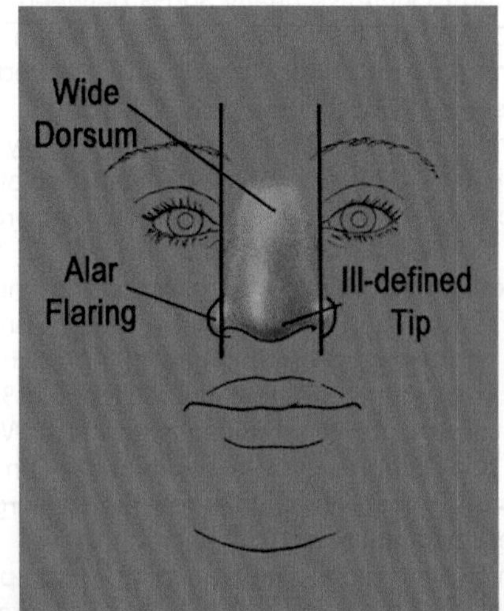

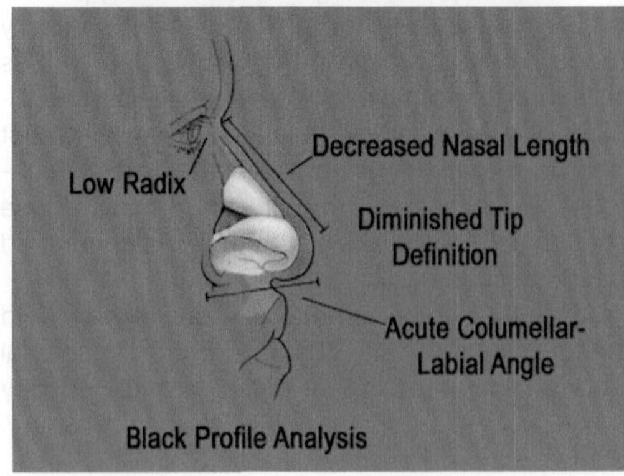

Fig. 2. Characteristic features of the African American nose. (*Above*) Frontal view. (*Below*) Lateral view. (*From* Gunter JP, Rohrich RJ, Adams Jr WP. Dallas rhinoplasty: nasal surgery by the masters. 2nd edition. St Louis (MO): Quality Medical Publishing Inc; 2007. p. 1110–1; with permission.)

to evaluate the ethnic rhinoplasty patient. Similarly, it is an error on the part of the surgeon to assume that the ethnic patient presenting for rhinoplasty desires to modify his or her nose to resemble that of the Caucasian or Northern European ideal. On the contrary, the surgeon must establish the aesthetic objectives of each patient individually. In past decades, arguably many ethnic patients presenting for rhinoplasty desired to look more like the "accepted standard of beauty," a more Caucasian-appearing nose. However, the modern ethnic patient seeking rhinoplasty more likely desires to attain an attractive nose that retains its ethnic character. It is the surgeon's responsibility to determine the exact aesthetic objective during the preoperative consultation to determine if the goals are realistic and to avoid any postoperative problems.

While there have been ideal standards described for the Caucasian female nose,[21–24] an ideal standard for the African American, Indian, Hispanic, or Arabic aesthetic has yet to be established. Porter and Olson[25] outlined objective values and proportions of African American female noses using anthropometric measurements. Similarly, Milgram and colleagues[26] provided anthropometric analysis of female Latinas from the Caribbean, Central America, and South America. However, considerable variability remains in these heterogeneous populations. Thus, a general knowledge and understanding of the more common anatomic and morphologic characteristics in patients of varying ethnicities will assist the surgeon in operative planning.

For example, classic descriptions of the African American nose include a short columella with decreased columella/lobule ratio, broad flat dorsum, slightly flaring alae, alar base width wider than the intercanthal distance, smaller nasolabial angle, increased nasofacial angle, rounded tip with ovoid nares, and greater variability in the nasal base shape.[25,27,28] Inadequate nasal projection is frequent, with nasal projection approximately 0.5 times the nasal length, as opposed to 0.67 times the ideal nasal length in Caucasians.[24] Bimaxillary protrusion is also common, and the upper lip is typically full with a prominent Cupid's bow.[27,28] Keeping these general differences in mind is important for the rhinoplasty surgeon embarking on nose reshaping in the African American patient, or any non-Caucasian patient with variable anatomy.

The senior author uses the following overall goals to obtain consistent aesthetic results in the non-Caucasian rhinoplasty patient (**Fig. 1**)[27,28]:

1. Nasal-facial harmony
2. A narrower, straight dorsum
3. Enhanced tip projection and definition
4. Slight alar flaring
5. Normal interalar distance.

Using these guidelines and slight modifications based on the individual patient will allow the rhinoplasty surgeon to achieve harmonious aesthetic results and avoid racial incongruity.

THE AFRICAN AMERICAN, INDIAN, AND ARABIC NOSES

The dispersion of the African diaspora throughout Europe, Asia, and the Americas occurred mostly during the Arab and Atlantic slave trades beginning in the ninth and fifteenth centuries, respectively.[29] This dispersion represented one of the largest migrations in human history, and is also

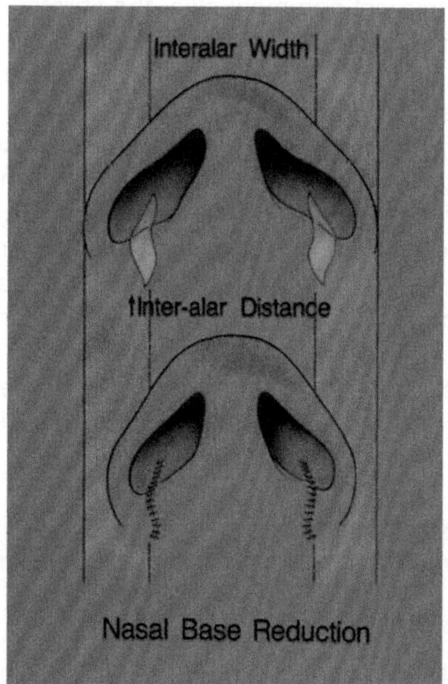

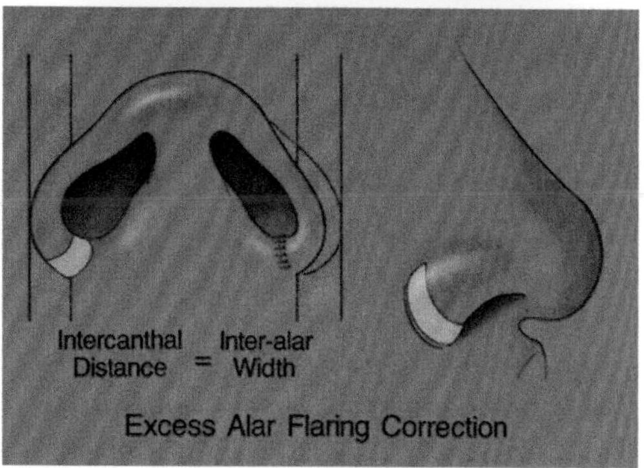

Fig. 3. (*Above*) Increased interalar distance. (*Below*) Excessive alar flaring. (*From* Gunter JP, Rohrich RJ, Adams Jr WP. Dallas rhinoplasty: nasal surgery by the masters. 2nd edition. St Louis (MO): Quality Medical Publishing Inc; 2007. p. 1115; with permission.)

responsible for the confluence of multiple races and ethnicities throughout the world. Populations around the globe have African influences, and this likely contributes to the anatomic similarities among African Americans, Latinos, Arabs, and people from the West Indies.

These populations historically were generalized as platyrrhine, referring to the broad nature of the nose, as opposed to leptorrhine, a term used to describe the narrow nose of the Caucasian.[30] Although these classifications are no longer applicable to a single race or ethnicity, these historical origins account for some of the similar anatomic features found among African American, Indian, Arabic, and Hispanic patients.

Anatomic Variations

There are 5 categories in which anatomic distinctions between the Caucasian nose and ethnic nose are most common: skin, the fibrofatty layer, alar cartilages, alar bases, and the bony pyramid.[27,28,30–36] In these patients the skin, especially at the tip, is typically thicker, more sebaceous, relatively inelastic, and with increased subcutaneous fibrofatty tissue (2–4 mm in thickness),[37] which causes an ill-defined tip (**Fig. 2**).

While the alar cartilages of these patients are similar in size to those of Caucasian patients[7,38] (Rohrich RJ, Schwartz R. Alar cartilage anatomy in the African American nose—a cadaver study, unpublished data, 2008), the angle between the medial and lateral crura (the "soft triangle") is often obtuse and filled with fat and skin. In some cases, the nasal spine may be underdeveloped, and this frequently contributes to diminished tip projection.

Alar base abnormalities are frequent and can be categorized into the following 3 entities (**Fig. 3**)[27,28,31–33]:

1. Increased interalar distance with the alar bases being lateral to the medial canthal lines
2. Excessive alar flaring characterized by a portion of the ala extending more than 2 mm lateral to the alar attachment of the cheek
3. A combination of alar flaring and increased interalar distance.

The bony pyramid is frequently characterized by a wide nasal base, low nasal dorsum, and deepened nasofrontal angle, particularly in African Americans[27,28,30,31] (see **Fig. 2**). There is an occasional lack of vertical projection of the ascending process of the maxilla, which exacerbates the appearance of a widened nasal base. In this case, the flattened nasal appearance is caused by a low dorsal bridge rather than a wide nasal base. As a result, dorsal augmentation is usually recommended as opposed to osteotomies and infractures of the bony base in this scenario.[27,28]

Variations more commonly seen in Arabic and Indian patients include a significant dorsal hump, nostril-tip imbalance and nostril asymmetries, droopy nasal tip with acute nasolabial angle, as well as an underprojected and hyperdynamic nasal tip.[32–36] A low nasal dorsum is less common

Table 1
Common characteristics of the Middle Eastern nose[a]

Characteristic	No. of Patients (%)
Amorphous, bulbous nasal tip	66 (93)
Thick sebaceous skin (fibrofatty soft-tissue envelope), especially at the tip	64 (90)
Wide bony and middle nasal vaults	61 (86)
Significant dorsal hump	60 (85)
Nostril-tip imbalance and nostril asymmetries	58 (82)
Droopy nasal tip with acute nasolabial (and columella-labial) angle (<80°)	57 (80)
Underprojected nasal tip	56 (79)
High septal angle	51 (72)
High, shallow radix	46 (65)
Cephalically and vertically malpositioned lower lateral crura	44 (62)
Hyperdynamic nasal tip (hyperactive depressor septi nasi muscle)	24 (34)
Weak and insufficient lateral, middle, and medial crura (nasal base platform)	N/A[b]

Abbreviation: N/A, not applicable.

[a] The total number of patients is 71.

[b] Crural morphology was observed intraoperatively and was not quantified.

Reproduced from Rohrich RJ, Ghavami A. Rhinoplasty for middle Eastern noses. Plast Reconstr Surg 2009;123(4):1343–54.

Table 2
Features infrequently seen in the Middle Eastern nose[a]

Feature
Low dorsum
Inadequate nasal length
Overprojected tip
Thin skin envelope with visible cartilage framework
Bifid tip
Distinct soft triangle facets
Round, transversely oriented nostrils
Obtuse nasolabial angle (and columellar labial angle)
Excess nostril show on frontal view

[a] Frequency for each trait was less than 20%.
Reproduced from Rohrich RJ, Ghavami A. Rhinoplasty for Middle Eastern noses. Plast Reconstr Surg 2009;123(4): 1343–54.

in Arabic patients, but a wide nasal base and thick sebaceous skin, especially at the tip, is very characteristic.[32–36]

Rohrich and Ghavami[33] recently reviewed 71 Middle Eastern rhinoplasty patients from North African countries (Morocco, Algeria, Libya, and Egypt), Gulf countries (Saudi Arabia, United Arab Emirates, Kuwait, Iran, and Oman), and other regional ethnic groups (Turkey, Lebanon, Syria, Armenia, Afghanistan, Pakistan, and India). This review determined the more common characteristics of the Middle Eastern nose, as well as infrequently seen features of the Middle Eastern nose, listed in **Tables 1** and **2**, respectively (**Fig. 4**).

THE HISPANIC NOSE

As with the African American and Middle Eastern populations, there is significant variability in the anatomic characteristics of Hispanic patients, which is mostly due to the variable heritage of Hispanic patients around the world. Several interpretations of the Hispanic nose have been discussed by Ortiz-Monasterio and Olmeda[38–42] on the mestizo nose, Sanchez[43] on the Chata nose, and Milgram and colleagues[26] who provided an anthropometric analysis of female Latinas from the Caribbean, Central America, and South America. More recently, Daniel[9] described 4 Hispanic nasal types based on analysis of 25 consecutive Hispanic rhinoplasty patients in his practice. He found that irrespective of national origin, 3 common nasal deformities exist in Hispanic patients, with a potential fourth type similar to the Black or African American nose. For simplicity, he associated each type with more traditional terminology. This classification included the Castilian nose, sharing more commonalities with the European nose, the Mexican-America nose, the mestizo nose, and the Creole or Chata nose.[8,9]

With such diversity within the Hispanic population, these patients demonstrate variable

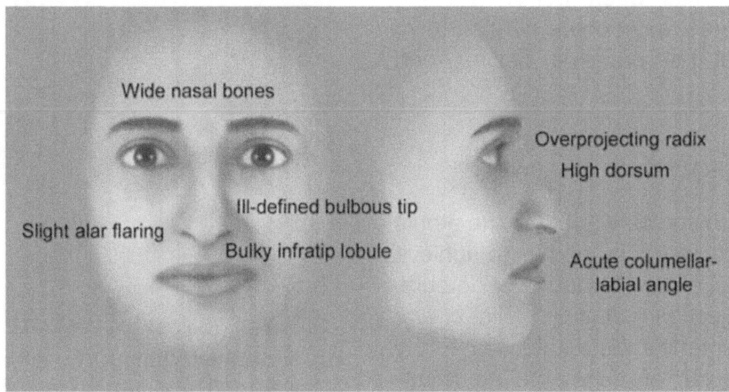

Fig. 4. Most common characteristics of the Middle Eastern nose. (*From* Gunter JP, Rohrich RJ, Adams Jr WP. Dallas rhinoplasty: nasal surgery by the masters. 2nd edition. St Louis (MO): Quality Medical Publishing Inc; 2007. p. 1142; with permission.)

Table 3
Summary of common characteristics among ethnic Rhinoplasty patients

	African/Indian/Arabic	Hispanic/European
Skin thickness	Thick	Variable
Nasal tip	Ill-defined	Variable
Dorsum	Low	Variable
Nasal base	Wide	Broad
Alar flaring	Excess	+/−

anatomic and morphologic features that exist along the spectrum between African and European noses. These patients display variable skin thickness, variable nasal tip projection, variable nasal dorsum, and frequently a broader nasal base but variable degrees of alar flaring (**Table 3**).[8,9,26,38–43]

FACIAL ANALYSIS

After reviewing the spectrum of literature that exists on the ethnic nose, it is evident that there can be no single algorithm to successfully treat the ethnic rhinoplasty patient. The diversity that exists even among the same ethnic groups is expansive. Given this realization, it is vital that the rhinoplasty surgeon master the art of facial analysis to appropriately identify the deformities in each patient and develop an individualized treatment algorithm.

Performing a thorough nasal analysis is requisite to ensure nasal-facial harmony and balance, and to ensure that the patient retains his or her ethnicity. A complete anatomic component evaluation[32,33] should be performed including skin and soft tissue envelope, bony pyramid and nasal dorsum, cartilage framework and nasal tip, alar base, and the nostrils. Once a thorough facial and nasal analysis has been performed, the surgeon can devise an appropriate surgical plan taking into account the patient's desires and expectations.

OPERATIVE TECHNIQUES

The basic tenets of rhinoplasty apply to the ethnic rhinoplasty patient as well. The goal is to achieve nasal-facial harmony, a straight-narrower dorsum, increased tip projection/definition, slight alar flaring, and normal interalar distance.[27,28,32,33] By applying the principles of augmentation rhinoplasty to the more ethnic nose, the senior author has attained reproducible results using the following techniques[27,28,32,33]:

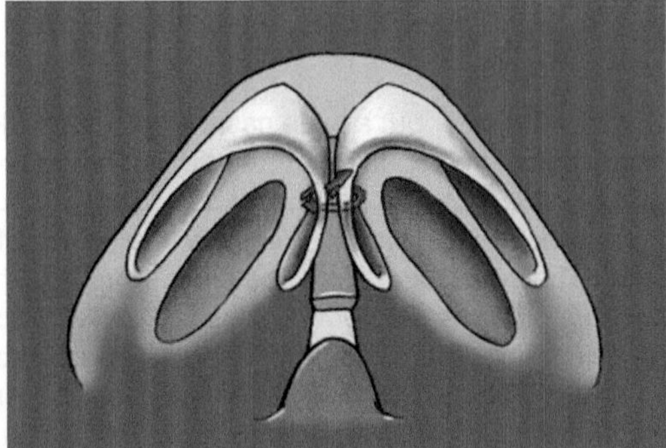

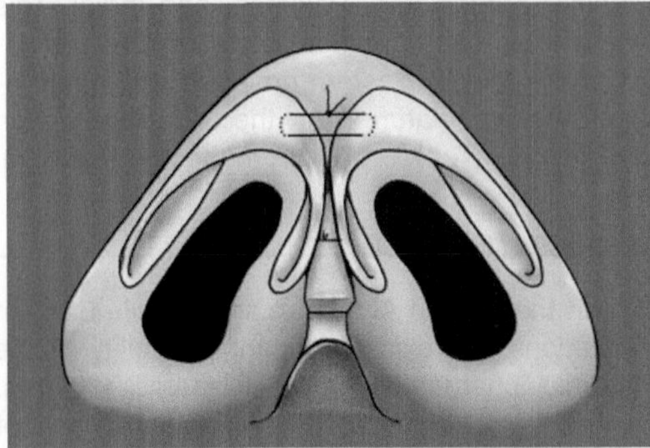

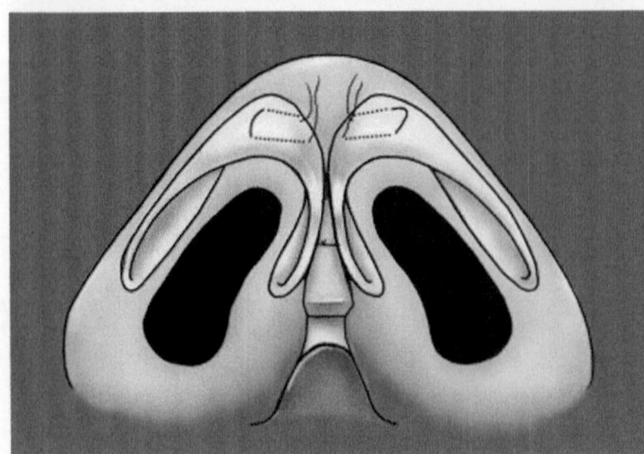

Fig. 5. Suture techniques for enhancing tip projection. (*Above*) Intercrural suture; (*center*) interdomal; (*below*) transdomal. (*Reproduced from* Rohrich RJ, Muzaffar AR. Rhinoplasty in the African American patient. Plast Reconstr Surg 2003;111(3):1322–39; with permission.)

1. Increasing tip projection
   a. Midcolumellar autogenous cartilage strut
   b. Suture plication of medial crura using interdomal and transdomal sutures (**Fig. 5**)
   c. Tip grafts: infratip lobular (Sheen), onlay (Peck), and combined infratip lobular/onlay (Gunter) (**Fig. 6**)
2. Increasing tip definition
   a. Transdomal suture techniques
   b. Multiple tip grafts, especially infratip lobular (Sheen) grafts
3. Dorsal augmentation
   a. Autologous tissue (septum or rib)
4. Graduated dorsal component reduction
5. Alar base surgery
   a. Correction of alar flaring with alar base resection
   b. Decreasing interalar distance by nostril sill excision and advancement.

By having a well-thought and organized approach to rhinoplasty, the surgeon is more likely to attain facial harmony and consistent aesthetic results. By using the following 6 principles,[27,28,32–36] the senior author can achieve consistent results in African American, Indian, Arabic, and Hispanic rhinoplasties:

1. External transcolumellar approach
2. Accurate intraoperative anatomic diagnosis
3. Meticulous hemostasis
4. Routine use of autogenous tissue or allografts for dorsum/tip augmentation
5. Minimum skin defatting
6. Meticulous wound closure.

The senior author has adopted an external approach to allow direct binocular vision for accurate anatomic diagnosis and optimal correction of the predetermined anatomic deformity.[44–46] His specific approach is described here in detail.[27,28,32,33]

After general anesthesia has been induced, the external nose and septum are injected using 10 mL of 0.5% lidocaine with 1:200,000 epinephrine, and the internal nose is packed bilaterally using 3.5-in neuropledgets moistened with oxymetazoline (Afrin; Schering-Plough Health Care Products Inc).

Bilateral infracartilagenous incisions along the caudal edge of the lower lateral cartilages are terminated medially at the narrowest portion of the columella. These incisions are connected using a transcolumellar stair-step incision.[47] This technique allows precise wound closure, and the underlying cartilages supply splinting to prevent scar contracture.

Before elevation of skin, methylene blue dots are placed along both sides of the incisions bilaterally to assist with more accurate wound closure. Next, the skin is elevated by dissecting the columellar skin away from the caudal edges of the medial crura. Dissection continues superiorly to the level of the infratip lobule, and then transitions laterally over the lateral crura and medially toward the soft triangle. The soft triangle is intentionally dissected last to avoid any damage to the genu of the lower lateral cartilage. Accurate anatomic dissection is maintained by hugging the perichondrium of the lower lateral

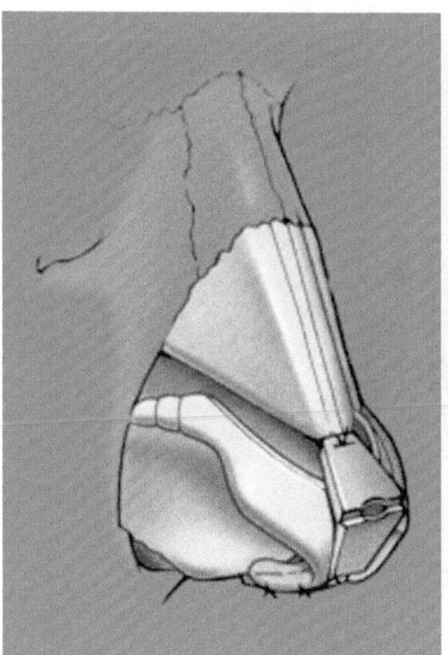
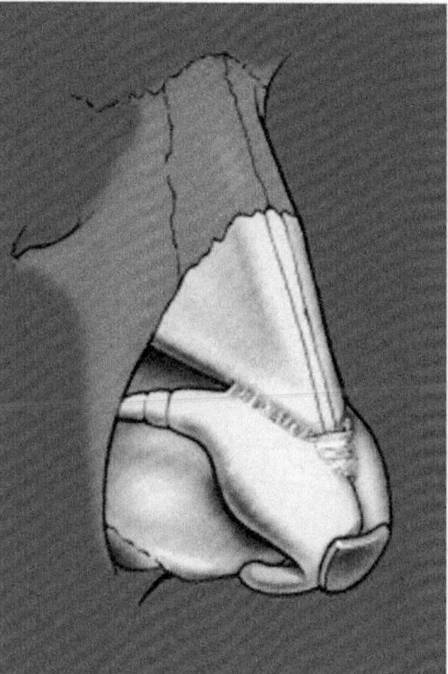
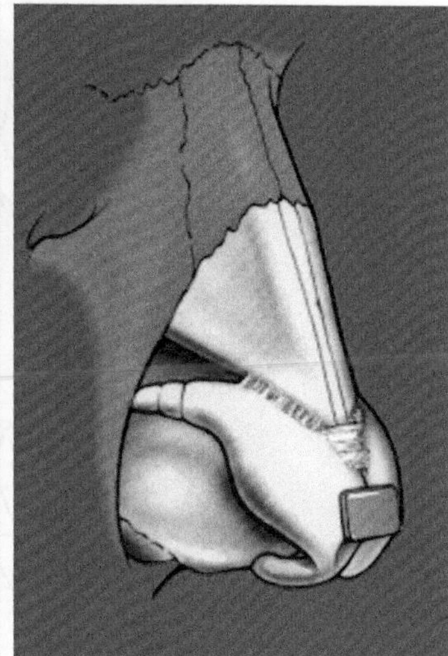

Fig. 6. Tip grafts useful in enhancing tip projection and definition. (*Left*) Combined infratip-onlay graft (Gunter type). (*Center*) Infratip lobular graft (Sheen type). (*Right*) Onlay graft (Peck type). (*Reproduced from* Rohrich RJ, Muzaffar AR. Rhinoplasty in the African American patient. Plast Reconstr Surg 2003;111(3):1322–39; with permission.)

cartilage. Loose fibrofatty tissue from the prominent supratip can be removed, but subdermal defatting is prohibited to avoid disrupting the blood supply and causing vascular embarrassment.[4,5,27,28]

The dissection continues over the upper lateral cartilages and the cartilaginous and bony dorsum up to the root of the nose. The soft tissues are then elevated from the nasal framework, and the tip cartilages are thoroughly evaluated. The nasal tip deformity and diminished tip projection are assessed, and the desired tip projection is determined; this will dictate the appropriate dorsal height.

Next, the dorsum is evaluated. Most African American rhinoplasty patients will require dorsal augmentation. First, any irregularities of the bony dorsum must be rasped to provide a smooth bed to place a dorsal graft. When augmentation is indicated, it must be performed after septal reconstruction or septal graft harvest, but before setting the final tip projection.[48]

On the contrary, most Middle Eastern or Arabic patients usually will require dorsal hump reduction. Using a graduated component dorsal hump reduction[49] is essential because excessive dorsal hump reduction can lead to significant racial incongruity. This reduction is performed by smoothing the bony dorsum with a rasp, followed by excision of the cartilaginous dorsum. Again, this must be performed before tip refinement.

If septal work is necessary for either straightening the septum or harvesting autologous cartilage grafts, the septum can be approached from

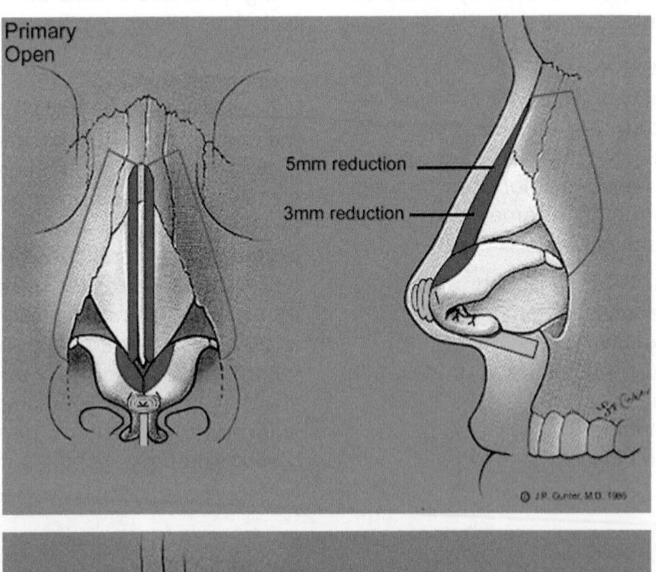

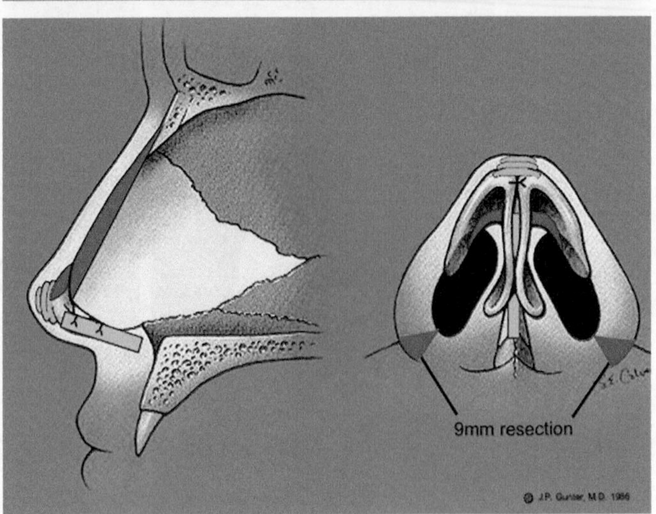

Fig. 7. Gunter graphics for case 1, a patient with primary nasal deformity with a high dorsal hump, wide bony base, and underprojecting, ill-defined tip. (Gunter diagrams, J.P. Gunter, MD) (*From* Gunter JP, Rohrich RJ, Adams Jr WP. Dallas rhinoplasty: nasal surgery by the masters. 2nd edition. St Louis (MO): Quality Medical Publishing Inc; 2007. p. 1128; with permission.)

the anterior septal angle through the open approach or through a separate transfixion incision. The authors' preference is to approach the septum using the open approach via the anterior septal angle. This method requires separating the medial crura to obtain adequate exposure. The septum is then separated from the upper lateral cartilages. If inferior turbinate hypertrophy is present, submucous resection of the anterior inferior turbinates is also performed at this time. If lateral osteotomies are required to properly align or narrow the nasal base, this should be done after septal cartilage harvest but before dorsal augmentation and final tip reconstruction.

To establish final tip projection or definition, a graduated approach is used.[50,51] First, a columellar strut is placed as the foundation for the desired tip. A long, Bowie knife-type strut in the columella increases the tip projection and augments the diminished columellar-labial angle. The columellar strut is secured in front of the nasal spine and between the feet of the medial crura using 5-0 clear polydioxanone sutures (PDS, Ethicon). This stage is followed by tip suturing techniques,[50–52] including interdomal and transdomal sutures. Excess fibrofatty tissue is excised over the dome area of the lower lateral cartilages, but again the subdermal plexus must be preserved to maintain adequate blood supply to the tip. Finally, tip cartilage grafts are placed, either an infratip graft (Sheen), an onlay graft (Peck), or combined grafts (Gunter). Additional double- and even triple-layer onlay grafts may be required to attain the desired tip projection.

Correction of alar-columellar disharmony[53] is critical, particularly in the Middle Eastern patient, and often presents as a "hanging columella" deformity.[32,33] Excess columellar show can be

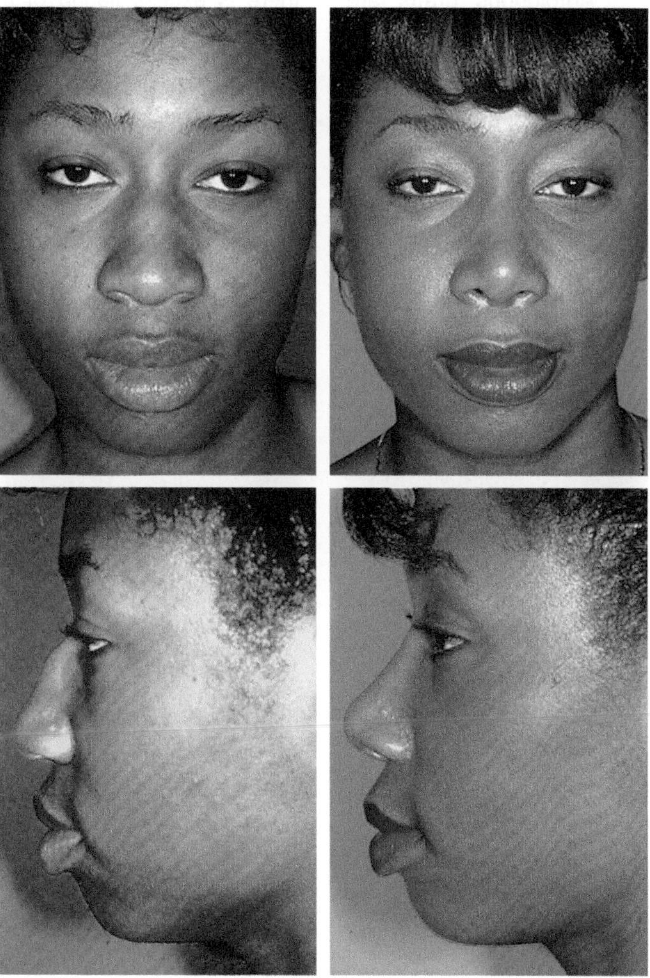

Fig. 8. Preoperative (*left*) and 2-year postoperative (*right*) frontal and side views of patient from case 1. (*From* Gunter JP, Rohrich RJ, Adams Jr WP. Dallas rhinoplasty: nasal surgery by the masters. 2nd edition. St Louis (MO): Quality Medical Publishing Inc; 2007. p. 1129; with permission.)

corrected using medial crural septal sutures, which will also assist in tip rotation.[50–52] Strict care must be taken to avoid overcorrection of the nasolabial angle, as there may be a tendency to overcorrect given the presence of severe caudal tip position preoperatively.

Another feature commonly seen in Arabic and some Hispanic patients is hypertrophy of the depressor septi nasi muscle.[32,33] This feature results in a hyperdynamic nasal tip that rotates caudally and deprojects, which can further exaggerate the dorsal deformity. Transection/transposition of the depressor septi nasi muscle[54] can increase the upper lip length and improve its aesthetic appearance by reducing the plunging nasal tip. Botulinum toxin type A injection preoperatively to the depressor septi nasi muscle is also being evaluated as an adjunctive treatment option.[55]

A graduated approach should be used for dorsal augmentation.[48] Autologous grafts are strongly preferred. If less than 4 mm of dorsal augmentation is required, the authors prefer to use septal cartilage or auricular cartilage dorsal onlay grafts. If more than 4 mm of dorsal augmentation is required, an anatomically contoured rib cartilage graft is preferred. In these cases, Alloderm (LifeCell Corp, Branchburg, NJ) or Enduragen (Porex Corp, Fairburn, GA) can be used for camouflage of the graft to soften the lateral edges, and it will absorb over approximately 1 year.

After final inspection of the augmented nasal framework, the skin is redraped and the external appearance evaluated. The nose is inspected on the frontal and basal view for correction of any alar rim abnormalities. Should an alar rim deformity be present on basal view, such as alar notching or alar rim collapse, a nonanatomic alar contour graft should be placed.[56–58] The skin is redraped, analysis of the nasal contour is again accessed, and all incisions closed. The infracartilagenous incisions are closed using 5-0 chromic gut, and the transcolumellar incision is closed using interrupted 6-0 nylon.

The nose is again inspected on the basal view for correction of any alar base abnormalities. If there is excess flaring of the alar rims (greater than 2 mm outside of the medial canthal lines), alar base resection is recommended.[59–61] This resection should be kept below the alar groove to avoid injury to the lateral nasal arteries. The lower incision is made 1 mm above the alar-cheek junction and curved medially into the nostril to

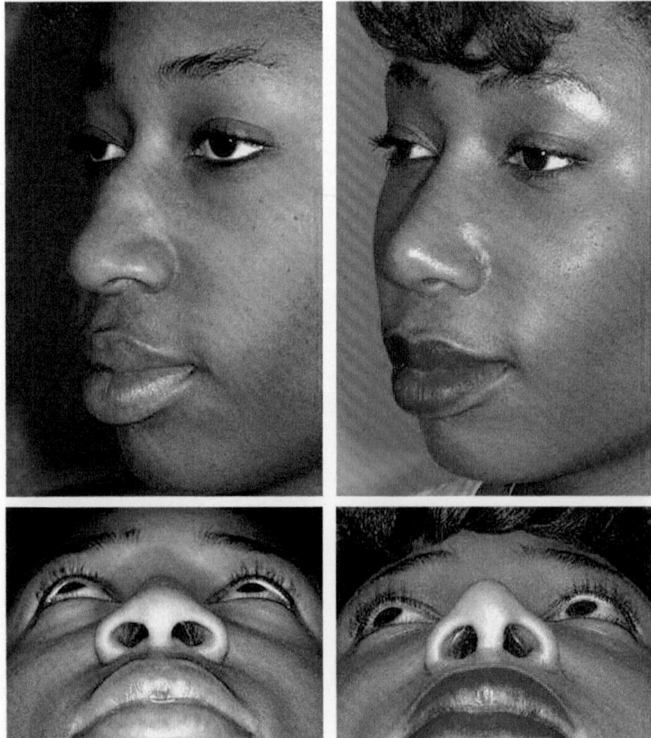

Fig. 9. Preoperative (*left*) and 2-year postoperative (*right*) oblique and submental views of patient from case 1. (*From* Gunter JP, Rohrich RJ, Adams Jr WP. Dallas rhinoplasty: nasal surgery by the masters. 2nd edition. St Louis (MO): Quality Medical Publishing Inc; 2007. p. 1129; with permission.)

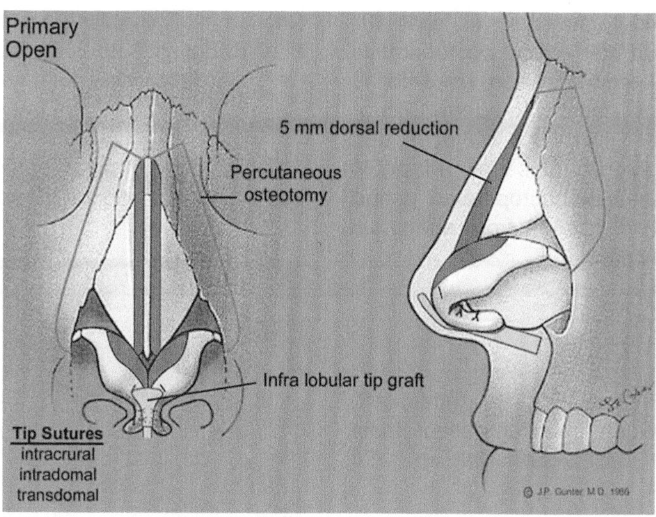

Fig. 10. Gunter graphic for the patient in case 2. (Gunter diagrams, J.P. Gunter, MD) (*From* Gunter JP, Rohrich RJ, Adams Jr WP. Dallas rhinoplasty: nasal surgery by the masters. 2nd edition. St Louis (MO): Quality Medical Publishing Inc; 2007. p. 1151; with permission.)

prevent alar notching. Once the required amount of tissue is resected from the alar base, the discrepancy between the upper and lower incisions is corrected by using buried 5-0 polyglactin 910 suture (Vicryl, Ethicon), followed by 6-0 nylon using the "halving" principle.[27,28]

If the abnormality is an increase in interalar distance, a nostril sill resection and advancement is performed.[59–63] These incisions are also closed using the "halving" principle, and all sutures are removed in 3 to 4 days.

Once the nose has been inspected from frontal, lateral, and basal views for symmetry, the nasal splints and dressings are applied. This application is particularly critical in the ethnic rhinoplasty patient as they tend to have prolonged postoperative edema. If septal work has been performed, bilateral septal splints are inserted and secured in place anteriorly using through-and-through 3-0 nylon sutures. An external dressing consisting of Steri-Strips (3M Corporation, St Paul, MN) and a conforming metal (Denver-type) splint is placed on the nasal dorsum for at least 1 week. Nasal packing is avoided. Postoperatively, patients are instructed to keep their eyes and nose covered with a chilled Swiss Therapy Eye Mask (Invotec,

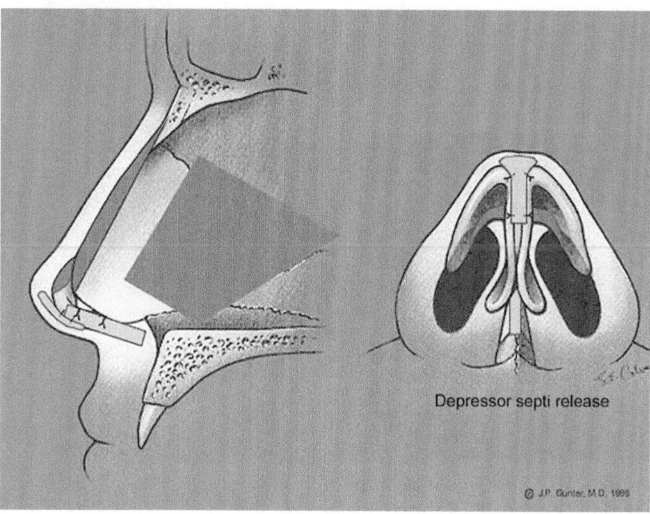

Fig. 11. Gunter graphic for the patient in case 2. (Gunter diagrams, J.P. Gunter, MD) (*From* Gunter JP, Rohrich RJ, Adams Jr WP. Dallas rhinoplasty: nasal surgery by the masters. 2nd edition. St Louis (MO): Quality Medical Publishing Inc; 2007. p. 1151; with permission.)

Jacksonville, FL), and to maintain at least 40° elevation of the head to reduce postoperative swelling. Silicone sheeting is also used for 3 months as tolerated to assist with edema. Perioperative antibiotics are given for 2 to 3 days, and methylprednisolone (Medrol Dosepak, Pfizer) is prescribed in the immediate postoperative period as well. Patients are to abstain from strenuous activity for at least 2 weeks.

CASE REPORTS

(*Reprinted from* Rohrich RJ, Muzaffar AR. Rhinoplasty in the African American patient. Plast Reconstr Surg;111(3):1322–39; Rohrich RJ, Ghavami A. Rhinoplasty for Middle Eastern noses. Plast Reconstr Surg 2009;123(4):1343–54).

Case 1

This healthy female patient presented with complaints of a dorsal hump and a wide, poorly

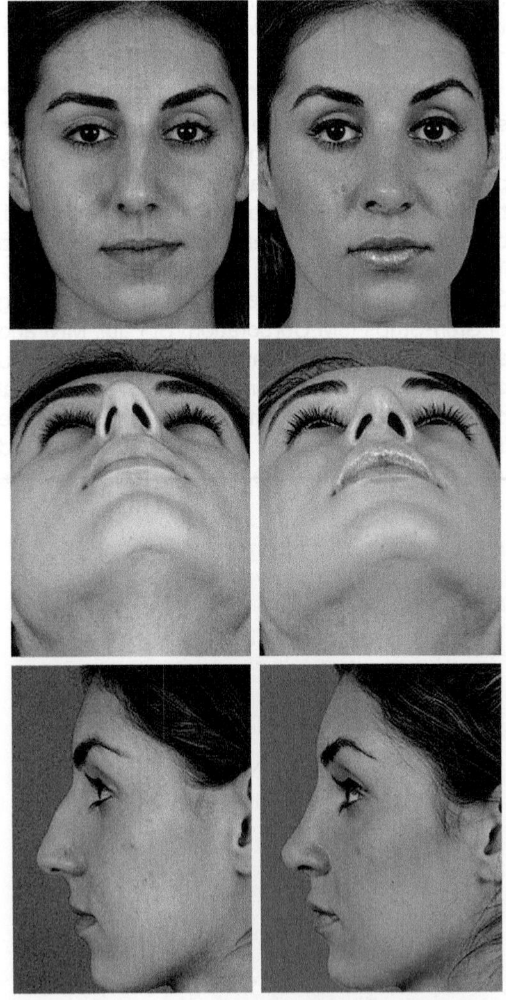

Fig. 12. Case 2. Preoperative (*left*) and 1-year postoperative (*right*) views. (*From* Gunter JP, Rohrich RJ, Adams Jr WP. Dallas rhinoplasty: nasal surgery by the masters. 2nd edition. St Louis (MO): Quality Medical Publishing Inc; 2007. p. 1152; with permission.)

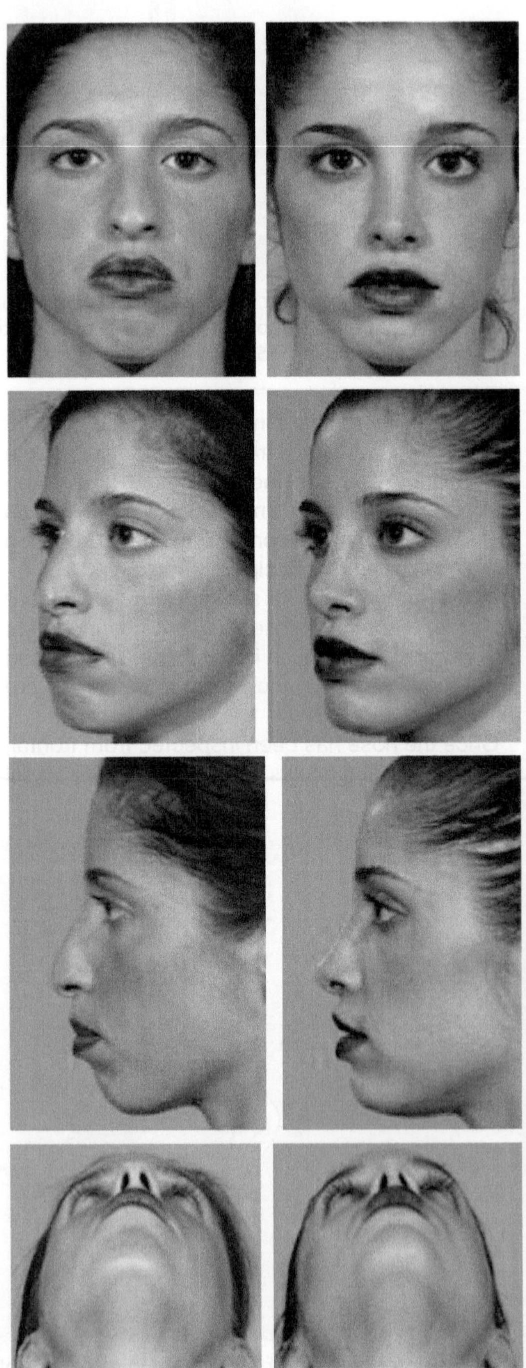

Fig. 13. Case 3. (*Left*) Preoperative and (*right*) postoperative views.

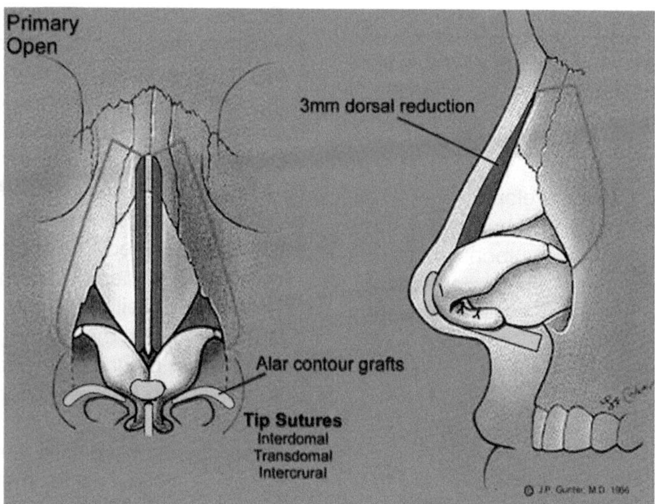

Fig. 14. Gunter graphic for the patient in case 3. (*Courtesy of* JP. Gunter, MD; with permission.)

defined nose. The frontal view demonstrated wide bony and alar bases with poor tip definition. On lateral view, the high dorsal hump was evident, in addition to the hanging ala/hidden columella. The basal view confirmed the alar flaring and bulbous appearance of the nasal tip, with columellar-lobular disproportion. Intranasal examination was normal.

Our operative goals were to: (1) reduce the dorsal hump, (2) narrow the bony pyramid, (3) correct the alar flaring, and (4) refine the nasal tip. The surgical plan (**Fig. 7**) was as follows:

1. Open approach with stair-step transcolumellar incision and bilateral infracartilaginous incisions
2. Component reduction of the dorsum
3. Cephalic resection of lower lateral cartilages
4. Columellar strut stabilized with intercrural sutures (5-0 polydioxanone suture)
5. Graduated tip suturing techniques using interdomal and transdomal sutures
6. Onlay tip graft ×3 suture stabilized to the tip with 5-0 polydioxanone suture
7. Lateral osteotomies (low to high)
8. Alar base resection (9 mm).

The preoperative analysis and diagnoses were confirmed intraoperatively with direct visualization of the nasal framework through and open approach. Comparison views of the preoperative and 2-year postoperative appearance demonstrate correction of these deformities (**Figs. 8** and **9**).

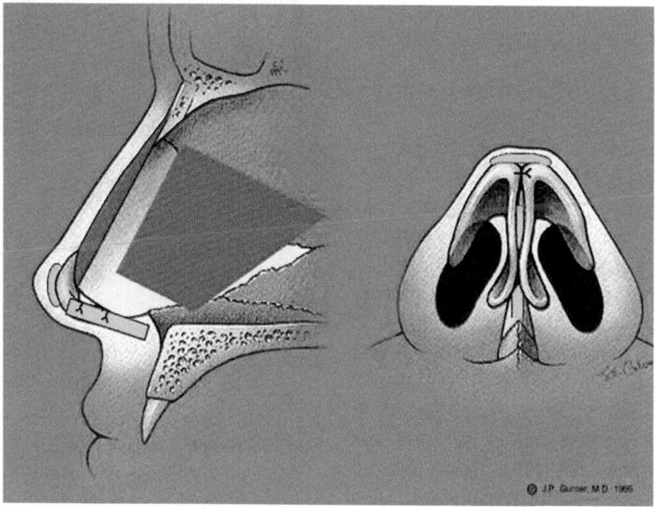

Fig. 15. Gunter graphic for the patient in case 3. (*Courtesy of* JP. Gunter, MD; with permission.)

Case 2

An 18-year-old woman with Fitzpatrick type III skin presented with complaints of nasal deviation, a dorsal hump, and a wide poorly defined nasal tip. Nasal analysis included the following:

- Moderately thick skin envelope
- Narrow midvault and dorsal hump (4–5 mm)
- An underprojected and bulbous nasal tip with minimally asymmetric alar cartilages
- Alar-columellar imbalance with retracted columella
- Septal deviation
- Nostril asymmetry
- Hyperactive depressor septi nasi muscle

The operative plan included the following **Figs. 10** and **11**:

- Open rhinoplasty approach by means of a transcollumellar incision with infracartilagenous extensions
- Septoplasty and cartilaginous graft harvesting
- 5-mm component dorsal reduction
- Cephalic trim leaving symmetric alar cartilages and a 6-mm rim strip
- A floating columellar strut graft
- Medial crural, interdomal, and transdomal sutures
- Depressor septi muscle release and transposition
- Infralobular graft
- Low-to-low percutaneous osteotomy

Twelve-month postoperative photographs are shown in **Fig. 12**.

Additional cases and the associated Gunter diagrams are displayed in **Figs. 13–18**.

POSTOPERATIVE COMPLICATIONS

Previous investigators have described unsatisfactory results following rhinoplasty,[64–66] and complications in the ethnic rhinoplasty patient are no different. However, there are several postoperative sequelae worth emphasizing as they are more notably in the ethnic rhinoplasty patient.

Protracted edema, sometimes up to 12 months, may persist in the ethnic rhinoplasty patient, mostly due to the thick sebaceous nature of the skin and the multiple incisions involved with the external approach.[27] Meticulous intraoperative hemostasis, prolonged postoperative splinting, perioperative steroids, and use of postoperative silicone gel sheeting or night-taping programs using elastic tape (Blenderm, 3M Corporation, St Paul, MN) can help to minimize prolonged lobule edema.[66]

Excess external scarring is of significant concern in the ethnic rhinoplasty patient, particular those with Fitzpatrick IV to VI skin types, as these patients have a greater propensity for keloid and hypertrophic scar formation. However, with meticulous wound closure and early suture removal at 7 to 10 days in the alar base resections and 6 to 7 days in the transcollumellar incision, the senior author has avoided this complication.[27]

Asymmetries, particularly in the alar base resections and nostril sill excisions, are another frequent complication. Asymmetry is usually due to poor preoperative planning and operative execution, but usually can be easily identified and corrected intraoperatively.[27]

Nasal tip necrosis is a dreaded complication, particularly when using the external approach and when extensive alar base resections are

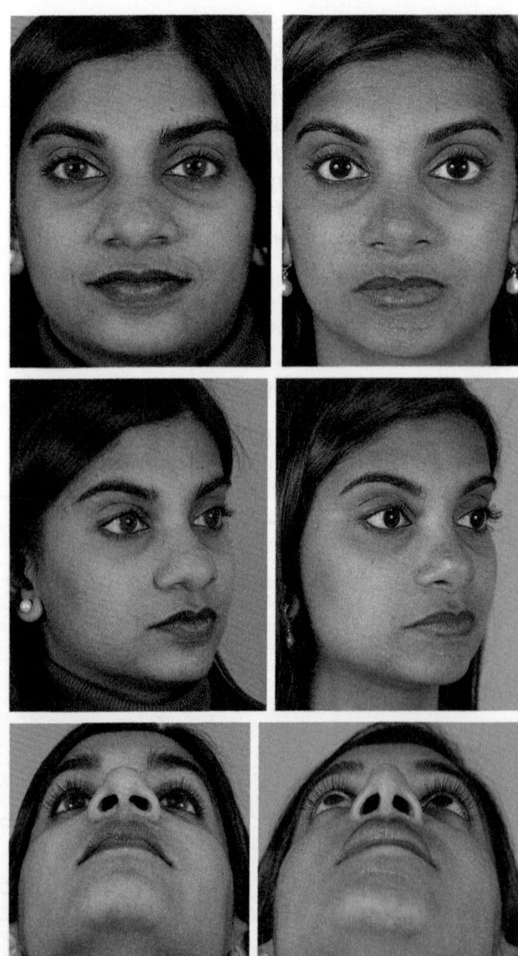

Fig. 16. Case 4. (*Left*) Preoperative and (*right*) postoperative views. (*From* Gunter JP, Rohrich RJ, Adams Jr WP. Dallas rhinoplasty: nasal surgery by the masters. 2nd edition. St Louis (MO): Quality Medical Publishing Inc; 2007. p. 1158–9; with permission.)

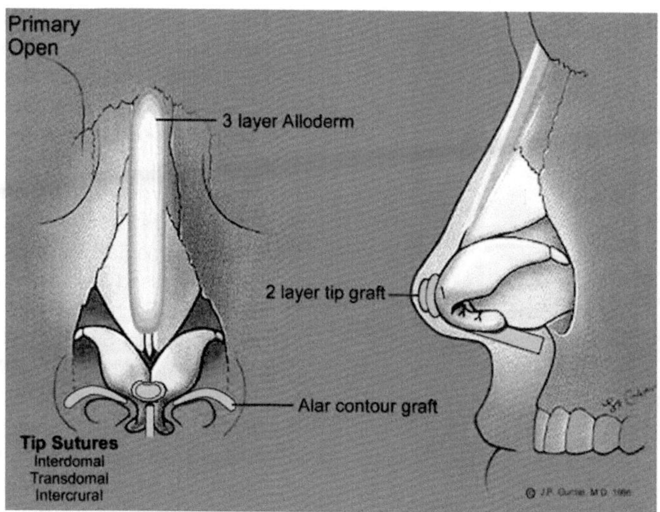

Fig. 17. Gunter graphic for the patient in case 4. (*Courtesy of* JP. Gunter, MD; with permission.)

required. As mentioned previously, alar base resections must not violate the alar groove to maintain adequate blood supply to the nasal tip.[67] In addition, onlay tip grafting can contribute to excessive skin tension at the nasal tip causing tip ischemia or dehiscence of the transcollumellar incision.[27]

Perhaps the most menacing complication in ethnic rhinoplasty is racial incongruity (**Fig. 19**). Incongruity is typically caused by nasal infracture accompanied by excessive alar base or nostril sill resection, resulting in a disproportionate narrowing of the dorsum with respect to the lobule. To avoid this ominous complication, the following 3 methods should be employed[27]:

1. Adjustment of the infracture proportionate to the lobule size or avoidance of nasal pyramid infracture in the majority of ethnic noses.
2. Performance of alar base or interalar sill reductions at the end of the operative procedure or as a subsequent stage if the surgeon is in doubt of the necessity for this procedure.
3. Simultaneous use of columellar strut and cartilaginous tip graft to increase the tip height and definition and lessen the emphasis of the alar width and flaring.

Employing these techniques as well as respecting the unique ethnic characteristics in each patient will avoid racial incongruity and the associated postoperative problems.

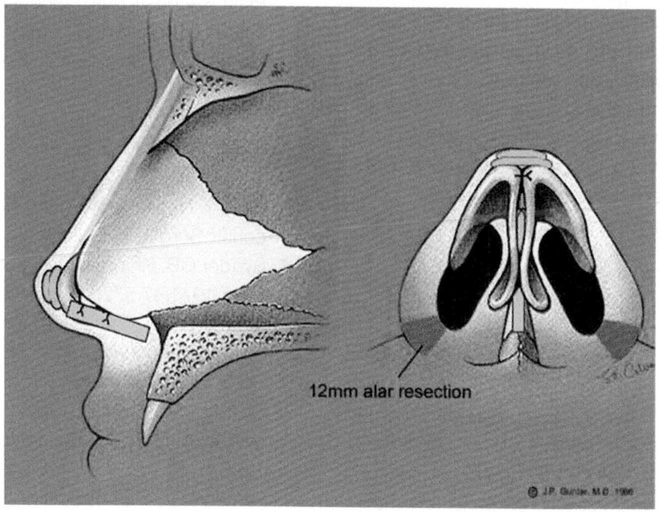

Fig. 18. Gunter graphic for the patient in case 4. (*Courtesy of* JP. Gunter, MD; with permission.)

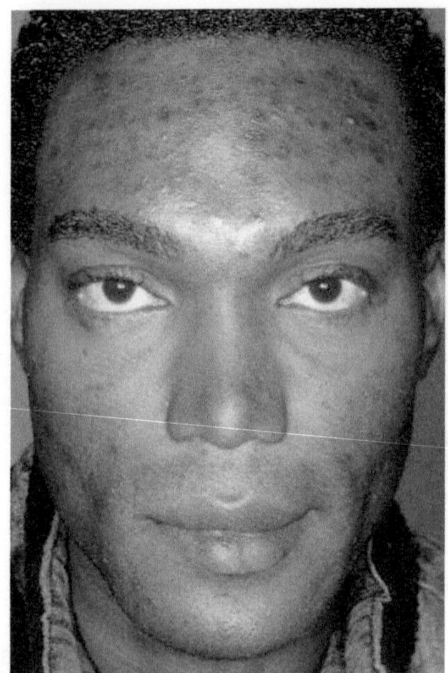

Fig. 19. Example of racial incongruity.

SUMMARY

Although successfully performing rhinoplasty in the ethnic patient can be challenging, the astute rhinoplasty surgeon can achieve consistent aesthetic results by following a few key principles. First, the surgeon must perform a complete preoperative nasal-facial analysis. Based on this analysis, the surgeon can determine the appropriate ethnic refinement and develop an individualized approach for each patient. Next, the authors recommend using an open approach to fully appreciate the anatomy, evaluate the deformity, and perform the appropriate augmentation. The use of autogenous grafts is preferred, and produces more consistent and predictable results. Lastly, the surgeon should incorporate nasal tip/dorsum augmentation, as well as alar base surgery. Understanding the unique anatomic characteristics found in various races and ethnicities, and using these key technical principles should produce a consistent, racially congruent, and aesthetically pleasing result in the ethnic rhinoplasty patient.

REFERENCES

1. United States. National population projections by age, sex, race, and Hispanic origin: 2008 to 2050, U.S. census bureau. Available at: http://www.census.gov/population/www/projections/2008projections.html. 2008. Accessed December 14, 2008.
2. National Clearinghouse of Plastic Surgery Statistics. Report of the 2007 statistics, American Society of Plastic Surgeons. Available at: http://www.plasticsurgery.org/Media/Statistics/2007_Statistics.html 2008. Accessed December 14, 2008.
3. American Academy of Facial Plastics and Reconstructive Surgery 2007 membership survey: trends in facial plastic surgery. Available at: http://www.aafprs.org/media/stats_polls/aafprsMedia2008.pdf. 2008. Accessed December 14, 2008.
4. Ofodile FA, Bokhari F, Ellis C. The African-American nose. Ann Plast Surg 1993;31:209.
5. Ofodile FA, Bokhari F. The African-American nose. Part II. Ann Plast Surg 1995;34:123.
6. Ofodile FA. Nasal bones and pyriform apertures in African-Americans. Ann Plast Surg 1994;32:21.
7. Ofodile FA, James EA. Anatomy of alar cartilages in African-Americans. Plast Reconstr Surg 1997;100:699.
8. Daniel RK. Hispanic rhinoplasty in the United States, with emphasis on the Mexican-American nose. Plast Reconstr Surg 2003;112:244.
9. Daniel RK. The Hispanic-American nose. In: Rohrich RJ, Gunter JP, Adams WB, editors. Dallas rhinoplasty: nasal surgery by the masters. 2nd edition. St Louis (MO): Quality Medical Publishing; 2007. p. 1197–220.
10. Bernstein L. Esthetics in rhinoplasty. Otolaryngol Clin North Am 1975;9:705.
11. Converse JM. Corrective rhinoplasty. In: Converse JM, editor. Reconstructive surgery. 2nd edition. Philadelphia: WB Saunders; 1977. p. 1040.
12. Sheen JH, Sheen AP. Aesthetic rhinoplasty. 2nd edition. St. Louis (MO): Quality Medical Publishing; 1998.
13. Gunter JP. Facial analysis for the rhinoplasty patient. Dallas Rhinoplasty Symp 1997;14:45.
14. Millard DR. Adjuncts in mentoplasty and rhinoplasty. Plast Reconstr Surg 1965;36:48.
15. Falces E, Wesser D, Gorney M. Cosmetic surgery of the non-Caucasian nose. Plast Reconstr Surg 1970;45:317.
16. Avelar JM. Personal contribution to the surgical treatment of Negroid noses. Aesthetic Plast Surg 1976;1:81.
17. Rees T. Nasal plastic surgery in the Negro. Plast Reconstr Surg 1969;43:13.
18. Synder GB. Rhinoplasty in the Negro. Plast Reconstr Surg 1971;47:572.
19. Matory WE Jr, Falces R. Non-Caucasian rhinoplasty: a 16-year experience. Plast Reconstr Surg 1986;2:239.
20. Rohrich RJ, Kenkel JM. The definition of beauty. In: Matroy WE Jr, editor. Ethnic considerations in facial aesthetic surgery. Philadelphia: Lippincott-Raven; 1998.
21. Farkas LG. Anthropometry of the head and face in medicine. New York: Elsevier; 1981.

22. Patterson CN, Powell DG. Facial analysis in patient evaluation for physiologic and cosmetic surgery. Laryngoscope 2004;84:1974.
23. Rogers BO. The role of physical anthropology in plastic surgery today. Clin Plast Surg 1974;1:439.
24. Byrd HS, Hobar PC. Rhinoplasty: a practical guide for surgical planning. Plast Reconstr Surg 1993;91:642.
25. Porter JP, Olson KL. Analysis of the African American female nose. Plast Reconstr Surg 2003;111:620.
26. Milgram LM, Lawson W, Cohen AF. Anthropometric analysis of the female Latino nose. Arch Otolaryngol Head Neck Surg 2003;122:244.
27. Rohrich RJ, Muzaffar AR. Rhinoplasty in the African-American patient. Plast Reconstr Surg 2003;111: 1322.
28. Rohrich RJ. Rhinoplasty in the black patient. In: Daniel RK, editor. Aesthetic plastic surgery. 2nd edition. Boston: Little Brown; 1993. p. 659–76.
29. Olson S. Mapping human history: genes, race, and our common origins. New York (NY): Houghton Miffin Company; 2003.
30. Kontis TC, Papel ID. Rhinoplasty in the African-American nose. Aesthetic Plast Surg 2002;26(Suppl 1):S12.
31. Rohrich RJ, Friedman RM. Black male. In: Marchac D, Granick MS, Solomon MP, editors. Male aesthetic surgery. Boston: Butterworth-Heinemann; 1996. p. 418.
32. Rohrich RJ, Ghavami A. The Middle Eastern nose. In: Rohrich RJ, Gunter JP, Adams WB, editors. Dallas rhinoplasty: nasal surgery by the masters. 2nd edition. St Louis (MO): Quality Medical Publishing; 2007. p. 1139–66.
33. Rohrich RJ, Ghavami A. The Middle Eastern nose. Plast Reconstr Surg 2009;123:4.
34. Bizrah MB. Rhinoplasty for Middle Eastern patients. Facial Plast Surg Clin North Am 2002;10:381.
35. Beheri GE. Rhinoplasty in Egyptians. Aesthetic Plast Surg 1984;8:145.
36. Guyuron B. The Middle Eastern nose. In: Matory WE Jr, editor. Ethnic considerations in facial aesthetic surgery. Philadelphia: Lippincott-Raven; 1998. p. 412.
37. Gonzales-Ulloa M. The fat nose. Aesthetic Plast Surg 1984;8:135.
38. Ortiz-Monasterio F, Olmedo A. Rhinoplasty on the mestizo nose. Clin Plast Surg 1977;4:89.
39. Ortiz-Monasterio F, Olmedo A, Ortiz Oscoy L. The use of cartilage grafts in primary aesthetic rhinoplasty. Plast Reconstr Surg 1981;67:597.
40. Ortiz-Monasterio F, Olmedo A. Rhinoplasty in the mestizo nose. Secondary rhinoplasty in the thick skinned nose. In: Rees TD, Baker DC, Tabbal N, editors. Rhinoplasty: problems and controversies. St. Louis (MO): CV Mosby; 1988. p. 372–83.
41. Ortiz-Monasterio F. Rhinoplasty in the non-Caucasian nose. In: Gruber RP, Peck GC, editors. Rhinoplasty: state of the art. St. Louis (MO): Mosby-Year Book; 1993. p. 391.
42. Ortiz-Monasterio F. Rhinoplasty. Philadelphia: WB Saunders; 1994.
43. Sanchez AE. Rhinoplasty in the "Chata" nose of the Caribbean. Aesthetic Plast Surg 1980;4:169.
44. Toriumi DM, Johnson CM. Open structure rhinoplasty: featured technical points and long-term follow-up. Facial Plast Clin 1993;1:1.
45. Flowers RS. The surgical correction of the non-Caucasian nose. Clin Plast Surg 1977;4:89.
46. Adams WP Jr, Rohrich RJ, Hollier LH, et al. Anatomic basis and clinical implications for nasal tip support in open versus closed rhinoplasty. Plast Reconstr Surg 1999;103:255.
47. Foda HM. External rhinoplasty for the Arabian nose: a columellar scar analysis. Aesthetic Plast Surg 2004;28:312.
48. Gunter JP, Rohrich RJ. Augmentation rhinoplasty: dorsal onlay grafting using shaped autogenous septal cartilage. Plast Reconstr Surg 1990;86:39.
49. Rohrich RJ, Muzaffar AR, Janis JE. Component dorsal hump reduction: the importance of maintaining dorsal aesthetic lines in rhinoplasty. Plast Reconstr Surg 2004;114:1298.
50. Rohrich RJ. Graduated approach to tip projection in rhinoplasty. Dallas Rhinoplasty Symp 1997;14:129.
51. Ghavami A, Janis JE, Acikel C, et al. Tip shaping in primary rhinoplasty: algorithmic approach. Plast Reconstr Surg 2008;122:1229.
52. Daniel RK. Open tip suture techniques. Part I: primary rhinoplasty. Plast Reconstr Surg 1999;103:1491.
53. Gunter JP, Rohrich RJ, Friedman RM. Classification and correction of alar-columellar discrepancies in rhinoplasty. Plast Reconstr Surg 1996; 97:643.
54. Rohrich RJ, Huynh B, Muzaffar AE, et al. Importance of the depressor septi nasi muscle in rhinoplasty: anatomic study and clinical application. Plast Reconstr Surg 2000;105:376.
55. Ghavami A, Janie JE, Guyuron B. Regarding the treatment of dynamic tip ptosis using botulinum toxin A. Plast Reconstr Surg 2006;118:L263.
56. Gunter JP, Friedman RM. Lateral crural strut graft: technique and clinical applications in rhinoplasty. Plast Reconstr Surg 1997;99:943.
57. Rohrich RJ, Raniere J Jr, Ha RY. The alar contour graft: correction and prevention of alar rim deformities. Plast Reconstr Surg 2002;109:2495–505.
58. Guyuron B. Alar rim deformities. Plast Reconstr Surg 2001;107:856 46.
59. Millard DR. External excisions in rhinoplasty. Plast Reconstr Surg 1965;36:48.
60. Millard DR. Alar margin sculpturing. Plast Reconstr Surg 1967;40:337.
61. Ship AG. Alar base resection for IVSP flaring nostrils. Br J Plast Surg 1975;28:77.
62. Daniel RK. Rhinoplasty: large nostril/small tip disproportion. Plast Reconstr Surg 2001;107:1874.

63. Guyuron B, Ghavami A, Wishnek SM. Components of the short nostril. Plast Reconstr Surg 2005;116:1517.
64. Davis PK, Jones SM. The complications of silastic implants: experience with 137 consecutive cases. Br J Plast Surg 1971;24:405.
65. Klabunde EH, Falces E. Incidence of complications in cosmetic rhinoplasties. Plast Reconstr Surg 2001; 107:561.
66. Gryskiewicz JM. Principles of postop care in rhinoplasty. In: Proceedings of 18th Annual Dallas Rhinoplasty Symposium. Dallas, Texas; 2001.
67. Rohrich RJ, Gunter JP, Friedman RM. Nasal tip blood supply: an anatomic study validating the safety of the transcolumellar incision in rhinoplasty. Plast Reconstr Surg 1995;95:795.

Secondary Rhinoplasty and the Use of Autogenous Rib Cartilage Grafts

C. Spencer Cochran, MD[a,b,*], Jack P. Gunter, MD[a,c]

KEYWORDS

• Rhinoplasty • Revision rhinoplasty • Secondary rhinoplasty
• Rib cartilage graft • Costal cartilage

Rhinoplasty is generally considered to be one of the most difficult procedures in cosmetic surgery, and the incidence of postoperative nasal deformities that require secondary rhinoplasty varies from 5% to 12%.[1] Deformities arising from an earlier rhinoplasty can range in severity from mild asymmetry of the nasal tip or dorsum to severe distortion and collapse of the osseocartilaginous framework. Regardless of the severity, the causes of postoperative rhinoplasty deformities are most frequently related to: (1) displacement or distortion of anatomic structures, (2) inadequate surgery resulting in under-resection of the nasal framework, or (3) over-resection caused by overzealous surgery.

Success in secondary rhinoplasty, therefore, relies on an accurate clinical diagnosis and analysis of the nasal deformities, a thorough operative plan to address each abnormality, and a meticulous surgical technique. Reconstruction of the osseocartilaginous framework is the foundation for obtaining consistent aesthetic and functional results in secondary rhinoplasty. Septal cartilage is generally considered to be the preferred grafting material for most applications in rhinoplasty, but secondary rhinoplasty frequently necessitates alternative sources of grafting material when there are severe structural deformities of the nasal framework or when insufficient amounts of septal cartilage are available.[2,3] In some cases, auricular cartilage may be suitable; however, rib cartilage provides the most abundant source of grafts and has proved to be the most reliable in the authors' hands when addressing major secondary deformities.

Although adequate results may be obtained with the endonasal technique in certain circumstances, the limited dissection and exposure offered by the endonasal approach often does not permit accurate assessment, intraoperative diagnosis, and appropriate treatment of complex anatomic problems. The authors, therefore, prefer addressing most secondary rhinoplasty deformities by the external approach to help ensure consistent aesthetic and functional results.

CLINICAL ANALYSIS AND OPERATIVE PLANNING

A thorough nasal analysis and precise anatomic diagnosis of each deformity (**Table 1**) is a key step for achieving optimal results in secondary rhinoplasty. Preoperative evaluation begins by defining the deformity, which is accomplished by a detailed history, physical examination, and complete aesthetic, facial, and nasal analysis. The nose should be examined and analyzed from top to bottom. Starting superiorly, the height, the

[a] Department of Otolaryngology-Head and Neck Surgery, University of Texas Southwestern Medical Center at Dallas, 5323 Harry Hines Boulevard, Dallas, TX 75390, USA
[b] Gunter Center for Aesthetics and Cosmetic Surgery, 8144 Walnut Hill Lane, Suite 170, Dallas, TX 75231, USA
[c] Department of Plastic Surgery, University of Texas Southwestern Medical Center at Dallas, Dallas, TX, USA
* Corresponding author. Gunter Center for Aesthetics and Cosmetic Surgery, 8144 Walnut Hill Lane, Suite 170, Dallas, TX 75231.
E-mail address: drcochran@gunter-center.com (C.S. Cochran).

Clin Plastic Surg 37 (2010) 371–382
doi:10.1016/j.cps.2009.11.001

Table 1
Common postoperative rhinoplasty deformities

Dorsum	Tip
Over-resection	Asymmetry
Dorsal irregularity	Alar collapse
"Polly-beak" deformity	Alar retraction
"Inverted-V" deformity	Hanging columella
Saddle deformity	Retracted columellar-labial angle
	Over-rotation of tip

width, and the symmetry of the dorsum should be noted. The nasofrontal angle normally begins at the supratarsal crease and may be noted to be lower in patients with an over-resected dorsum. The contour of the dorsum should be assessed and any irregularity should be noted. The width of the bony pyramid and upper lateral cartilages should be inspected for asymmetry, collapse, and for the presence of an "inverted-V" deformity. The supratip area is evaluated for the presence of a "polly-beak" deformity or absence of an appropriate supratip break. The nasal tip is evaluated in terms of its projection and its rotation. The lower lateral cartilages are assessed for their symmetry, width, position, and symmetry of the tip-defining points. The alar rims are inspected for collapse or retraction. The columella is examined for increased or decreased show. The columellar-lobular and columellar-labial angles are evaluated to ascertain the desired angulation. The internal nasal examination evaluates patency of the nasal valves, position and integrity of the septum, and state of the turbinates.

Another important aspect of the preoperative evaluation is the assessment of the patient's psychological status and stability. It has been estimated that 5% of patients seeking cosmetic surgery have body dysmorphic disorder, which is a preoccupation with a slight or imagined defect with some aspect of their physical appearance that leads to significant disruption of daily functions.[4] It is important to distinguish patients with a legitimate cosmetic or functional concern from patients who are hyperconcerned about minor imperfections of their nose.

After the patient has been deemed a good psychological candidate and the deformities defined, the goals of the surgery should be established and an operative plan formulated to address each abnormality. The operative goals are individualized for each patient according to the deformity. The goals may be to augment the dorsum, to straighten a dorsally deviated septum, to lower the supratip area, to correct tip asymmetry and alar collapse, to decrease columellar show, and so forth. If the existing osseocartilaginous framework is under-resected, the amount and location of further reduction are determined. If the nasal framework has been over-resected, the missing tissues and the need for augmentation are determined. Secondary surgery is usually deferred until 12 months after the previous rhinoplasty.

ASSESSMENT OF GRAFTING REQUIREMENTS

A key component of operative planning in secondary rhinoplasty includes assessment of the grafting requirements and determination of the potential source of grafting materials that will be required. Secondary rhinoplasty often necessitates significant numbers of grafts, such as spreader graft, lateral crural strut grafts, and dorsal onlay grafts when structural deformities result from previous procedures.[2] The authors prefer autogenous cartilage for any nasal framework replacement. Successful use of irradiated homologous rib cartilage has been reported in the past,[5] but problems with infection, absorption, and warping have limited its routine use in secondary rhinoplasty (Dingman RO, personal communication, 1980).

Septal cartilage is generally the preferred grafting material in primary and secondary rhinoplasty. The integrity of the nasal septum, and thus its availability for use as cartilage grafts, can be assessed during the office consultation and examination by gently palpating the septum with a cotton tip applicator. There are several advantages to using septal cartilage. A large amount of septal cartilage and septal bone can be harvested from the same operative field without the morbidity of an additional donor site. Compared with auricular cartilage, septal cartilage is more rigid, provides better support, and does not have convolutions. Septal cartilage is preferably used as a columellar strut, spreader grafts between the upper lateral cartilages and the septum, and lateral crural strut grafts to support or replace parts of the lower lateral cartilage complexes. When a sufficient quantity is available, it may also be used as a dorsal onlay graft for minimal amounts of dorsal augmentation.

Severe deformities or a paucity of available septal cartilage requires an alternative source of grafting material. The auricle can provide a modest amount of cartilage for nasal reconstruction.[6] Using a postauricular approach, the amount of harvested conchal cartilage can be maximized without compromising ear protrusion by preserving sufficient cartilage in 3 key areas: (1) the inferior crus of the antihelix, (2) the root of the helix, and (3) the area where the concha cavum transitions into the posterior-inferior margin of the external auditory canal. A vertical incision is created on the posterior aspect of the auricle, and dissection is carried down through the perichondrium. A 27-gauge needle dipped in methylene blue is percutaneously placed every half centimeter along the inner aspect of the antihelical fold to tattoo the cartilage along the planned excision path to maximize the amount of harvested cartilage while ensuring that sufficient antihelical contour is maintained. Dissection proceeds along the anterior and the posterior surface of the conchal bowl, and a kidney-bean shaped piece of conchal cartilage is harvested while leaving sufficient cartilage at the aforementioned key areas for support.

Because of its flaccidity and convolutions, auricular cartilage is best used when these characteristics are desired. Auricular cartilage is usually used for reconstructing the lower lateral cartilage complex, for small onlay grafts, or for placement in the columella to provide tip support. However, it is a second choice to septal cartilage because of the inherent difficulty in obtaining and maintaining the desired shape and contour. While initial results of dorsal augmentation with auricular cartilage are often satisfactory, surface irregularities can become apparent with the passage of time. Furthermore, the irregular contour and the limited supply of auricular cartilage often preclude its use.

Autogenous rib cartilage provides the most abundant source of cartilage for graft fabrication and is the most reliable when structural support or augmentation is needed, and therefore has been the authors' graft material of choice for secondary rhinoplasty when sufficient septal cartilage is not available.[2,7]

Various types of alloplastic materials have been used in rhinoplasty, including: (1) solid silicone, (2) high-density porous polyethylene (Medpor, Porex Surgical Inc, College Park, GA, USA), and (3) expanded polytetrafluoroethylene (Gore-Tex, W.L. Gore Associates, Flagstaff, AZ, USA). Alloplastic materials have the advantages of being easy to use, readily available, and having an unlimited supply. Unfortunately, because of their permanent nature, many of these alloplastic materials are fraught with long-term complications, such as infection, migration, extrusion, and palpability.[8–11] Thus, autogenous tissue continues to be the authors' preferred source of grafts.

HARVESTING RIB CARTILAGE

Rib cartilage is a versatile grafting material in secondary rhinoplasty. The grafting requirements and planned uses dictate the choice of the rib to be harvested. It is often possible to construct all required grafts from a single rib, and the surgeon should choose the cartilaginous portion of a rib that provides a straight segment. The authors prefer to harvest cartilage from the fifth, sixth, or seventh rib, depending on the rib that is the longest and straightest. If additional grafts are needed, a part or the entire cartilaginous portion of an adjacent rib may be harvested.

The rib cartilage graft may be harvested from either the patient's left or right side; however, harvesting from the patient's left side facilitates a 2-team approach. In female patients, the incision is marked several millimeters superior to the inframammary fold and measures 5 cm in length (**Fig. 1**). In males, the incision is usually placed directly over the chosen rib to facilitate the dissection.

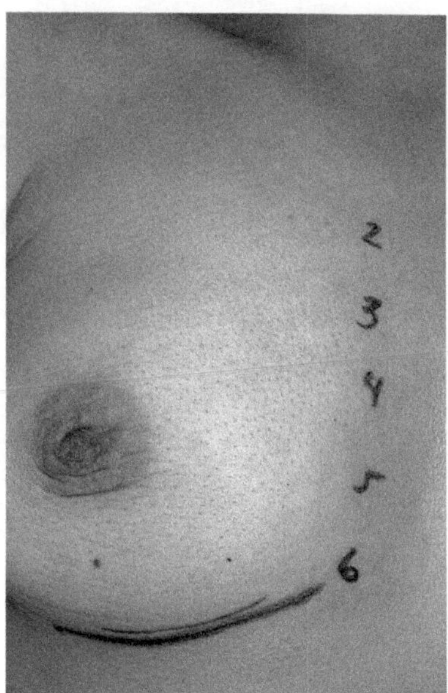

Fig. 1. Rib cartilage harvest incision (*thin line*) placed slightly superior to inframammary fold (*thick line*).

To decrease the chances of postoperative wound infections, the chest is prepared and draped separately from the nose, and separate surgical instruments are used to prevent cross-contamination. A 5-cm skin incision is created along the inframammary fold with a 15-blade scalpel, and the subcutaneous tissue is divided with electrocautery. Once the muscle fascia is reached, the surgeon palpates the underlying ribs and divides the muscle and fascia with electrocautery directly over the chosen rib. The dissection should be carried medially until the junction of the rib cartilage and sternum can be palpated. Identification of the lateral extent of dissection is facilitated by the subtle change in color of the rib at the bony-cartilaginous junction; the cartilaginous portion is generally off-white in color, whereas the bone demonstrates a distinct reddish-gray hue.

After the selected rib is exposed, the perichondrium is incised along the long axis of the rib. A Dingman elevator is used to elevate the perichondrium superiorly and inferiorly from the cartilaginous rib (**Fig. 2**). Perpendicular cuts are also made in the perichondrium at the most medial and lateral aspects of the longitudinal incision to facilitate reflection of the perichondrium. If needed, a 1.5-cm by 5-cm strip of perichondrium can be harvested from the anterior surface of an adjacent rib for use as a camouflaging graft .

The subperichondrial dissection continues circumferentially as far posteriorly as possible. A curved rib stripper is then used to complete the posterior dissection (see **Fig. 3**). It is important to ensure that the rib stripper remains between the rib and perichondrium to decrease the chances of causing a pneumothorax, and the rib stripper is slid medially and laterally along the rib until the undermining is complete.

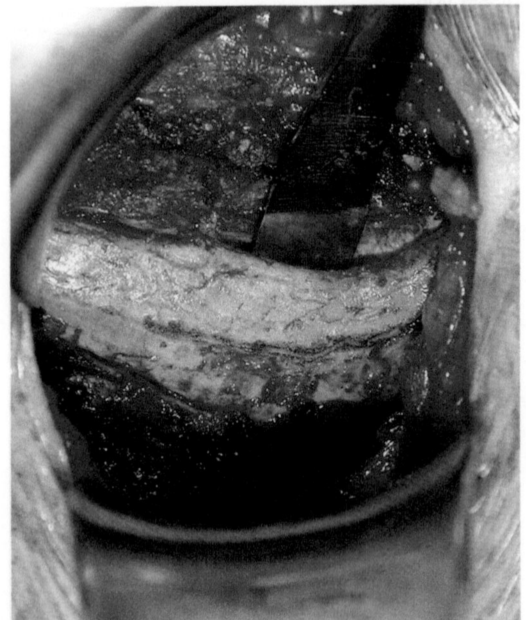

Fig. 2. Perichondrium is elevated superiorly and inferiorly from the cartilaginous rib.

The cartilaginous rib is cut medially near its attachment to the sternum and laterally where it meets the bony rib by making a partial thickness incision perpendicular to the long axis of the rib using a number 15 blade at the aforementioned junctions. The cartilaginous incision can then be completed with a Freer elevator using a gentle side-to-side movement. Once the cartilage segment is released medially and laterally, the graft is easily removed from the wound and placed in sterile saline until the surgeon is ready to fabricate the grafts. If more grafting material is required, a portion of an adjacent rib or an entire rib can then be harvested in a similar fashion.

After the rib cartilage has been harvested, the donor site is checked to ensure that no pneumothorax has occurred. This is accomplished by filling the bed of the wound with saline solution while the anesthesiologist applies positive pressure into the lungs. If no air leak is detected, a pneumothorax can be excluded. The wound is then closed in layers using 2-0 Vicryl sutures. Particular attention should be directed at reapproximating the perichondrium and then the muscle fascia layers tightly to prevent a palpable or visible chest wall deformity. This tight closure also helps "splint" the wound and reduces postoperative pain. Skin closure is performed using deep dermal and subcuticular 4-0 Monocryl sutures.

If a pneumothorax has been diagnosed, it usually represents an injury only to the parietal pleura and not to the lung parenchyma itself.

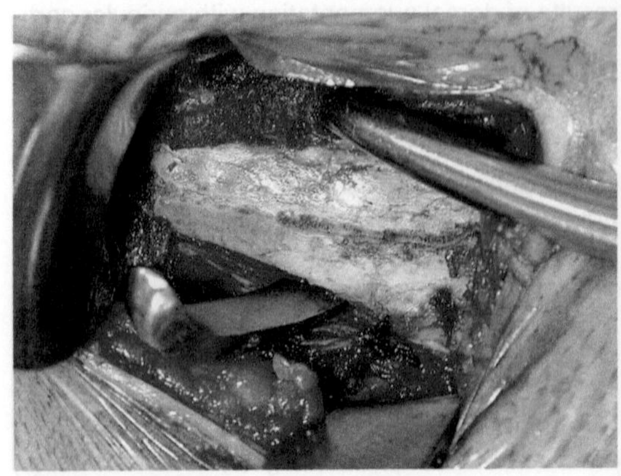

Fig. 3. A curved rib stripper is used to complete the posterior dissection.

This does not mandate chest tube placement. A red rubber catheter can be inserted through the parietal pleural tear into the thoracic cavity. The incision should then be closed, as described earlier, in layers around the catheter. Positive pressure is then applied and the catheter is clamped with a hemostat until the catheter is removed. At the end of the operation, the anesthesiologist applies maximal positive pressure into the lungs and holds this as the catheter is placed on suction and removed. A postoperative chest radiograph should be taken if there is any concern about the effectiveness of reestablishing negative pressure within the pleural space.

Because older patients may have calcification of their ribs that preclude their use as grafts, a computed tomography scan of the sternum and ribs with coronal reconstructions is recommended in those patients in whom there is a high index of suspicion (**Fig. 4**). Despite appropriate preoperative screening, patients will occasionally present with premature calcification of the cartilaginous rib. This is limited, and occurs commonly at the junction of the osseous and cartilaginous portions of the rib or along the periphery. Small foci of calcification may also be found within the body of the rib cartilage itself. These foci can impair the preparation of individual grafts and can act as a site of weakness that gives the cartilage a tendency to fracture. The authors have found that the use of a powered drill with a diamond burr can prove useful in contouring these areas of calcification. If the cartilage were unexpectedly found to be so extensively calcified at the time of the operation that it is unusable, the use of irradiated donor cartilage would then be considered.

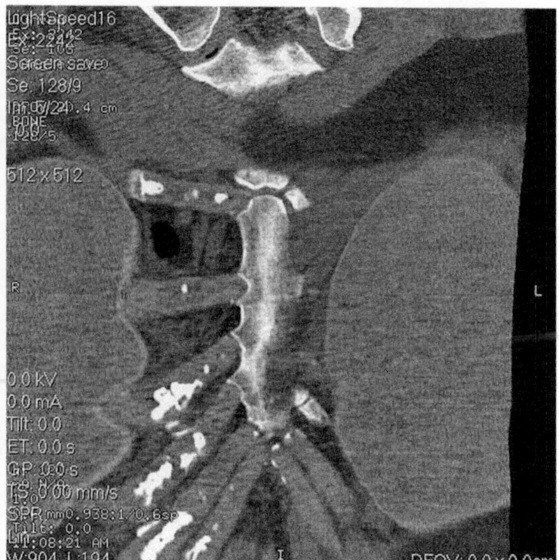

Fig. 4. A computed tomography scan of the sternum and ribs with coronal reconstructions showing calcifications with the ribs.

OPERATIVE SEQUENCE FOR SECONDARY RHINOPLASTY

Although an individualized approach is applied to each case and variations in operative steps and sequence occur, the general steps of open secondary rhinoplasty proceed in the following sequence: (1) incisions, (2) elevation of the soft tissue envelope, (3) confirmation of preoperative diagnosis and reassessment of grafting requirements, (4) septoplasty and septal cartilage harvest, (5) establishment of desired tip projection and reconstruction of the nasal tip complex, (6) dorsal modification and osteotomies, (7) final tip cartilage positioning and shaping, (8) wound closure, and (9) application of splints and dressings.

Incisions

With the patient under general anesthesia the external nose and septum are injected with 1.0% lidocaine with 1:100,000 epinephrine, and the internal nose is packed with quarter-inch gauze strips soaked with a vasoconstricting medication such as oxymetazoline hydrochloride. Bilateral marginal incisions along the caudal edge of the lower lateral cartilages are terminated medially at the narrowest part of the columella and connected with a transcolumellar incision. If the initial rhinoplasty performed was by the endonasal approach, an inverted-V or chevron-shaped incision is used. This broken line closure allows for precise wound closure and decreased scar visibility. If the preceding rhinoplasty performed was by the open approach, the same incision is used to minimize scarring. For wide or unattractive transcolumellar scars, the previous scar can be excised; however, any resultant shortening of the columellar skin may hinder closure and place excess tension on the incision.

Elevation of the Soft Tissue Envelope

The thin columellar skin is elevated from the caudal edges of the medial crura and elevation of the soft tissue envelope proceeds towards the domes. The dissection continues over the lateral crura in either a medial to lateral or lateral to medial direction. Care should be taken to avoid unnecessary retraction or injury to the soft tissue envelope, and in particular, the columellar skin, as the blood supply may be tenuous because of previous disruption caused in previous surgeries. The normal tissue planes are frequently non existent having been replaced with variable amounts of scar tissue, and the surgeon should be cautious not to perforate the skin overlying the lower lateral cartilage complexes.

It is important to preserve the integrity of the domal segments (when they are present) as dissection continues over the tip because any usable portion of the lower lateral cartilages facilitates reconstruction of the tip complex. Once the tip is exposed, dissection continues over the dorsal septum and upper lateral cartilages. When the nasal bones have been reached, a Joseph elevator is used to lift the periosteum off the nasal bones superiorly to the level of the nasofrontal angle. Retraction of the undermined area allows exposure of the entire osseocartilaginous framework.

Confirmation of Preoperative Diagnoses and Reassessment of Grafting Requirements

After the soft tissue envelope is elevated from the underlying nasal framework, the nasal cartilages are evaluated and correlated with the preoperative diagnosis. The extent of the upper lateral cartilages and nasal tip deformity are determined, and any cartilages displaced or distorted by scar tissue are dissected free. A crucial step in the operative sequence is the assessment of adequate tip projection, because any reduction or augmentation of the dorsum should be performed with the final tip projection in mind.

A useful means of assessing the graft requirements is to use silicone sizers, which can be used to estimate the shape and size of the columellar strut and dorsal onlay graft when indicated. The sizers are prefabricated by the surgeon from molds of anatomically shaped dorsal onlay grafts and columellar struts carved in a paraffin wax block in an assortment of shapes and sizes. Room Temperature Vulcanizing silicone is mixed and poured into the molds and left for 24 hours to polymerize before trimming to their final form. The sizers are then sterilized before being placed in the operative field. With a columellar sizer in place, various dorsal sizers are then placed on the dorsum and the skin redraped until the desired combination is determined.

Septal Cartilage Harvest and Septoplasty

If septal work is required, the septum may be approached from above after the upper lateral cartilages have been divided from the septum. The upper lateral cartilages can be freed from the dorsal septum after submucoperichondrial tunnels are created bilaterally using an elevator beginning at the septal angle. Alternatively, the septum may be approached by a separate transfixion incision.

The mucoperichondrium is elevated on one side, and the appropriate septal modification or septal cartilage harvest is performed. If septal cartilage is to be harvested, care should be taken to preserve an "L-shaped" septal strut measuring at least 1 cm in width. If the caudal septum is deviated or dislocated from the maxillary crest or nasal spine area, it should be reduced to the midline and fixated with a figure-of-8 suture. It may be necessary to separate the medial crura to gain better exposure, but their attachment to each other, which aids in support of the tip, must be reestablished before the end of the operation.

It is not uncommon during secondary rhinoplasty to find that the integrity and strength of the septal "L-strut" may have been compromised because of previous surgery. If the septal "L-strut" has been weakened or over-resected during previous surgery, dorsal spreader grafts placed along either side of the septum allow for stabilization. Similarly, a weak "L-strut" can be straightened and strengthened with a piece of the bony septum that is sutured along the deformed segment after suture holes are created in the bone with a 1-mm drill bit (**Fig. 5**).

Spreader Graft Placement

After the desired tip projection is estimated and septal work has been completed, the cartilaginous-bony dorsum is evaluated and any needed

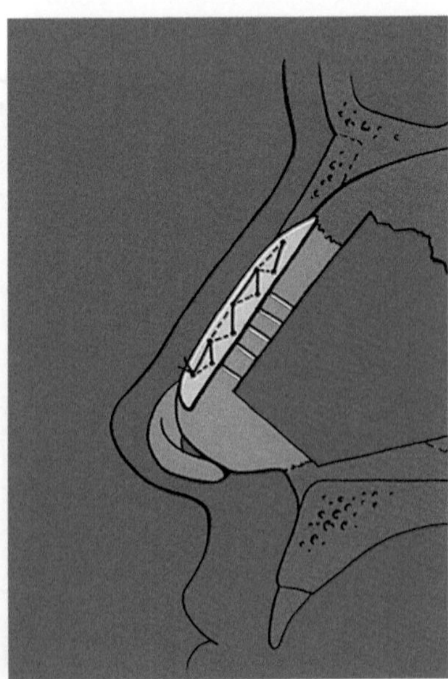

Fig. 5. A weak septal "L-strut" can be straightened and strengthened with a piece of the bony septum that is sutured along the deformed segment.

augmentation or reduction of the dorsum is performed. Reduction of the bony dorsum is usually performed with a rasp, and any remaining contour irregularities of the bony dorsum can be smoothed using a drill with a coarse diamond burr. The dorsal septum and upper lateral cartilages can then be trimmed to the desired height with a scalpel or sharp angled scissors.

Frequently, patients undergoing secondary rhinoplasty require placement of dorsal spreader grafts. Spreader grafts are usually paired, longitudinal grafts placed between the dorsal septum and the upper lateral cartilages (**Fig. 6**). Spreader grafts are used to straighten a deviated dorsal septum, to improve the dorsal aesthetic lines, to correct upper lateral cartilage collapse, and to reconstruct an open roof deformity.[12]

The length and the shape of the spreader grafts may vary depending on the indication. The grafts may extend above the level of the dorsal septum to slightly augment the dorsum or extend caudally beyond the septal angle as extended spreader grafts to lengthen the nose. The grafts should be suture-fixated to the septum before reapproximation of the upper lateral cartilages to the septum-spreader graft complex. Failure to reapproximate the upper lateral cartilages to the dorsal septum can cause an inverted-V deformity and contribute to internal valve obstruction.

Dorsal Augmentation

With the midvault reconstructed, the dorsum may then be augmented as necessary. Autogenous rib cartilage has been the authors' graft material of choice for dorsal augmentation when sufficient septal cartilage is not available. Before graft preparation, the dorsum of the nose must be prepared to receive the dorsal graft. The recipient bed on the dorsum must be made as flat and as smooth as possible to give the greatest surface area for the dorsal onlay graft to contact. A uniform surface of the dorsal recipient bed aids in the graft adhering solidly to the osseocartilaginous framework; this prevents postoperative movement of the graft after healing is complete, as is often seen in grafts placed in soft tissue envelopes. Soft tissue irregularities and scar tissue should be judiciously removed from the undersurface of the soft tissue envelope to prevent overlying irregularities.

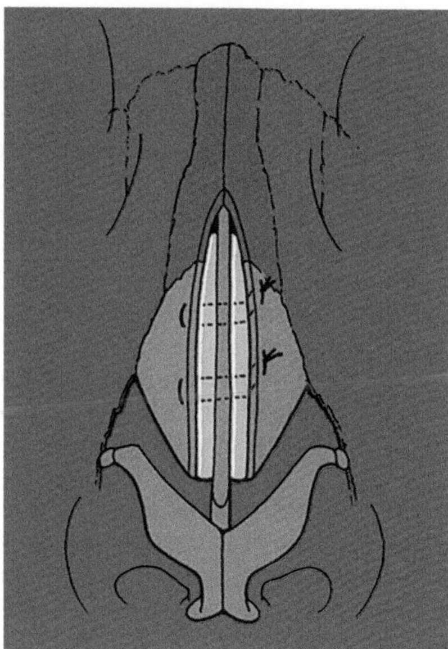

Fig. 6. Spreader grafts are placed between the dorsal septum and the upper lateral cartilages.

For minimal amounts of dorsal augmentation or for camouflaging irregularities of the dorsum, soft tissue grafts, such as perichondrium or temporalis fascia, may suffice. For slight amounts of dorsal augmentation, septal cartilage grafts can be effective provided that adequate cartilage is available. For more significant augmentation, rib cartilage is necessary to construct the dorsal onlay graft (**Fig. 7**).

The major disadvantage of using rib cartilage is its tendency to warp. In response to this, the senior author (J.P.G.) has devised a technique in which the dorsal onlay graft and columellar strut are reinforced with a centrally placed Kirschner wire (K-wire) to decrease warping and to provide a more stable and predictable result.[13] To avoid warping of smaller grafts, the authors follow the principle of carving balanced cross sections originally described by Gibson and Davis[14] and later substantiated by Kim and colleagues.[15]

The harvested rib segment that is selected for the dorsal onlay graft is manually stabilized in a specifically designed K-wire guide jig, and a smooth 0.028-in K-wire is drilled longitudinally through the center of the graft. The 0.028-in K-wire is removed and replaced with a threaded 0.035-in K-wire to better stabilize the graft and avoid migration of the K-wire. The same routine is used for placing an internal K-wire in the columellar strut if rib cartilage is used.

The cartilage grafts with the internal K-wires are then carved into similar but slightly larger shapes than the selected sizers. The K-wire in the dorsal onlay graft should be placed within 2 to 3 mm of the cephalic end of the graft and cut flush with the caudal end. The K-wire in the columellar strut should extend three-quarters of the length of the graft, with 8 to 10 mm of the K-wire left exposed at the graft base that will be seated into a drill hole created in the maxilla.

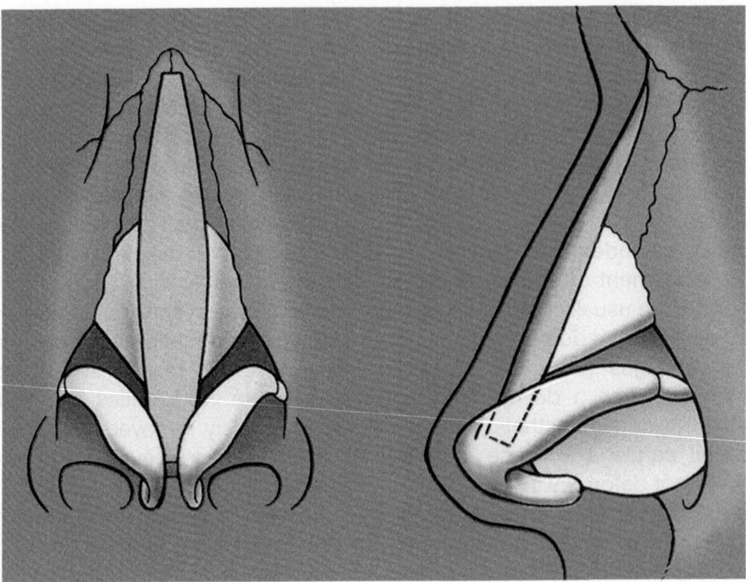

Fig. 7. Augmentation with rib cartilage dorsal onlay graft.

The grafts are then placed in their anatomic position to see what further shaping is required. Carving proceeds carefully from this point usually by scraping the grafts with the sharp edge of a number 10 blade perpendicular to the graft surface until the exact desired size, shape, and contour is obtained.

Next the dorsal onlay graft is placed and secured. Fixation of the cephalic end of the dorsal graft is achieved by placing a temporary 0.028-in smooth K-wire percutaneously through the graft into the nasal bones near the nasofrontal angle. This percutaneous K-wire is removed in the office with a wire twister 1 week postoperatively when the external splint is removed. The graft is secured to the nasal dorsum caudally, by a suture that passes around or through the graft and through the upper lateral cartilages and nasal septum-spreader graft complex in the area of the septal angle. Any remaining tip work and indicated osteotomies, if not previously performed, are then completed.

Tip Reconstruction Using the Tripod Concept

Once the nasal dorsum has been addressed, attention is redirected to the tip, where the estimated tip projection is confirmed, final tip projection is established, and reconstruction of the tip cartilages is performed. The Tripod Concept that relates nasal tip support and shape to the paired lower lateral cartilage complexes is a useful premise for nasal tip reconstruction and for correcting deformed lower lateral cartilages.

Each lower lateral cartilage complex consists of a medial crus (including the intermediate crus) and a lateral crus. These paired complexes can be visualized as a tripod, with each lateral crus forming a separate lateral (cephalic) leg and the adjoining medial crura forming the caudal third leg.[16] Using this concept to anatomically simulate the paired lower lateral cartilage complexes allows reestablishment of this tripod, and is the goal for any nasal-tip reconstruction.

To be successful, the reconstructed tripod structure must have the strength to support the tip and prevent the alar sidewalls from collapsing, and the shape to provide the nasal tip with an aesthetically pleasing, natural appearance. Septal, auricular, and rib cartilage can all be used, with each having its own inherent advantages and disadvantages.

Support for the central leg of the tripod should be reconstructed first. In some cases tip support and projection can be achieved with septal extension grafts or extended spreader grafts. These grafts are suture fixated to the septum in the area of the septal angle and extend into the tip lobule complex; they require the presence of a stable caudal septum. Reestablishing tip support and projection can effectively be achieved through the use of a columellar strut. Septal cartilage is appropriate for most columellar struts. However, a rib cartilage columellar strut reinforced with a central K-wire allows for maximal tip support and precise control of tip projection and rotation (**Fig. 8**).

To prepare for placement of a rib cartilage columellar strut with K-wire stabilization, a pocket is

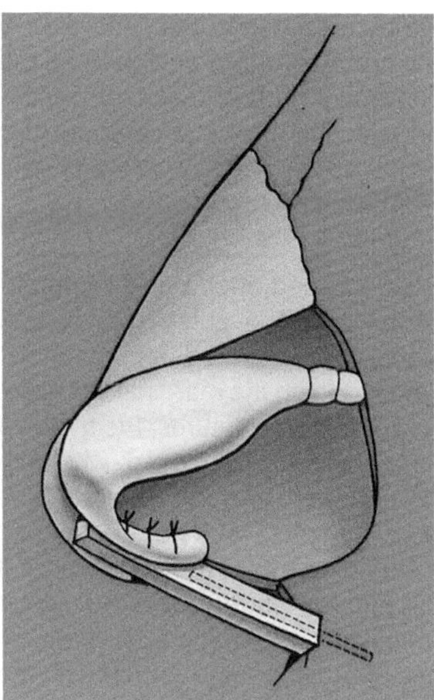

Fig. 8. A rib cartilage columellar strut reinforced with a central K-wire allows for maximal tip support and precise control of tip projection and rotation.

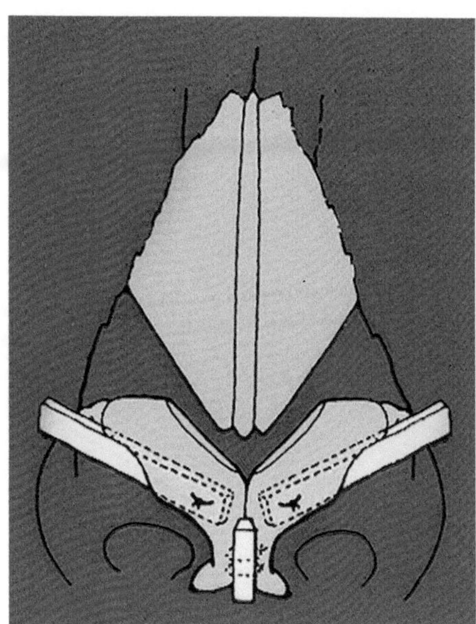

Fig. 9. Lateral crural strut grafts are grafts placed in an undermined pocket between the undersurface of the lateral crus and the vestibular skin.

dissected between the medial crura to expose the nasal spine that is removed with a rongeur. A drill with a 1.0-mm wire passer bit is used to place a 1.0-mm drill hole just lateral to the maxillary midline, thus avoiding damage to the incisive foramen. The hole is drilled to a depth of 11 to 12 mm and lays parallel to and 2 to 3 mm inferior to the nasal floor. After drilling this hole a 0.028 smooth K-wire is placed in the drill hole to make certain that it is contained in the bone of the palate and has not perforated intraorally or intranasally. If it does, a new drill hole is placed on the opposite side of the midline of the maxilla. The K-wire in the columellar strut should extend three-quarters of the length of the graft with 8 to 10 mm of the K-wire left exposed at the graft base, which will be seated into the drill hole created in the maxilla.

The method used for rebuilding the lateral legs of the tripod (lateral crura) depends on several factors, the most important of which are (1) how much usable cartilage is present in the tip, and (2) what cartilage (septal, auricular, or rib) is available for grafting. For tip deformities in which the lower lateral cartilages are present but are collapsed or mildly deformed, lateral crural strut grafts fashioned from septal or auricular cartilage are used to reestablish the shape and stability of the lateral legs of the tripod.[17] Lateral crural strut grafts are grafts that are placed in an undermined pocket between the undersurface of the lateral crus and the vestibular skin, and stabilized by suturing it to the crus (**Fig. 9**). These grafts are used to correct alar retraction, alar rim collapse, and concave, convex, or malpositioned lateral crura. The lateral crural strut grafts are extended laterally to overlap the piriform aperture and end in an undermined pocket inferior to the alar groove. If the pocket is created superior to the alar groove, it will sometimes produce a visible bulge above the ala. The authors use a columellar strut in almost all cases of nasal tip reconstruction to stabilize the caudal leg and thereby resist displacement by scar tissue contraction or swelling.

When the lateral crura are absent or so deformed that they cannot be used, correction is more challenging, and autogenous rib cartilage has proved to be the cartilage of choice. If the lateral crura are not usable but the medial crura and domes are intact, a columellar strut is sutured between the medial crura to strengthen the caudal leg of the tripod. Next, the vestibular skin is undermined off the undersurfaces of the domes. The lateral crural strut grafts are sutured to the undersurface of each dome to replace the missing lateral crura (**Fig. 10**).

If the medial and lateral crura are absent or unusable, autogenous rib cartilage is carved as a "shaped" columellar strut to act as the caudal leg of the tripod, to simulate the contour of the caudal margins of the medial crura and medial portion of the domes along the columella-infratip lobule.

The lateral legs of the tripod are reconstructed in a fashion similar to those used when the domes

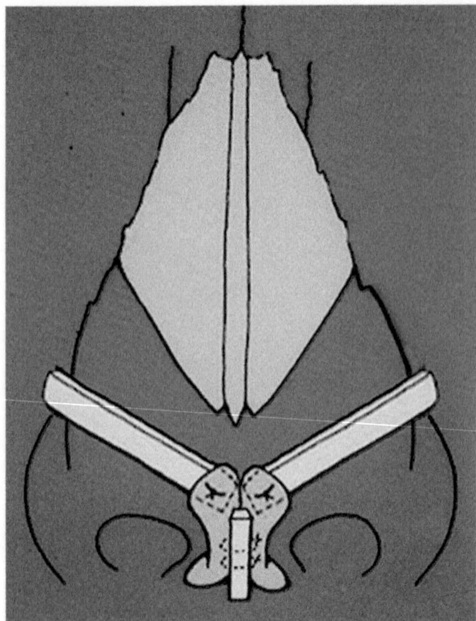

Fig. 10. Lateral crural strut grafts are sutured to the undersurface of each dome to replace missing lateral crura.

are present. The only difference is that instead of suturing the medial ends of the lateral crural strut grafts to the undersurface of the domes, the surgeon sutures the grafts to the tip of the "shaped" columellar strut to replace the missing lateral crura (**Figs. 11** and **12**). It is preferable and easier to suture the lateral crural strut grafts to the undersurface of the domes, assuming they are present, than to the tip of the columellar strut.

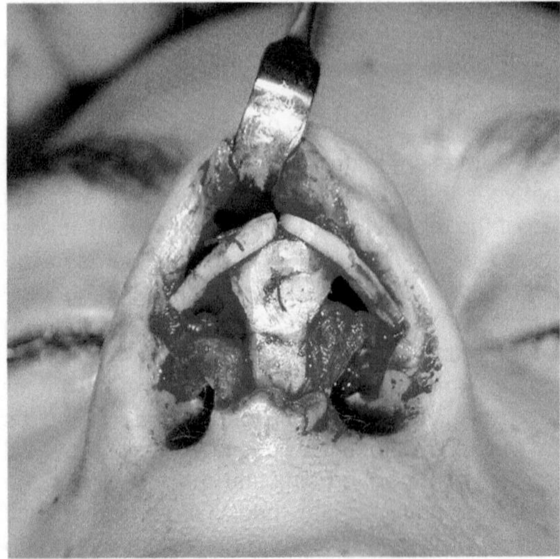

Fig. 11. Lateral crural strut grafts suture to the tip of a "shaped" columellar strut to replace the missing lower lateral cartilages.

If the domes are absent, the "shaped" strut and the lateral crural strut grafts should be tapered. A soft tissue onlay graft of fascia or perichondrium is also an effective means of camouflaging irregularities of the tip cartilages and grafts edges.

Wound Closure and Splints

The skin is redraped after a final inspection of the nasal framework. The external appearance and nasal interior are evaluated, and the incisions are closed. After closing the marginal incisions with interrupted 5-0 chromic sutures, the transcolumellar incision is meticulously closed with interrupted 6-0 nylon sutures. No subcutaneous sutures are necessary. If septal work has been performed, bilateral septal splints are placed and sutured in place with through-and-through 3-0 nylon sutures. Nasal packing is avoided if hemostasis is adequate. Steri-Strips and an aluminum cast are placed on the nose and allowed to remain for 1 week.

DISCUSSION

The major advantage of the open approach in the management of secondary nasal deformities lies in the complete, undistorted anatomic exposure of the nasal framework. This exposure allows for a precise anatomic diagnosis and correction of the deformity with original tissues and supplemental cartilage grafts. The bony and cartilaginous structures can be continuously assessed intraoperatively. The final anatomic alignment and symmetry of the nasal framework become more predictable. Despite all the advantages of the open approach, it is not indicated for every secondary nasal deformity. Minor asymmetries or under-resection can sometimes be corrected endonasally, but for major deformities the open approach is preferred.

The major potential disadvantage of the open rhinoplasty technique is the transcolumellar scar. However, using a broken line incision across the columella, with strict attention to operative techniques during closure, results in a scar usually indistinguishable at conversational distances. Wound separation and delayed secondary healing are rare occurrences. The open approach also increases the operative time and may prolong tip edema. The increased operating time is necessary for the suture stabilization required for any grafting and repositioning of the anatomic structures and accurate closure of the transcolumellar incision.

Autogenous rib cartilage provides the most abundant source of cartilage for graft fabrication and is the most reliable when structural support or augmentation is needed; therefore, rib cartilage

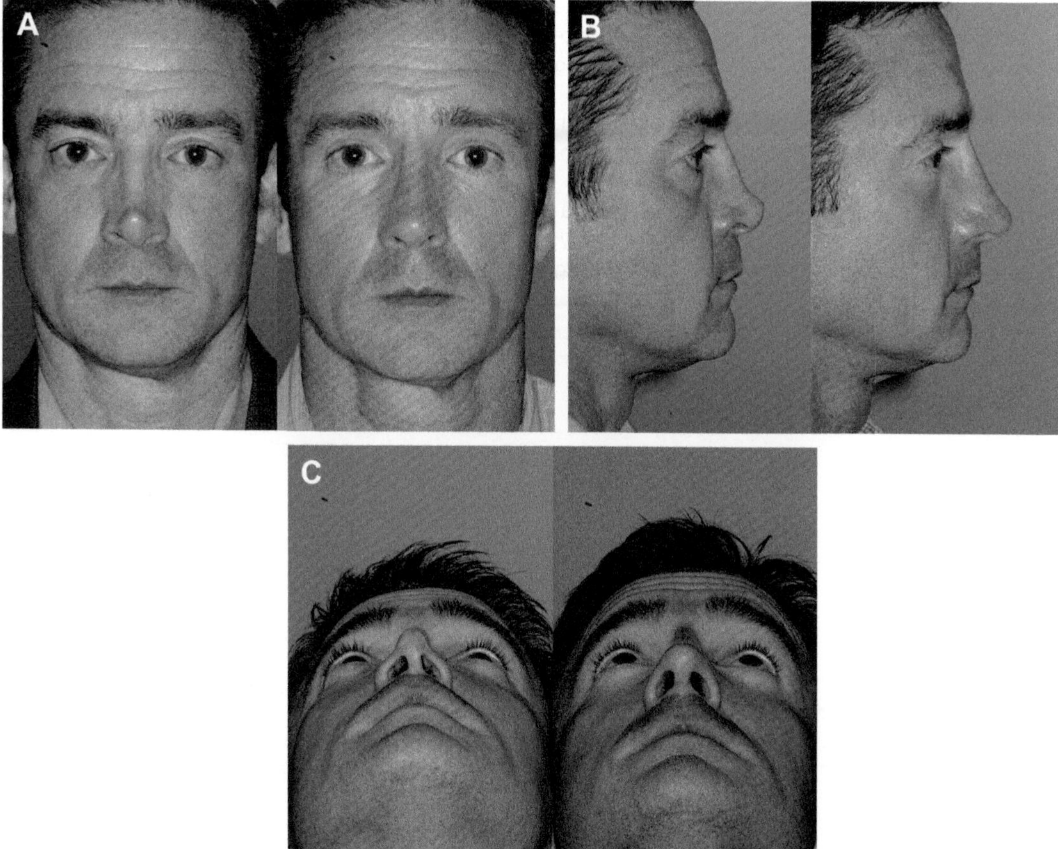

Fig. 12. (*A–C*) Pre- versus postoperative views of a patient who underwent secondary rhinoplasty. Rib cartilage was used to augment his dorsum and reconstruct his tip using the Tripod Concept.

has been the authors' graft material of choice for secondary rhinoplasty when sufficient septal cartilage is not available.

Major postoperative nasal deformities having a distorted nasal framework with aesthetic and functional compromise are a difficult problem. The complexity of secondary nasal deformities requires strict adherence to the basic principles as outlined, an understanding of the individual's aesthetic nasal analysis, and a systematic treatment plan. Use of the open approach for major postoperative nasal deformities has produced more consistent aesthetic and functional results in the management of these multifaceted problems.

REFERENCES

1. Rees TD, Krupp S, Wood-Smith D. Secondary rhinoplasty. Plast Reconstr Surg 1970;46:332.
2. Gunter JP, Rohrich RJ. Augmentation rhinoplasty: onlay grafting using shaped autogenous septal cartilage. Plast Reconstr Surg 1990;86:39.
3. Peer LA. Cartilage grafting. Br J Plast Surg 1955;7:250.
4. Veale D, De Haro L, Lambrou C. Cosmetic rhinoplasty in body dysmorphic disorder. Br J Plast Surg 2003;56(6):546–61.
5. Clark JM, Cook TA. Immediate reconstruction of extruded alloplastic nasal implants with irradiated homograft costal cartilage. Laryngoscope 2002;112(6):968–74.
6. Murrell GL. Auricular cartilage grafts and nasal surgery. Laryngoscope 2004;114(12):2092–102.
7. Gunter JP, Rohrich RJ. External approach for secondary rhinoplasty. Plast Reconstr Surg 1987;80:161.
8. Hiraga Y. Complications of augmentation rhinoplasty in the Japanese. Ann Plast Surg 1980;4:495.
9. Davis PKB, Jones SM. The complications of Silastic implants: experience with 137 consecutive cases. Br J Plast Surg 1971;24:405.
10. Godin MS, Waldman R, Johnson CM. The use of expanded polytetrafluoroethylene (Gore-Tex) in rhinoplasty. Arch Otolaryngol Head Neck Surg 1995;121:1131.

11. Raghavan U, Jones NS, Romo R III. Immediate autogenous cartilage grafts in rhinoplasty after alloplastic implant rejection. Arch Facial Plast Surg 2004;6:192–6.
12. Sheen JH. Spreader graft: a method of reconstructing the roof of the middle nasal vault following rhinoplasty. Plast Reconstr Surg 1984;73(2):230–9.
13. Gunter JP, Clark CP, Friedman RM. Internal stabilization of autogenous rib cartilage grafts in rhinoplasty: a barrier to cartilage warping. Plast Reconstr Surg 1997;100:162.
14. Gibson T, Davis WB. The distortion of autogenous cartilage grafts: its causes and prevention. Br J Plast Surg 1958;10:257.
15. Kim DW, Shah AR, Toriumi DM. Concentric and eccentric carved costal cartilage: a comparison of warping. Arch Facial Plast Surg 2006;8(1):42–6.
16. Anderson JR. A reasoned approach to nasal base surgery. Arch Otolaryngol 1984;110:349–58.
17. Gunter JP, Friedman RM. Lateral crural strut graft: technique and clinical applications in rhinoplasty. Plast Reconstr Surg 1997;99:943–52.

Secondary Rhinoplasty in Unilateral Cleft Nasal Deformity

Tom D. Wang, MD

KEYWORDS

• Cleft-lip • Revision rhinoplasty • Alar-columellar web

The cleft-lip nasal deformity presents a formidable challenge in rhinoplasty. The 3 main factors contributing to this deformity are congenital anatomic deficiency or aberrancy, surgical scarring from previous reconstructive attempts, and changes related to growth.

Various techniques have been proposed for the correction of this problem. The sheer number of methods described in the literature serves as a testament to the intrinsically difficult nature of this deformity. All these techniques attempt to address some aspect of the problem. However, complete correction of all nasal deficiencies remains an elusive goal for many.

UNILATERAL CLEFT NASAL DEFORMITY

The unilateral deformity results from tissue deficiency of the cleft lip, deficiency in the bony premaxilla, and abnormal muscle pull on the nasal structures. The unilateral secondary nasal deformity may comprise most, if not all, of the following features:

1. The dome on the cleft side is retrodisplaced and less well-projected.
2. The columella on the cleft side is foreshortened.
3. The medial crus slumps laterally.
4. The lower lateral cartilage (LLC) and the alar rim form a caudal hood.
5. There is an alar-columellar web.
6. There is insufficient vestibular skin in the region of the vestibular dome.
7. The nostril orientation can vary due to lateralized alar-base position and deficient nasal floor.
8. The alar-base displacement (lateral, inferior, and posterior) is universally present in the primary cleft deformity. This can be affected by primary lip repair, primary cleft rhinoplasty, and alveolar bone grafting.
9. The caudal septum is deflected into the noncleft side, but the severity of the deflection is variable.

Primary Unilateral Cleft Rhinoplasty

Primary nasal repair at the time of primary cleft-lip repair can help improve the cleft-lip nasal deformity by achieving better symmetry and improved overall long-term appearance of the nose. The primary lip repair is typically performed by the time the patient is 3 months old. All efforts are made to minimize nasal tissue trauma and scarring, which may unfavorably affect subsequent growth. In this regard, an effective method for primary unilateral cleft rhinoplasty involves unilateral LLC suspension via limited dissection.

Adequate correction from the primary procedure may lessen or eliminate the need for secondary cleft rhinoplasty.

Secondary Unilateral Cleft Rhinoplasty

Secondary nasal surgery includes intermediate and definitive rhinoplasty. Intermediate rhinoplasty is performed before nasal growth is completed and is based on 2 separate timing strategies.

Division of Facial Plastic and Reconstructive Surgery, Department of Otolaryngology-Head and Neck Surgery, Oregon Health and Science University, 3303 SW Bond Avenue, Mail Code: CH 5E, Portland, OR 97239-450, USA
E-mail address: wangt@ohsu.edu

Clin Plastic Surg 37 (2010) 383–387
doi:10.1016/j.cps.2009.12.013

Rhinoplasty is done between the ages of 4 and 6 years, sometimes concomitantly with lip revision, to minimize any peer psychological pressure. Waiting until 8 to 12 years of age and until after the completion of orthodontic alignment and alveolar bone grafting allows a better skeletal base for correction of severe nasal deformities. In general, the intermediate rhinoplasty techniques are more conservative than those of definitive rhinoplasty.

Definitive rhinoplasty is performed when maxillary and nasal growths are complete. This usually occurs between 16 and 18 years of age. Rhinoplasty performed in this time frame allows for more aggressive septoplasty, osteotomies, and cartilage grafting maneuvers. Each patient requires an individualized approach to timing of secondary rhinoplasty, based on the severity of soft tissue and skeletal deformities.

The author's preferred technique for secondary rhinoplasty is the sliding cheilorhinoplasty. This technique is designed to address the deficiencies present on the cleft side of the nose, including lowered dome height, LLC malposition, lateralized alar base, alar-columellar web, and vestibular lining deficit. This is accomplished using a laterally based chondrocutaneous flap of LLC, vestibular skin, and lip scar tissue, which is advanced superiorly and laterally. This procedure is usually performed through an external rhinoplasty approach with structural cartilage grafting to maintain nasal tip support and contour.

Technique

The sliding cheilorhinoplasty technique uses the existing upper lip scar as part of the advancement flap for increasing the vestibular internal lining. The vermilion is marked with methylene-blue tattoo marks (**Fig. 1**).

Two parallel incisions are then marked, which center on and encompass the unilateral upper lip scar that is to be revised. The width of this flap depends on the width of the original scar but should be at least 5 mm. The length of this flap is dictated by the amount of the lip scar that needs to be revised. The markings of these 2 parallel incisions are then extended into the nose. At the columella, the medial incision becomes continuous with the marginal incision. This incision is extended superiorly to encompass any alar webbing and is marked to create a rim margin that is symmetric to the contralateral normal rim.

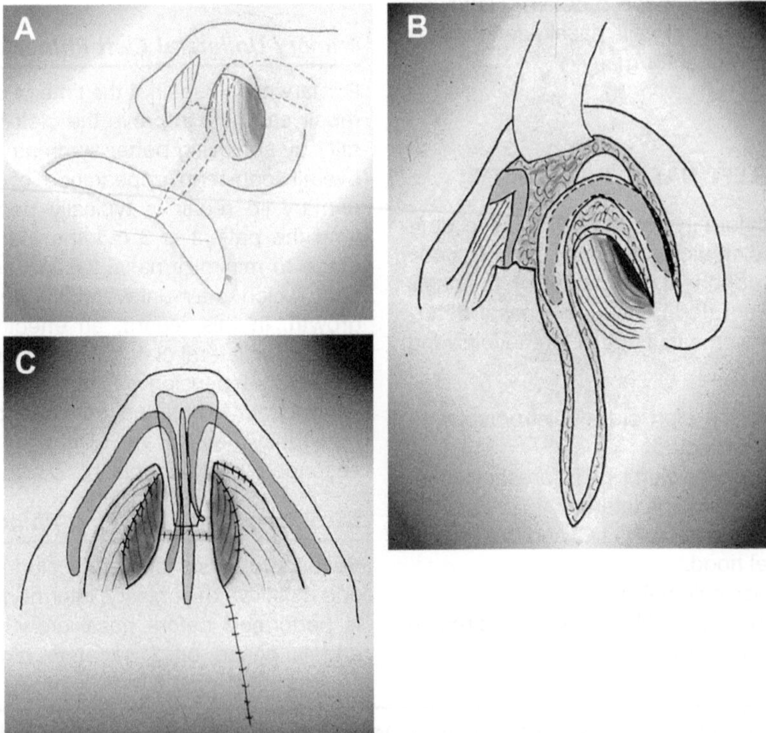

Fig. 1. (*A*) Outline of lip scar, chondrocutaneous flap, alar-web incision, and transcolumellar incision. (*B*) Laterally based chondrocutaneous flap elevated, along with external rhinoplasty exposure. (*C*) Chondrocutaneous flap advanced superior-laterally, secured with columellar strut and tip graft.

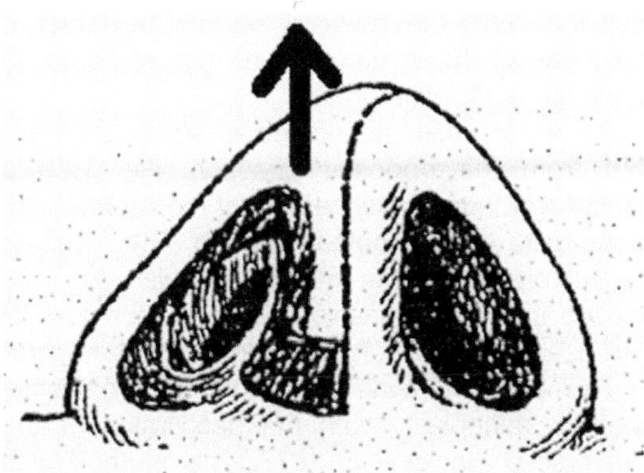

Fig. 2. Gillies and Kilner technique with superior advancement of hemicolumella.

This incision is then merged with the continuation of the marginal incision laterally.

The lateral lip incision transitions into an intercartilaginous incision intranasally, and is carried superiorly and then laterally, outlining the entirety of the LLC. The lateral attachment of the flap is maintained to preserve flap vascularity.

Local anesthetic solution is infiltrated for hemostasis. The amount that is least necessary for vasoconstriction should be used to minimize tissue distortion.

Starting from the lip incision, the flap is elevated and extended superiorly and laterally, encompassing the lip scar and the LLC. Again, the lateral attachment of the flap is maintained for flap vascularity. The remainder of the nasal dorsum and the contralateral LLC is then exposed via the standard external rhinoplasty approach.

Any septal work may be accomplished at this time, including septoplasty and harvesting of grafting material. Care should be taken to leave sufficient dorsal caudal support for the nose.

A columellar pocket is next created. A columellar strut, which is used to anchor the cleft side LLC to the contralateral normal LLC, may be carved from either the septal or auricular cartilage. Symmetry of vestibular dome height is crucial in the positioning of the LLC. This symmetry typically requires advancement of the medial crus of the cleft LLC superiorly to match the vestibular dome heights bilaterally. This superior flap advancement in turn uses the residual lip scar as an internal nasal vestibular lining. Once the appropriate vestibular dome position has been established, the medial crura of the LLCs are secured to the strut with horizontal mattress sutures.

The upper lip is then repaired with tension-bearing sutures placed within the orbicularis musculature.

Once the base of the nose has been stabilized, attention is directed toward the nasal tip. Cephalic trim of the LLC may be performed as indicated. A shield-type tip cartilage graft can be sutured into position to maintain tip projection and to augment tip support. This graft also has the added advantage of allowing camouflage of minor tip asymmetries.

Closure of all incisions is then performed. Slight infolding of the alar-columellar web tissue on reapproximation of the marginal incision improves alar

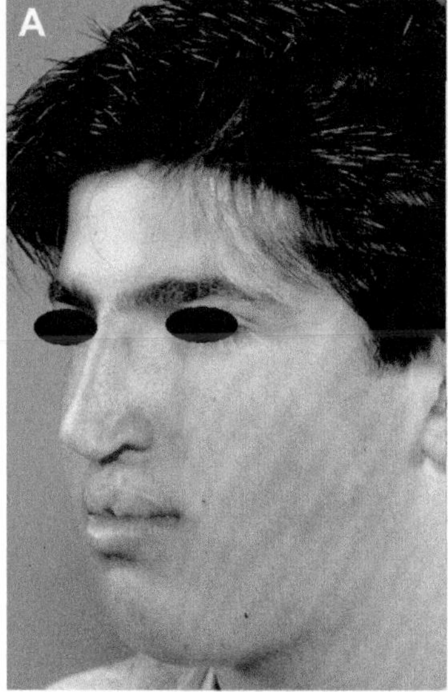

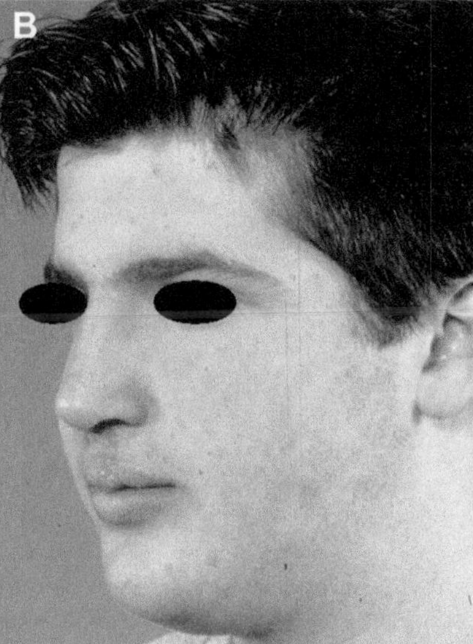

Fig. 3. (*A*) Secondary unilateral cleft nasal deformity. Note the tip asymmetry and alar-columellar web. (*B*) Note the correction of tip asymmetry and alar-columellar web.

margin symmetry. The routine intranasal and external dressings and splint are then applied.

DISCUSSION

Many different techniques have been described for correction of the unilateral cleft nasal deformity. In 1932, Gillies and Kilner introduced a superior advancement of the composite chondrocutaneous hemicolumella flap (**Fig. 2**). This technique used a midcolumellar incision. In 1964, Converse provided the first major modification of this technique by replacing the midcolumellar incision with a marginal incision. The medial crura composite flap was advanced superiorly and sutured to the contralateral dome. The defect at the base of the columellar was repaired with an auricular composite graft.

Potter, in 1954, advocated a similar concept, but from the opposite direction. He used a lateral-to-medial advancement of the lateral crural composite chondrocutaneous flap. The resultant defect created in the lateral vestibular skin was closed in a V-to-Y fashion. Potter's technique is still used by some surgeons today.

Tajima and Maruyama advanced the evolution in cleft-lip rhinoplasty with the description of the "reverse-U" incision in 1977. This method was an extension of the marginal incision into a rim incision at the point of the alar web. The skin of the

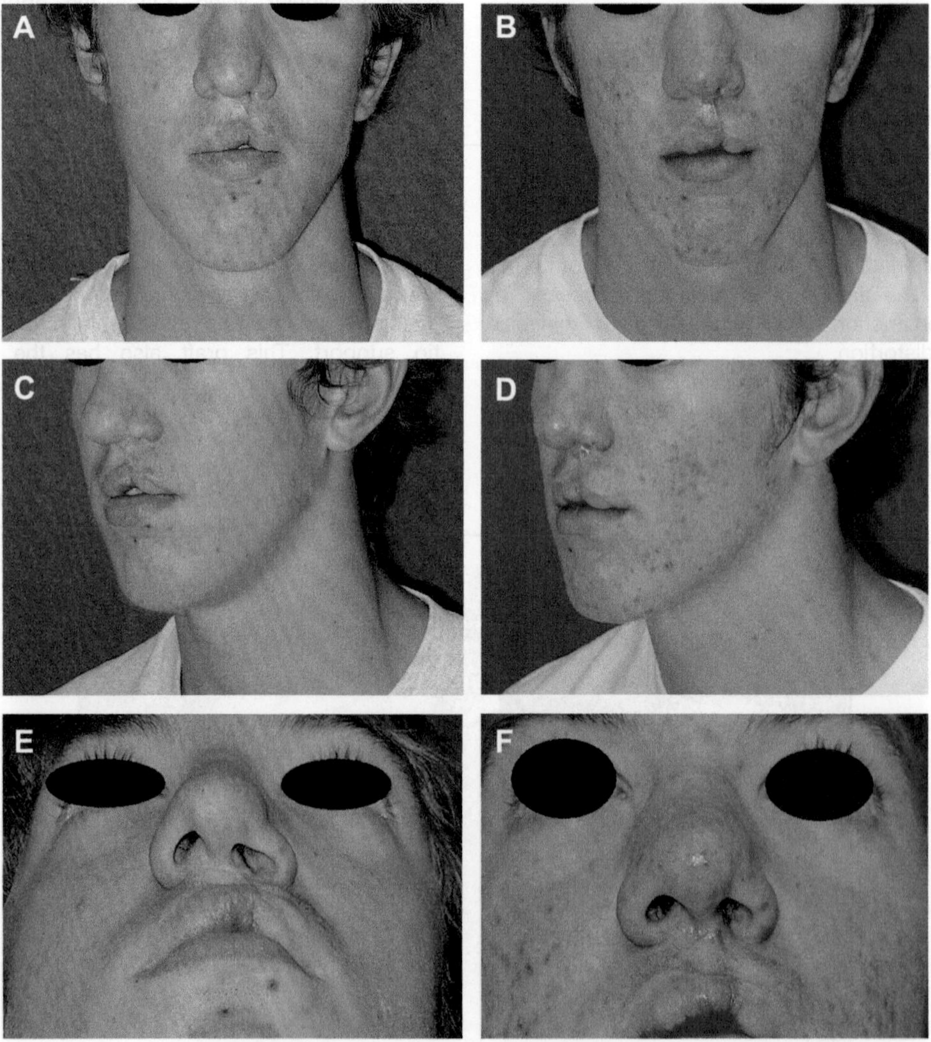

Fig. 4. (*A*) A patient with secondary cleft-lip nasal deformity is shown prerevision. Note the tip asymmetry, alar-columellar web, and poor upper lip alignment. (*B*) The same patient is shown after cleft-lip nose revision. Note the improvement in tip symmetry, alar web, and upper lip alignment. (*C*) Secondary cleft-lip nasal deformity is shown before revision. (*D*) After cleft-lip nose revision. (*E*) Prerevision, base view. (*F*) Post cleft-lip nose revision, base view.

web was incorporated with the vestibular skin and the LLC flap. The flap was then suspended cephalically and medially from the LLC to the ipsilateral upper lateral cartilage and the septum by sutures. Conversion of external skin of the alar web to nasal lining, which is done to correct the alar-columellar web, also corrects the deficiency of vestibular skin associated with the cleft-lip nasal deformity.

Effective repair of the cleft-lip nasal deformity addresses the insufficiency of vestibular skin with a simpler approach. The LLC is mobilized as a composite flap along with the vestibular skin. The direction of mobilization, that is, lateral-to-medial or medial-to-lateral, is of less importance than the advancement of a robust chondrocutaneous flap. The repositioned cartilage allows for increased stability of repair (**Figs. 3** and **4**).

An aggressive incisional approach to the alar-columellar web allows correction of this difficult area. The web skin can be either converted into vestibular lining or discarded according to the patient's needs.

The approach that is outlined in this article amalgamates many of the above-mentioned cleft-lip rhinoplasty concepts into a single unified technique. Increased stability and symmetry of the nasal tip is achieved by combining these techniques with the open rhinoplasty approach, a columellar strut, and a structural shield graft.

The multitude of surgical approaches to the cleft-lip nose is proof to the difficulty of this reconstructive problem. A thorough understanding of the deformity and the methods for its correction forms the foundation for successful reconstruction.

Problems in Rhinoplasty

Joseph M. Gryskiewicz, MD[a], Daniel A. Hatef, MD[b], Jamal M. Bullocks, MD[b], Samuel Stal, MD[b,*]

KEYWORDS

• Rhinoplasty • Complications • Problems • Infection

The aesthetic surgeon who wishes to reshape the nose to improve function and aesthetics must be thoroughly familiar with the consequences of these operations. There are numerous complicated maneuvers that are performed during the rhinoplasty sequence; each one can contribute to a successful outcome or an unwanted problem.

Patient education and the setting of appropriate expectations is the first step in decreased morbidity and reoperation rates in rhinoplasty. Education must focus on the goals and limitations of the procedure. A prepared patient will understand the difference between postoperative morbidity and a true problem.

The preoperative evaluation must be precise; anatomic analysis guides surgical goals. Previous medical history is important, because the perioperative use of medications such as steroids and vasoconstrictors is not without complication and interaction. Routine follow-up appointments must be scheduled to ensure patient confidence and to intercept early signs of complications. The patient should be told to purchase a bottle of oxymetazoline nasal (Afrin) or over-the-counter oxymetazoline spray and have it ready at the bedside postoperatively to facilitate early outpatient management of bleeding. An important part of patient education is preparation for this management of bleeding. Optimal postoperative care is facilitated by having the patients' contact information and keeping in touch with them in the early postoperative period.

In this review, the complications of rhinoplasty are examined in terms of their timing of presentation. An algorithmic approach to postoperative problems is discussed.

INTRAOPERATIVE COMPLICATIONS

Intraoperative injuries to the nasal tissues are uncommon and manageable when encountered. Fracture of the septum or the L-strut left after septoplasty is uncommon, but possible where extensive septal harvest has weakened its structural integrity. A recent review demonstrates that this occurs in about 1% of cases.[1] This history and the following findings on physical examination warn the surgeon of this possibility: (1) secondary cases where a previous hump reduction was performed, (2) short nasal bones with a dorsal hump, (3) the severely deviated nose with a deviated septum, and (4) severe fracture or comminution of the nasal bones or septum. Significant hump removal and septoplasty with osteotomies can lead to instability; the surgeon should be vigilant in cases where these maneuvers are required. When septal fracture is recognized, continued exposure must be cautiously exercised, as intact mucoperichondrium helps in stabilization of the fracture segments. Ultimately, fractures can be treated through several methods: (1) suture fixation of the septal parts, using the mucoperiosteum as support, (2) direct suture fixation of spreader grafts to the dorsal strut, (3) direct suture fixation

[a] Cleft Palate and Craniofacial Clinics, University of Minnesota, Academic Health Center School of Dentistry, MN, USA
[b] Division of Plastic Surgery, Department of Surgery, Baylor College of Medicine, 6701 Fannin Street, Suite 620, Houston, TX, USA
* Corresponding author.
E-mail address: sxstal@texaschildrenshospital.org (S. Stal).

Clin Plastic Surg 37 (2010) 389–399
doi:10.1016/j.cps.2009.11.003
0094-1298/10/$ – see front matter

to the dorsal osseocartilaginous junction, (4) percutaneous Kirschner wire (K-wire) fixation of the nasal bones to the L-strut, or any combination of sutures, grafts, and K-wires needed to maintain central structural stability.

Cribriform plate fracture can occur in patients with a history of trauma. In these patients, force should be used judiciously when dissecting the septum and performing dorsal osteotomies. Osteotomies can also result in skin tears if the osteotome is not thoughtfully guided during tapping. Also, an aggressive lateral osteotomy can enter the maxillary sinus or the lacrimal drainage system and cause several problems, such as enophthalmos, silent sinus syndrome, or mucocele formation.[2,3]

Nasal bones can collapse because of overaggressive infracturing or misplacement of an osteotomy. Failure to correct collapse results in a poor aesthetic appearance with visible asymmetry and palpable deformity. Adjacent internal valve collapse negatively affects the airway. If this is noted, an elevator should be used to replace the bones to their appropriate position, much as one would perform a closed reduction of a nasal fracture. Internal and external splinting should be used postoperatively.

IMMEDIATE POSTOPERATIVE COMPLICATIONS

Bleeding

Bleeding is the most common immediate complication. A thorough preoperative history will reveal any medications and herbal supplements that may put the patient at risk for postoperative bleeding. Aspirin should be discontinued 10 days before the procedure, as should any herbal supplements.[4] Several clinical pearls have been useful in decreasing bleeding in our hands: (1) appropriate preoperative injection using local anesthetic mixed with epinephrine into the subcutaneous tissue and topical Afrin or cocaine on the mucosa, with adequate time given for the onset of these drugs; (2) dissection in the correct tissue planes, that is, maintaining dissection in the submucoperichondrial plane, where appropriate. If dissection is too superficial, it will reach the nasal superficial musculoaponeurotic system (SMAS),[5] which is well vascularized,[6] resulting in bleeding and subsequent irritation of the nasal soft tissue.

Besides the use of bipolar cautery for hemostasis, bleeding can be minimized by not packing the nose at the end of the operation, as this can lead to some bleeding with removal.[4] Goldwyn[7] retrospectively reviewed 780 patients who underwent elective rhinoplasty, and demonstrated that there was a 3.6% incidence of excessive bleeding and a 0.9% incidence of severe bleeding. Bleeding was managed successfully by repacking the nose in the short term, cauterizing a bleeding site, or suturing an open area in the incision or at the columella-septum junction. No specific factors were statistically associated with the incidence of bleeding. However, other surgeons have demonstrated a significant benefit to packing the nose. Guyuron and colleagues[8] demonstrated in a randomized prospective study that packing the nose was superior to a septal quilting stitch-only, in terms of airway improvement, residual deviation, and drip pads used. Guyuron and both of the senior authors of this article (J. G. and S. S.) prefer soft Silastic Doyle splints when splinting is deemed necessary.

Mild epistaxis is easily managed with head elevation and digital pressure; for this reason, it is not of concern to the plastic surgeon. However, bleeding can be greatly distressing to the patient, and for this reason, the patient should be able to get in touch with the surgeon with great ease. The surgeon should have an algorithm for the situation whereby the patient calls emergently with the complaint of postoperative bleeding, as this will occur in a busy rhinoplasty practice. Early light epistaxis can be managed by either oxymetazoline (Afrin, Schering-Plough HealthCare Products Inc, Memphis, TN, USA), or ice with digital pressure, or a combination of both. The key is to allay the patient's fears and inquire as to the amount and color of the blood. Color is key, as patients consider even a drop of blood to be a great deal. If the blood is bright red, and bleeding is persistent despite ice and digital pressure at the nasal root, or oxymetazoline twice into each nostril and elevation of the head, the patient is instructed to come into the emergency room for immediate evaluation. In the emergency room, the head should continue to be elevated, and the patient's blood pressure should be checked. The bottom line in this situation is that the plastic surgeon must intervene and stop the bleeding. The bleeding source should be observed; this observation is facilitated by removing all clots. Quick Relief (Biolife, L.L.C., Sarasota, FL, USA) may be considered for minor epistaxis located more anteriorly. Epinephrine-soaked cottonoids should be inserted to minimize bleeding so that a thorough and direct examination can be performed. If anterior packing does not work, then posterior packing with a Foley or Rhino Rocket (Shippert Medical Technologies Corporation, Centennial, CO, USA) is the next step (**Fig. 1**). The Rhino Rocket is inserted and maintained for 24 to 48 hours and should be coated with Bactroban ointment (GlaxoSmithKline

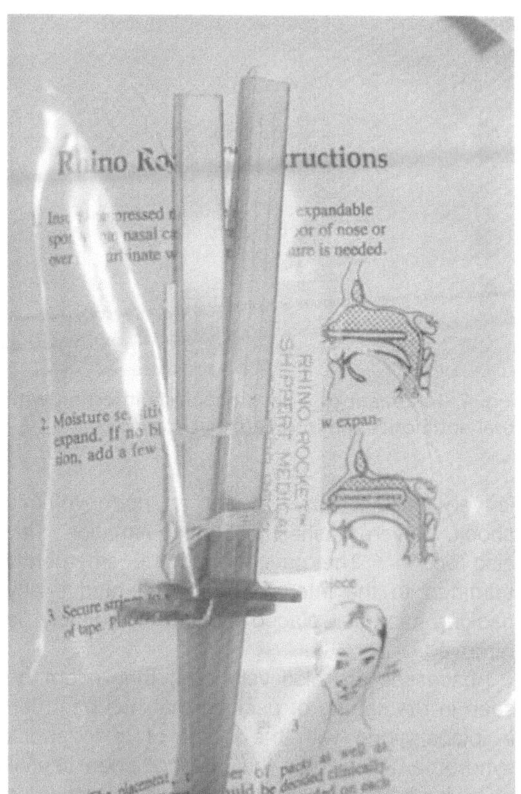

Fig. 1. Rhino Rockets being used to help control postoperative bleeding.

PLC, Brentford, Middlesex, UK) to ease its slide into the nostril. Ice packs should be applied, and the nose should be elevated. Activity must be limited. The patient should be educated concerning optimal care for the period that the Rhino Rocket is in place: this includes saline spray to the ends of the rockets every 2 hours while awake to keep them moist; 1 to 3 Afrin sprays every 12 hours in each nostril; and broad-spectrum oral antibiotics to prevent the development of toxic shock syndrome. When the rockets are pulled, they should be pulled a little bit at a time to prevent rebleeding. The surgeon should pull just hard enough to move the rocket a millimeter, and then wait 10 minutes; advance about 1 cm every 10 minutes until it is completely removed. Once it is out, 3 puffs of Afrin should be administered in each nostril. Afrin should be continued for 3 weeks postoperatively.

If the surgeon is perplexed by increased bleeding either intraoperatively or early postoperatively, or if bleeding persists for days, the administration of desmopressin (DDAVP) should be considered. DDAVP can be given during the case, at the end of a case, or in past anesthesia recovery in which the patient seems to be generally bleeding a great deal. DDAVP is a synthetic analogue of a natural antidiuretic form of vasopressin that upregulates coagulation by increasing plasma clotting factors.[9] Unrecognized coagulopathies can result in this type of postrhinoplasty bleeding, and a history of easy bruising or excessive surgical bleeding may inform the surgeon preoperatively.[10]

DDAVP is also indicated for patients with hemophilia A with factor VIII coagulant activity levels greater than 5%, and for patients with mild to moderate classic von Willebrand disease (Type I) with factor VIII levels greater than 5%. DDAVP injection has infrequently produced changes in blood pressure, causing either a slight elevation or transient decrease with a compensatory increase in heart rate. DDAVP may decrease coronary blood flow, causing angina, and should be avoided in patients with coronary artery disease. Patients should be monitored for chest pain. Patients should be cautioned to ingest only enough fluid to satisfy thirst, to decrease the potential occurrence of water intoxication and hyponatremia.

Under extreme circumstances consulting the appropriate service for embolization of the maxillary artery or posterior ethmoid artery should be considered, if either of these is felt to be the source in uncontrollable bleeding. With rare profuse bleeding after rhinoplasty, a return trip to the operating room should be considered but is rarely necessary. If reoperation is undertaken, a discrete bleeding source should be identified and controlled with suction cautery. Diffuse bleeding should be treated by the other methods described in this section.

Erythema

Redness of the skin can be a sign of different complications (**Fig. 2**). Erythema seen in the setting of revision rhinoplasty may be a red flag to the surgeon that rhinoplasty incision and dissection may have jeopardized the nasal soft tissue vascularity, causing congestion. Postoperative erythema can also signal an allergy to topical adhesives used as dressings. The surgeon is wise to remove the dressings and allow the area to resolve without the dressing. Lastly, erythema may be the result of an infectious inflammatory condition.

Infection

Infection is extremely rare, but when it occurs, it requires an emergent evaluation. The patient will typically present with regional erythema or

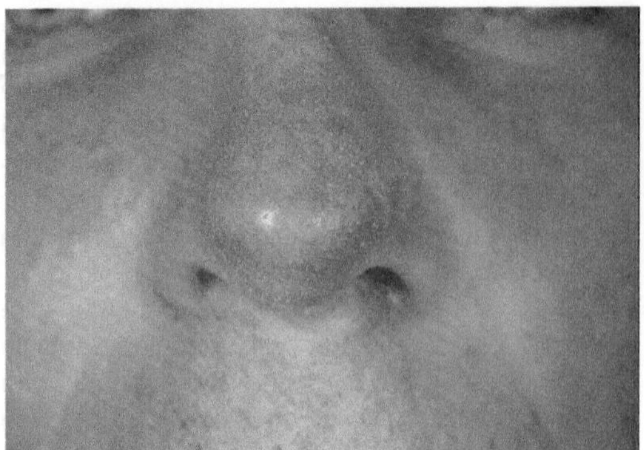

Fig. 2. Erythema presenting as the first sign of a postrhinoplasty infection. The patient was successfully managed on an outpatient basis with oral clindamycin and intranasal bacitracin.

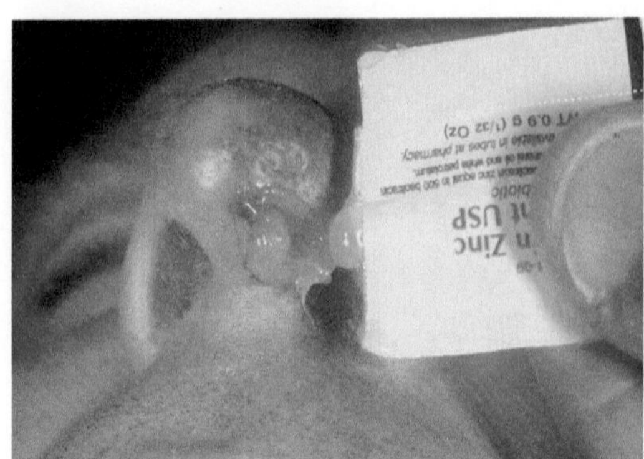

Fig. 4. Treatment of a postrhinoplasty infection with oral antibiotics and intranasal bacitracin.

cellulitis (**Fig. 3**). The patient may or may not be febrile, and purulence will not likely be present at an early presentation. The surgeon must rule out an allergic reaction to tape or ointment. If it is felt that the response represents a true infection, then the patient should be started on oral antibiotics, intranasal bacitracin (**Fig. 4**), and in severe presentations (**Fig. 5**) be admitted for intravenous antibiotics. As *Staphylococcus* species is the most common offender, Bactrim (trimethoprim/sulfamethoxazole), clindamycin, or levofloxacin should suffice. The remote risk of toxic shock syndrome is another reason not to pack the nose postoperatively.[11] Although toxic shock syndrome is very rare, it may present as normovolemic shock. Severe rashes and desquamation may also occur.[12] The patient must be emergently admitted to the intensive care unit, and if any packing has been placed it must immediately be removed.

Abscesses are also very rare; they might be seen in the setting of packing that has been left in place along with the onset of toxic shock syndrome. Abscesses that are not open should be incised and allowed to drain, and this includes suture abscesses, which may present many years later.

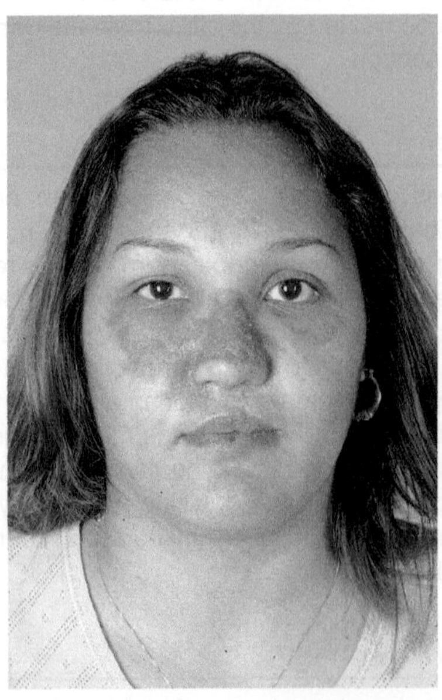

Fig. 3. Cellulitis after secondary cleft rhinoplasty. The patient was successfully treated with intravenous antibiotics.

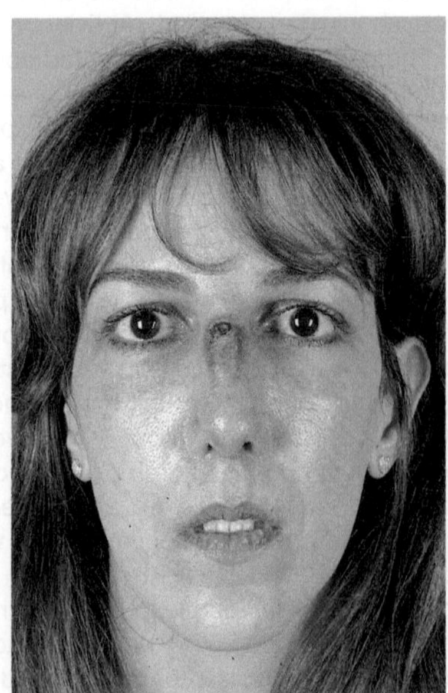

Fig. 5. Severe infection of a dorsal graft. The patient was treated with emergent operative intervention, removal of the dorsal graft, and intravenous antibiotics.

Edema

Edema, like ecchymosis, is to be expected after rhinoplasty. Patient education is key to minimizing postoperative anxiety for the patient: Patients must understand that the "final" result should not be expected for about a year or so.

In 2 randomized, prospective studies conducted in Turkey,[13,14] perioperative steroids were shown to decrease periorbital edema. In one study it was shown that the use of single-dose dexamethasone significantly decreased eyelid edema.[13] In another study, steroids given before osteotomy and in triple dosages were demonstrated to decrease periorbital edema.[14] However, in another prospective randomized study, steroids did not decrease postoperative edema.[15] A meta-analysis of existing prospective data demonstrates that steroids do significantly reduce edema after rhinoplasty.[16]

Skin Loss

Skin loss is an uncommon but unfortunate complication seen after rhinoplasty (**Fig. 6**). The patient shown in **Fig. 6** had 3 sutures placed in the supratip area to fix the skin to the dorsal septum. The use of an open approach, rhinoplasty in an active smoker, defatting of the tip, supratip skin-tacking sutures, or a combination of these may lead to an increased risk for this complication. An aggressive alar base reduction may also predispose an already at-risk patient to vascular embarrassment and skin loss, as this maneuver may delete the lateral nasal artery's primary contribution to tip perfusion.[17]

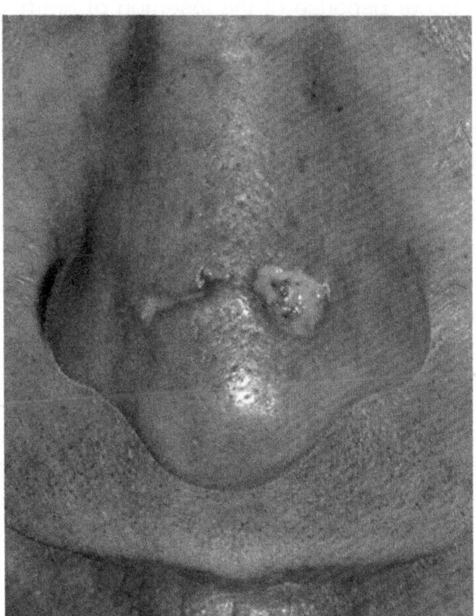

Fig. 6. Patient with skin loss after open rhinoplasty, defatting of the tip, and 3 sutures placed from septal perichondrium to dermis.

The Early Unsatisfactory Result

On initial removal of the splint, both surgeon and patient may be alarmed at the appearance of the nose (**Fig. 7**). The patient shown in **Fig. 7** was so horrified by her upturned nose she wore Band-Aids to camouflage her appearance. Most commonly, the nose has been set at the wrong nasolabial angle because the patient's profile was not correctly evaluated in the supine position at operation. Also, there is sometimes early displacement or graft migration, or malpositioning not recognized intraoperatively (**Fig. 8**). When it is obvious that the problem is not going to correct itself and the patient is going to be miserable for months to come while waiting for the revision surgery, an early return sometime during the first 7 to 12 days is reasonable.[18] After that period of time, however, the surgery can be fraught with a great deal of swelling, induration, and the deposition of fibrous tissue. These situations are also some in which the senior authors do not wait for the usual 10 to 12 months for a secondary correction. Early intervention should be an option for a variety of untoward occurrences,

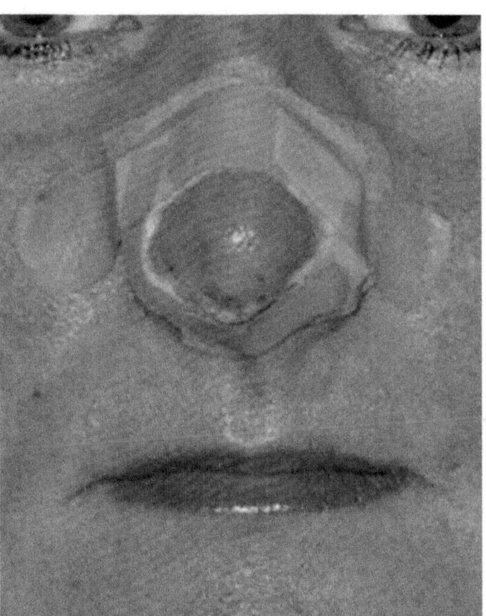

Fig. 7. Patient who was so horrified by her "upturned nose" that she wore Band-Aids to conceal the perceived deformity. Rather than allow this patient to languish with an incorrectly exaggerated nasolabial angle, she was returned to the operating room for early correction.

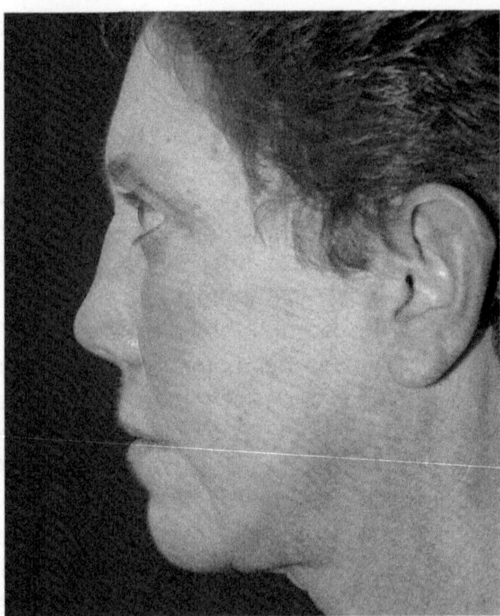
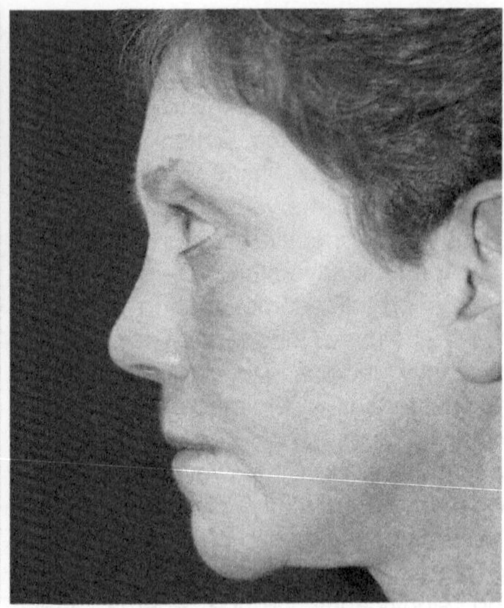

Fig. 8. Patient with early displacement of a radix graft that required an early return to the operating room for correction.

and patients can be returned to the operating room for correction.

INTERMEDIATE COMPLICATIONS

Anosmia

Anosmia can be seen after any sort of nasal surgery.[18] Anosmia is caused by iatrogenic cribriform plate fracture. In the setting of rhinoplasty in the previously traumatized nose, it is a good idea to ask patients about their ability to smell. In addition, nasal surgery can affect the patient's ability to smell without completely taking it away.[19] It has been shown using objective smell testing that around 10% of patients may have compromised olfaction after nasal surgery[20]; however, this has never been previously reported after cosmetic rhinoplasty.

Rhinorrhea

Rhinorrhea is a very rare complication after rhinoplasty. A recent review demonstrated that 3 of 256 patients (1.17%) presented with cerebrospinal fluid leaks after rhinoplasty.[21] This can be a devastating complication, signaling unrecognized injury to the cribriform plate or anterior cranial fossa.[22] These cerebrospinal fluid leaks are diagnosed with laboratory examination of the fluid demonstrating low glucose and high protein levels. Extensive immediate repair is usually not warranted, as many of these spontaneously resolve with antibiotics.[23] Chronic leakage requires surgical intervention with flap coverage. If signs of meningitis should appear, an immediate neurosurgical consult must be obtained for possible insertion of a lumbar drain.

Delayed Healing and Skin Loss

Delayed healing is one of the general sequelae that can be seen after rhinoplasty. If patients smoke, they should be forewarned that smoking exposes them to unnecessary risk for wound-healing problems.

The blood supply to the nose is so robust that loss of skin is a rare complication. Loss of skin can occur because of the insertion of grafts that are too large, and infection with subsequent skin loss. Care must be taken in secondary rhinoplasty not to undermine too widely; also, with the open incision, the columellar branches of the superior labial artery are out, so the nasal soft tissues are dependent on the lateral nasal artery and the subdermal plexus. It is pertinent not to jeopardize their vascularity, and this can be done by dissecting in the subperichondrial or supraperichondrial plane, as the clinically relevant arterial blood supply runs within the SMAS.[6,7] Tissue fillers injected as a touch-up into the nasal tip have caused skin necrosis.

Finally, excessive pressure from the tape and splint can lead to problems with wound healing and skin loss. This factor should be kept in mind during their application at the end of the procedure.

Septal Perforation

Small septal perforations that are recognized during surgery are managed with prolonged splinting. Late perforations are uncommon; however, in this situation it is important to rule out infection, especially if caused by atypical species. Reconstruction should be delayed until the mucosal surface is no longer inflamed. When these are small, a septal advancement or pivot can be done. Perforations too large to be closed in this manner can be managed with a flap of turbinate mucosa, a composite ear cartilage graft, or an Integra inlay. Large septal perforations should be reconstructed with large, well-vascularized, regional flaps, such as a nasolabial flap or a facial artery musculomucosal flap.[24]

Prolonged Swelling

Prolonged swelling can be seen in 2 ways. The first is edema that refuses to subside over time. A great deal of handholding must be done for the patient who has prolonged edema of this sort. Once again, preoperative education is a cornerstone to successful patient management. If patients are counseled preoperatively that they may have swelling of 6 to 12 months' duration, and that their final result will not be seen for at least 1 year, then these realistic expectations will go a long way in buying time for resolution of edema. The patient should understand that most often, the skin envelope of the nose will shrink down to its framework over time, but that this is a long process. In addition, if the procedure is being performed concomitantly with endoscopic nasal surgery, there will be a tendency for a greater time for resolution of edema.[25] Any patient undergoing combined procedures like this should be aware of this fact.

Another manner in which prolonged swelling may present is in the form of postoperative supratip deformity (**Fig. 9**). Although this is often a postoperative problem secondary to inadequate tip support and overreduction of the dorsum,[26,27] it can also present in an inflammatory form at a more acute time point. If the surgeon believes that the dorsal reduction is appropriate and projection/rotation of the cartilaginous framework of the tip is good, then the early supratip may be caused by scar and fibrosis.[28] This condition should be managed with aggressive taping of the supratip tissues for 10 to 14 days (**Figs. 10** and **11**), and at night massage of the tip should be carried out by the patient at home. If this regimen does not enable the swelling to subside, then dilute injections of Kenalog (10 mg/mL) can be implemented early postoperatively. One milligram (1/10 cc) added to an equivalent volume of xylocaine is injected into the subcutaneous tissue just deep to the dermis every 2 to 4 weeks (as needed) for up to 4 to 6 injections (**Fig. 12**), while avoiding injecting the dermis. Before each future injection, care should be taken to examine the injected area carefully for thin skin, prominent veins, color changes, or an actual depression. These potential sequelae should be discussed candidly with the patient. Further injections are to be discontinued if any of these sequelae occur.

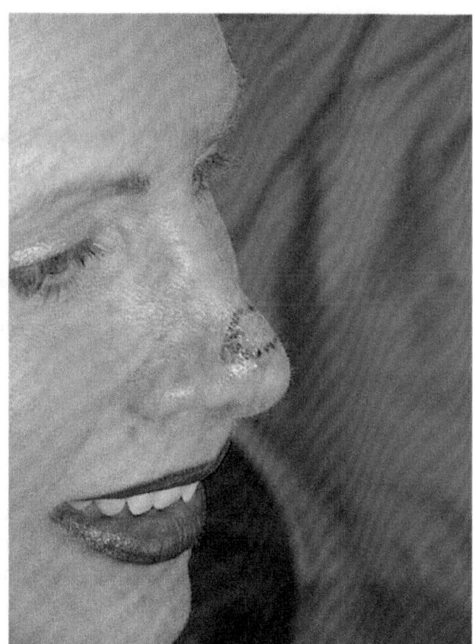

Fig. 9. Postoperative supratip deformity caused by fibrosis of the soft tissues in the tip.

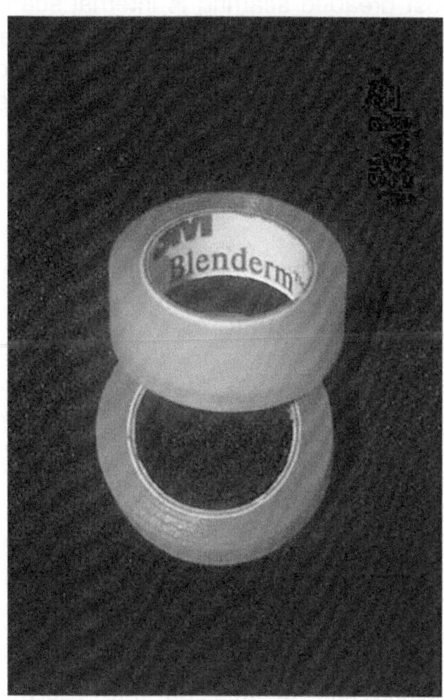

Fig. 10. Blenderm tape used for supratip taping.

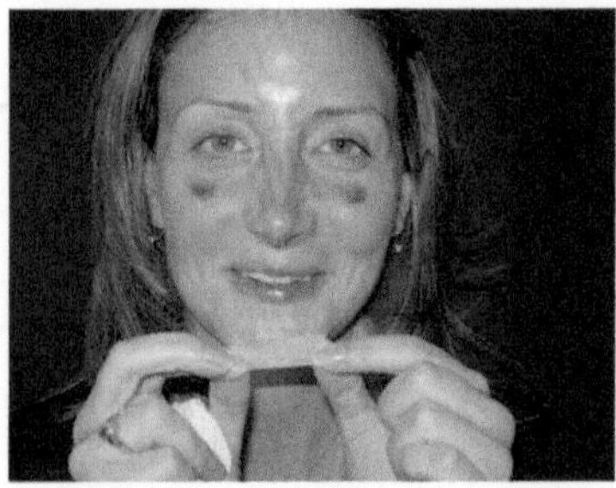
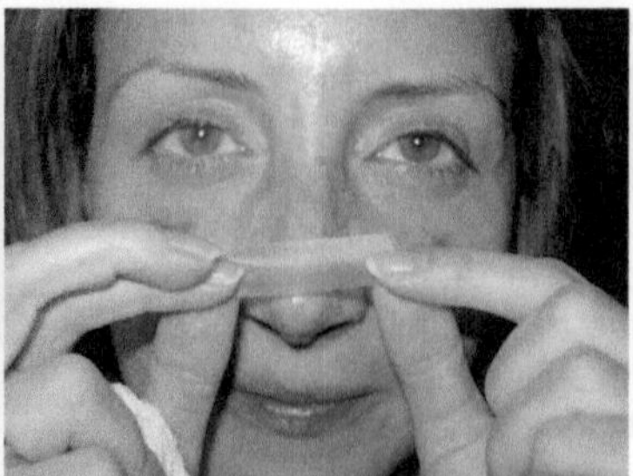
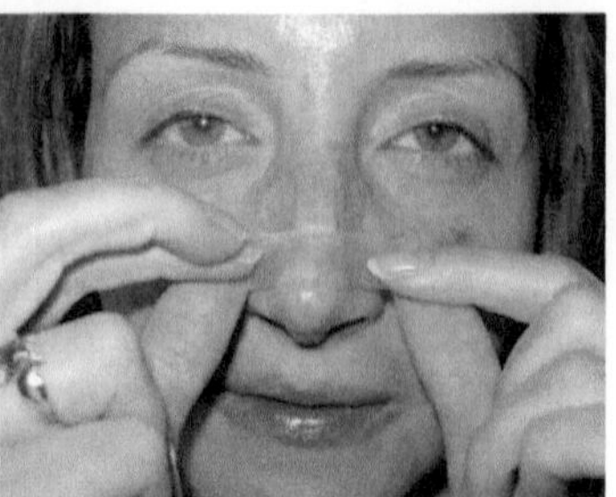

Fig. 11. Patient demonstrating postoperative taping method for supratip deformity.

LONG-TERM COMPLICATIONS

Scarring

Scarring can present in several forms. The columellar scar created during exposure in the open technique can notch when there is inordinate tension secondary to a large increase in tip projection/rotation (**Fig. 13**). Percutaneous osteotomies can also result in unsightly visible scars, caused by traumatic tattooing.[29] This scarring is avoided by carefully cleansing the osteotome before entry into the skin. Patients with fair skin and those with very dark skin can be at greater risk for issues with scarring. This factor should be taken into consideration when planning open rhinoplasty or external osteotomies. Internal scarring of the nasal soft tissues can lead to thinning of the skin, discoloration, and an operated appearance. This internal scar tissue can complicate secondary attempts at correction, causing distortion of dissection planes and potentially jeopardizing nasal skin. Perhaps the most dreaded scarring is internal scarring of the nasal mucosa. This can create problematic synechiae. The avoidance and correction of internal scarring are further covered under the discussion of nasal airway obstruction.

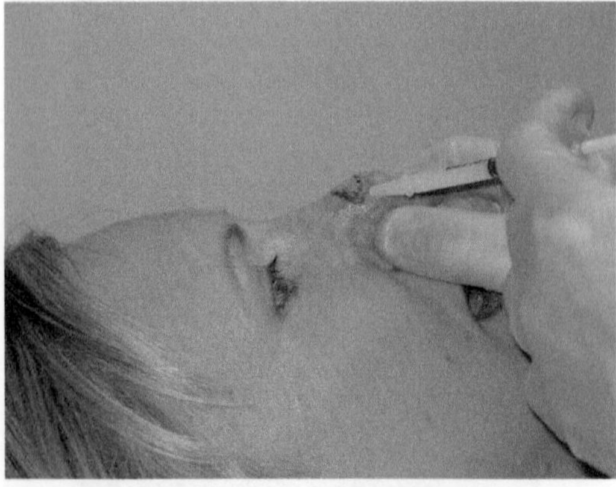

Fig. 12. Injection of Kenalog into subcutaneous tissues in the nasal tip.

Nasal Airway Obstruction

Nasal airway obstruction can present in 1 or more of the 3 nasal vaults. External nasal valve collapse secondary to cosmetic rhinoplasty can be caused by excessive scoring or lower lateral cartilage overresection, specifically overtransection during a "cephalic trim." An overly aggressive maneuver can weaken the lower lateral cartilage, to the point where the middle crura buckles into the airway on inspiration.[30] The external and internal nasal valves can be compromised by stenosis secondary to synechiae. Sheen[31] discusses the formation of vestibular stenoses subsequent to trimming of the caudal edge of the upper lateral cartilage. These trims left mucosal deficits, as mucosa was trimmed along with cartilage. Any form of injury to the vestibular lining can create these types of scars. Such injury can be avoided by injection of saline/local anesthetic into the vestibular skin; this elevates the skin from the undersurface of the cartilage through hydrodissection, and allows for room to dissect and place sutures.[32] Also, an "M flap" or an "M alar wedge resection" can be used by carefully designing these intranasal incisions, with the goal of decreasing scar contracture and alar deformities. Intraoperative recognition of these types of tears is important, as they can be suture repaired at this stage. If a patient presents with airway obstruction caused by synechiae formation, correction can be carried out using direct excision and scar revision; transposition flaps from the alar skin[33,34]; intranasal z-plasty with vestibular mucosa flaps, paranasal myocutaneous flaps,[35] labial mucosal flaps[36]; or mucosal grafts.

Finally, compromise of the bony vault can result from moving the nasal bones too far medially after an osteotomy. Also, a poorly executed lateral nasal osteotomy can move too far medially and cause this compromise. This mistake can be avoided by using caution to preserve Webster's triangle (the inferior/posterior portion of the pyriform rim).

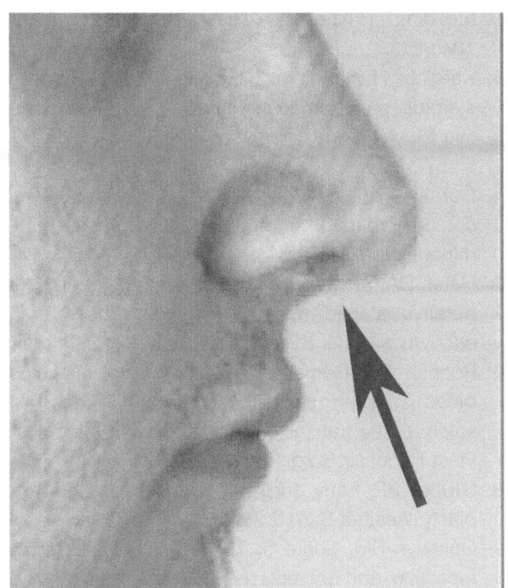

Fig. 13. Notching of columellar scar after open rhinoplasty.

Irregularities

No discussion on rhinoplasty complication would be complete without a discussion of postoperative irregularities of the dorsum and tip. The surgeon must allow for time to differentiate between true and relative "lumps". Often after swelling subsides, the problem is structural, and has not been noted at the time of surgery. Secondary rhinoplasty is an appropriate management strategy in several these aesthetic irregularities, such as saddle nose deformity caused by overresection of septum, graft malposition, rocker deformity, or an open roof.

Postrhinoplasty Cysts

Cysts may be caused by free mucosal grafts in an ectopic position, entrapment of mucosa along the osteotomy path, or by actual herniations of nasal mucosa into the subcutaneous tissue. One of the senior authors (J. G.) has encountered 2 postrhinoplasty cysts, and pathologic examination revealed inflammation without cyst elements consistent with a paraffinoma (bacitracin- or Vaseline-induced cyst) rather than respiratory epithelium or cyst components.[37]

A paraffinoma is caused from overly tight packing (usually Vaseline gauze) that displaces bacitracin or oil-based antibiotic ointments through the osteotomy sites or the tip-lobule incisions. Treatment is by intranasal or percutaneous excision of all remnants.

To avoid these problematic issues, there are several procedures that one of the senior authors has used:

(1) Assiduously preserve mucosal integrity by extramucosal dissection
(2) Avoid undermining osteotomy sites to prevent dead space
(3) Use perforating osteotomies to preserve mucosa and create a smaller path
(4) Clean the surgical field meticulously of any debris at the end of the procedure
(5) Do not use packing material
(6) If you must pack, do not overpack
(7) Avoid petroleum-based ointments; instead use water-soluble, water-based Bactroban (mupirocin ointment, 2%) on splints.

Implant Exposure

Implants may cause eventual erosion (**Fig. 14**). The patient shown in **Fig. 14** suffered an exposure of a Gore-Tex graft. This erosion can occur because of infection, capsular contracture, or placement under thin skin. Some investigators recommend avoiding their use in the tip, in the columella, or in regions that require rigid grafts, stating that this strategy decreases complications.[38] The best way to avoid this complication is to never place a prosthetic implant in the nose. If one is faced with a patient who presents with exposure, the implant should be expediently and completely removed. If purulence is present, cultures, a stat Gram stain, and antibiotics should be considered.

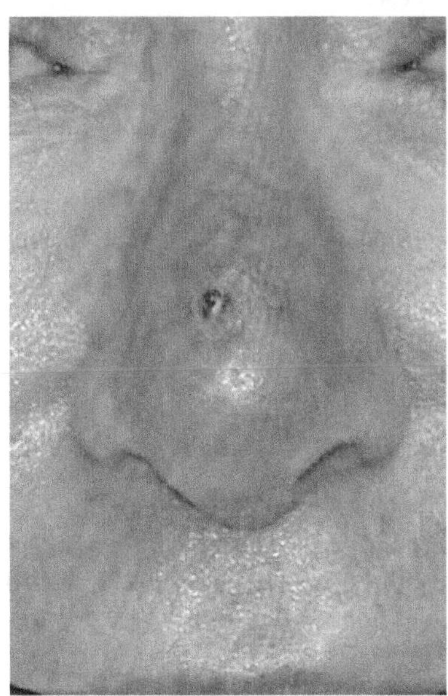

Fig. 14. Erosion of a dorsal Gore-Tex implant through the skin of the nasal dorsum.

Another implant should not be placed. The nose should be reconstructed with autogenous material once the skin softens and erythema clears, which will take at least 6 months and may require up to a year.

SUMMARY

Complications are unfortunate but they can frequently be avoided by meticulous technique, recognition of pitfall points, and early attention to perioperative morbidity. Reoperative rates can be minimized with good patient education and proper command of the postoperative situation, so that unnecessary procedures are not undertaken.

REFERENCES

1. Gunter JP, Cochrane CS. Management of intraoperative fractures of the nasal septal "L-strut": percutaneous Kirschner wire fixation. Plast Reconstr Surg 2006;117:395.
2. Osquthorpe JD, Calcaterra TC. Nasolacrimal obstruction after maxillary sinus and rhinoplastic surgery. Arch Otolaryngol 1979;105:264.
3. Eloy JA, Jacobson AS, Elahi E, et al. Enophthalmos as a complication of rhinoplasty. Laryngoscope 2006;116:1035.
4. Gruber RP, Aiach G. Open rhinoplasty. In: Goldwyn RM, Cohen MN, editors. Avoiding the unfavorable result in plastic surgery. 3rd edition. Philadelphia: Lippincott Williams & Wilkins; 2001. p. 950–81.
5. Letourneau A, Daniel RK. The superficial musculoaponeurotic system of the nose. Plast Reconstr Surg 1988;82:48.
6. Schaverien M, Pessa JE, Saint-Cyr M, et al. The arterial and venous anatomies of the lateral face lift flap and the SMAS. Plast Reconstr Surg 2009;123:1581.
7. Goldwyn RM. Unexpected bleeding after elective nasal surgery. Ann Plast Surg 1979;2:201.
8. Guyuron B. Is packing after septorhinoplasty necessary? A randomized study. Plast Reconstr Surg 1989;84:41.
9. Guyuron B, Vaughan C, Schlecter B. The role of DDAVP (Desmopressin) in orthognathic surgery. Ann Plast Surg 1996;37:516.
10. Guyuron B, Zarandy S, Tirgan A. von Willebrand's disease and plastic surgery. Ann Plast Surg 1994; 32:351.
11. Gall R, Blakley B, Warrington R, et al. Intraoperative anaphylactic shock from Bacitracin nasal packing after septorhinoplasty. Anesthesiology 1999;91:1545.
12. Umeda T, Ohara H, Hayashi O, et al. Toxic shock syndrome after suction lipectomy. Plast Reconstr Surg 2000;106:204.
13. Kara CO, Gokalan I. Effects of single-dose steroid usage on edema, ecchymosis, and intraoperative bleeding in rhinoplasty. Plast Reconstr Surg 1999; 104:2213.
14. Kargi E, Hosnuter M, Babuccu O, et al. Effect of steroids on edema, ecchymosis, and intraoperative bleeding in rhinoplasty. Ann Plast Surg 2003; 51:570.
15. Gurek A, Fariz A, Aydogan H, et al. Effects of different corticosteroids on edema and ecchymosis in open rhinoplasty. Aesthetic Plast Surg 2006;30:150.
16. Hatef, DA, Ellsworth, WA, Bullocks, JM, et al. Perioperative steroid use for minimizing edema and ecchymosis after rhinoplasty. Aesth Surg J, in press.
17. Rohrich RJ, Gunter JP, Friedman RM. Nasal tip blood supply: an anatomic study validating the safety of the transcolumellar incision in rhinoplasty. Plast Reconstr Surg 1995;95:795.
18. Gruber RP. Early surgical intervention after rhinoplasty. Aesthet Surg J 2001;21:4549–51.
19. Goldwyn RM, Shore S. The effects of submucous resection and rhinoplasty on the sense of smell. Plast Reconstr Surg 1968;41:427.
20. Pade J, Hummel T. Olfactory function following nasal surgery. Laryngoscope 2008;118:1260.
21. Prado AS, Fuentes P, Donoso R. A new treatment for injuries to the anterior cranial fossa after rhinoplasty. Plast Reconstr Surg 2006;117:721.
22. Bilgic MI, Karaca M, Karanfil H, et al. A rare but disturbing complication of rhinoplasty: Rhinorrhea. J Craniofac Surg 2008;19:1433.
23. Hallock GG, Trier WC. Cerebrospinal fluid rhinorrhea following rhinoplasty. Plast Reconstr Surg 1983;71: 109.
24. Heller JB, Gabbay JS, Trussler A, et al. Repair of large nasal septal perforations using facial artery musculomucosal (FAMM) flap. Ann Plast Surg 2005;55:456.
25. Sclafani AP, Schaefer SD. Triological thesis: concurrent endoscopic sinus surgery and cosmetic rhinoplasty: rationale, risks, rewards, and reality. Laryngoscope 2009. [Epub ahead of print].
26. Stucker FJ, Smith TE. The nasal bony dorsum and cartilaginous vault. Arch Otolaryngol 1976;102:695.
27. Sheen JH. A new look at supratip deformity. Ann Plast Surg 1979;3:498.
28. Guyuron B, DeLuca L, Lash R. Supratip deformity: a closer look. Plast Reconstr Surg 2000;105:1140.
29. Gryskiewicz JM. Visible scars from percutaneous osteotomies. Plast Reconstr Surg 2005;116:1771.
30. Bruintjes TD, van Olphen AF, Hillen B, et al. A functional anatomic study of the relationship of the nasal cartilages and muscles to the nasal valve area. Laryngoscope 1998;108:1025.
31. Sheen JH. In: Sheen JH, Sheen A, editors. Aesthetic rhinoplasty. St. Louis(MO): Q.M.P; 1997. p. 24–5.
32. Shaida AM, Kenyon GS. The nasal valves: changes in anatomy and physiology in normal subjects. Rhinology 2000;38:7.

33. Constantian MB. An alar base flap to correct nostril and vestibular stenosis and alar base malposition in rhinoplasty. Plast Reconstr Surg 1998;101:1666.
34. Aydogdu E, Akan M, Gideroglu K, et al. Alar transposition flap for stenosis of the nostril. Scand J Plast Reconstr Surg Hand Surg 2006;40:311.
35. Kotzur A, Gubisch W, Meyer R. Stenosis of the nasal vestibule and its treatment. Aesthetic Plast Surg 1999;23:86.
36. Blandini D, Tremolada C, Beretta M, et al. Iatrogenic nostril stenosis: aesthetic correction using a vestibular labial mucosal flap. Plast Reconstr Surg 1995;95:569.
37. Gryskiewicz JM. Paraffinoma or post-rhinoplasty mucous cyst of the nose: which is it? Plast Reconstr Surg 2001;108:2160.
38. Conrad K, Torgerson CS, Gillman GS. Applications of Gore-Tex implants in rhinoplasty reexamined after 17 years. Arch Facial Plast Surg 2008;10:224.

Index

Note: Page numbers of article titles are in **boldface** type.

Clin Plastic Surg 37 (2010) 401–405
doi:10.1016/S0094-1298(10)00009-X
0094-1298/10/$ – see front matter

S

T

U

V

Moving?

Make sure your subscription moves with you!

To notify us of your new address, find your **Clinics Account Number** (located on your mailing label above your name), and contact customer service at:

Email: journalscustomerservice-usa@elsevier.com

800-654-2452 (subscribers in the U.S. & Canada)
314-447-8871 (subscribers outside of the U.S. & Canada)

Fax number: 314-447-8029

Elsevier Health Sciences Division
Subscription Customer Service
3251 Riverport Lane
Maryland Heights, MO 63043

*To ensure uninterrupted delivery of your subscription, please notify us at least 4 weeks in advance of move.

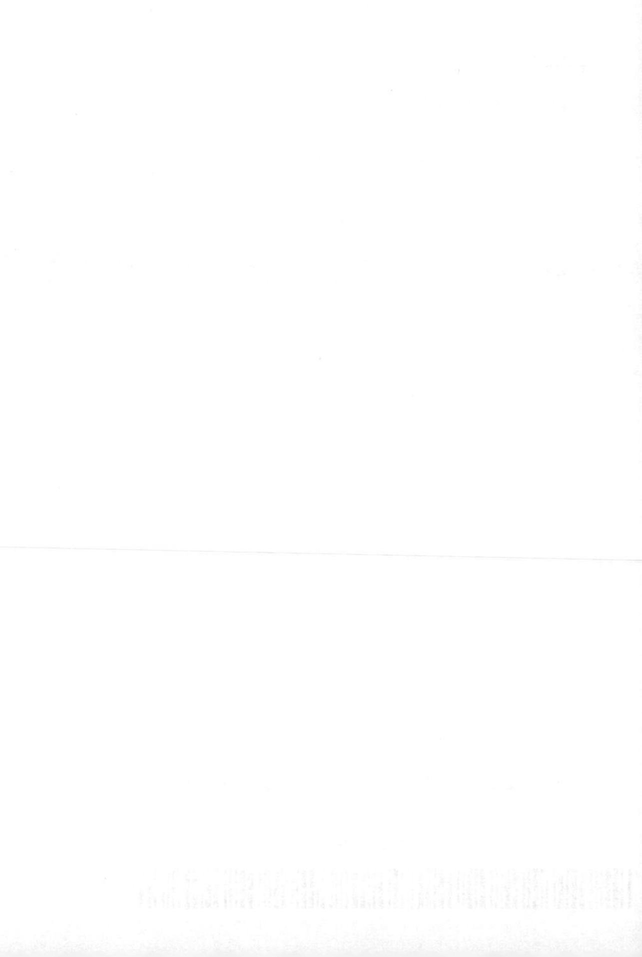

Printed and bound by CPI Group (UK) Ltd, Croydon, CR0 4YY

03/10/2024

01040353-0003